Anthropology of Tobacco

Tobacco has become one of the most widely used and traded commodities on the planet. Reflecting contemporary anthropological interest in material culture studies, *Anthropology of Tobacco* makes the plant the centre of its own contentious, global story in which, instead of a passive commodity, tobacco becomes a powerful player in a global adventure involving people, corporations and public health.

Bringing together a range of perspectives from the social and natural sciences as well as the arts and humanities, *Anthropology of Tobacco* weaves stories together from a range of historical, cross-cultural and literary sources and empirical research. These combine with contemporary anthropological theories of agency and cross-species relationships to offer fresh perspectives on how an apparently humble plant has progressed to world domination, and the consequences of it having done so. It also considers what needs to happen if, as some public health advocates would have it, we are seriously to imagine 'a world without tobacco'.

This book presents students, scholars and practitioners in anthropology, public health and social policy with unique and multiple perspectives on tobacco-human relations.

Andrew Russell is Associate Professor in Anthropology at Durham University, UK, where he is a member of the Anthropology of Health Research Group. His research and teaching spans the sciences, arts and humanities, and mixes both theoretical and applied aspects. He has conducted research in Nepal, the UK and worldwide. Earlier books include *The Social Basis of Medicine,* which won the British Medical Association's student textbook of the year award in 2010, and a number of edited volumes, the latest of which (co-edited with Elizabeth Rahman) is *The Master Plant: Tobacco in Lowland South America.*

Routledge Studies in Public Health

Anthropology of Tobacco

Ethnographic Adventures in Non-Human Worlds

Andrew Russell

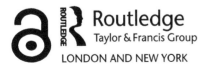

Routledge
Taylor & Francis Group
LONDON AND NEW YORK

First published 2019 by Routledge

2 Park Square, Milton Park, Abingdon, Oxon, OX14 4RN

605 Third Avenue, New York, NY 10017

Routledge is an imprint of the Taylor & Francis Group, an informa business

First issued in paperback 2020

British Library Cataloguing-in-Publication Data
A catalogue record for this book is available from the British Library

Library of Congress Cataloging-in-Publication Data
A catalog record has been requested for this book

ISBN: 978-1-138-48514-3 (hbk)
ISBN: 978-0-367-70945-7 (pbk)

Typeset in Bembo
by Integra Software Services Pvt. Ltd.

To Jane, Ben, Euan and (at Euan's insistence) Bertie, our non-human partner

Contents

Illustrations

Figures

Table

Acknowledgements

The tale changes in the telling, and this book is no exception. When I started writing I presumed my task was a fairly straightforward one. I intended pulling together some ethnographic and other kinds of research about tobacco I and others have done within my home discipline, anthropology. I assumed I would present findings and consider what they meant for how we understand tobacco, a commodity so familiar (and, some would say, dangerous) that it hardly needs any introduction. However, rather like the smoke of a fat cigar, as my work progressed so my subject matter has insinuated itself across a range of different disciplines, theoretical perspectives, geographical areas and time frames. I was moving into largely uncharted terrain in following tobacco's story, and travelling without guides is dangerous indeed. Numerous people have given me advice, information and admonishment along the way.

My colleague Claudia Merli found YouTube clips of contemporary *curanderos* (traditional healers) in Peru using tobacco smoke in curing rituals and saying things (in Spanish) like 'tobacco has the energy to clean and cure'. Such intriguing statements led me to convene a symposium with Elizabeth Rahman in July 2013 that brought together scholars to share observations and information about tobacco production and use amongst indigenous Amazonian and other groups from lowland South America. The contributions to the edited volume arising from that symposium have all been incredibly useful in formulating many of the ideas contained in this one, so many thanks to Elizabeth, Juan Alvaro Echeverri, Bernd Brabec de Mori, Renzo S. Duin, Paolo Fortis, Françoise Barbira Freedman, Pete Gow, Nick Kawa, Augusto Oyuela-Caycedo, Alejandro Reig and Juan Pablo Sarmiento Barletti.

As a result of recognizing common interest, Jane Macnaughton and I set up a Smoking Special Interest Group (SSIG) that has been generously supported by the Wolfson Research Institute for Health and Wellbeing and hosted at the Institute for Medical Humanities at Durham University. Members of that group whose insights have been invaluable include Jane herself, Susan Carro-Ripalda, Kwanwook Kim (whose *hyeonmi-nokcha* – Korean brown rice green tea – became a mainstay of this book's production), Sue Lewis and Frances Thirlway. The SSIG then morphed into a Wellcome Trust-funded Senior Investigator Award led by Jane Macnaughton (Durham) and Havi Carel (Bristol). Particularly valuable input from that group has been provided by Krzysztof Bierski, David Fuller, Phil Horky, Alice Malpass, Sarah McLusky, Fredrik Nyman, Rebecca Oxley, Mary Robson, Arthur Rose and Corinne Saunders. Current and former colleagues, students and friends in the Anthropology Department at Durham, and especially the Anthropology of Health Research Group, have been unfailing in their support, particularly Catherine Alexander, Helen Ball, Luisa Elvira Belaunde, Sandra Bell, Gillian Bentley, Mark Booth, Hannah Brown, Ben Campbell, Matei Candea, Peter Collins, Iain Edgar, Kate Hampshire, Serena Heckler, Ben Kasstan, Jeremy Kendal, Elisabeth Kirtsoglou, Steve Lyon, Nayanika Mukherjee, Tehseen Norani, Ian Rickard, Felix Ringel, Ernesto Schwartz-Marin, Bob Simpson, Courtney Tinnion and Tom Widger. Other people in the University who have given special help at various times include Elizabeth Archibald, David Chappel, Christina Dobson, Catherine Dousteyssier-Khoze, Ray Hudson, David Hunter, James Mason, Richard Sugg, Pat Waugh and Angela Woods.

My contacts with the Making Smoking History in the NE group and the Smoke Free Durham Local Alliance have been particularly enriching, so thank you to Andy Lloyd, Catherine McConnell, Ailsa Rutter, Martyn Willmore and Peter Wright. Others working in the field of tobacco control in the UK and internationally have been very supportive, such as Deborah Arnott, Alison Cox, Eugene Milne and Francis Thompson. A trip to Uruguay with members of W-WEST ('Why Waste Everything Smoking Tobacco') Glasgow was particularly instructive. Other UK-based friends and colleagues who have been particularly helpful include Shirley Ardener, Matthew Bury, Caroline Davidson, Marie-Bénédicte Dembour, Jordan Goodman, Ian Harper, Will Hawthorne, Andy Jones, Sue Smith, Peter Welford and Nigel Wright. Outlines and extracts from the book have been presented in a number of public forums where feedback has been invaluable – these include the Café Scientifique, Stockton, the Institute for Public Health, Bengalaru, and the Indian Institute of Human Settlement, Bengalaru. There are also innumerable other people with whom I have had conversations about smoking. Not all would want to be named, but you know who you are!

This book would never have got started without the support of a Leverhulme Research Fellowship (2014) and would never have got finished without the support of the Wellcome Trust 'Life of Breath' project (grant number 103339). Other sources of funding for my research have included the

National Prevention Research Initiative (a consortium supported by the British Heart Foundation; Cancer Research UK; Chief Scientist Office, Scottish Government Health Directorate; Department of Health; Diabetes UK; Economic and Social Research Council; Health & Social Care Research & Development Office for Northern Ireland; Medical Research Council;

Welsh Assembly Government; and World Cancer Research Fund), Cancer Research UK, Durham University's Wolfson Research Institute for Health and Wellbeing, the Faculty of Social Sciences and Health, the Centre (now Institute) for Medical Humanities, a Matariki Network Universities Mobility Grant, a Santander Mobility Grant and an award from the National Teaching Fellowship Scheme.

Needless to say all idiosyncrasies of fact, fiction, omission and over-interpretation remain my own.

Introduction: re-imagining tobacco

Tobacco: a non-human ethnography

This is a book about tobacco, but not as you may have thought of it before. Anthropology is conventionally about people, but anthropologists are becoming increasingly interested in re-examining the significance of non-humans in the lives of the human, and the important relationships and exchanges that occur. As they do so they are developing new ways of thinking about how humans, animals, plants and other non-human entities or 'things' become entangled in each other's existences rather than, as was most often the case in the past, treating the non-human as, at best, a backdrop to humanity's position centre stage, with all the dire consequences that entails.[1] This book is an attempt to put such approaches to work in looking afresh at the place of tobacco in history and contemporary life.

In doing so I shall take a 'thing' (tobacco) and turn it 'uncommon', in the sense of presenting it as "unusual, unsettling, even virtually inconceivable, and in not being *held in common* by everyone, all the time".[2] Salmond usefully defines and describes 'things' as "the forms in which whatever we study as ethnographers comes to command our attention. They may appear as material objects; as practices or concepts; as events, institutions or beliefs; as gifts, mana, traps, actants, spirits or dividuals; or as structures, perspectives, networks, systems or scales".[3] I admire the breadth of Salmond's analysis, but propose a further push in the direction of things ontological, in the logic of which it isn't that things "may appear as material objects", things in some cases at least *are* material objects.[4] I take a more Latourian view regarding the hybridity of things to try and circumvent some of problems that straddle this borderland, the relationship of knowledge to reality.

Most of the extensive literature that exists on the production, distribution and use of tobacco regards it as essentially a passive commodity. Such a history tends to begin in the colonial era with the plant's 'discovery' by Europeans in the 15th and 16th centuries. Brought from the 'New World' to the 'Old', its appealing medicinal and psychoactive properties turned it into a valued commodity, one which mariners and merchants rapidly transported to the four corners of the earth. With some notable exceptions, in most places it became extremely popular. One of the first truly global commodities, companies and corporations prospered on its cultivation, production, distribution and use. As time went on, new technologies were invented to enable industrial-scale processing of the plant and a concomitant increase in its availability and consumption. New scientific discoveries led to concerns about the health hazards attributed to the long-term use of tobacco. Public health officials thus moved to reduce public access and tobacco's allure, turning what had so quickly become a taken-for-granted presence in domestic and public spaces into a product mired in controversy.

To use social science parlance, accounts such as this are anthropocentric, focused solely on 'human agency', with tobacco provided with a 'less-than-human' role. In what follows I propose a less diffident role for tobacco in people's lives. Taking a much longer and more complex historical, biographical view and comparing this with stories deriving from tobacco's presence in the world today, I invite a re-imagination of tobacco as being more than the innocent victim in a colonial history of its exploitation by people.[5] The final chapter of a classic book comparing tobacco and sugar is entitled 'How Havana Tobacco Embarked on its Conquest of the World'.[6] A review of another classic work, on tobacco shamanism in South America talks of "an indigenous American weed whose own conquest of the Old World began with the European conquest of the New".[7] What if we take statements like this in a literal rather than metaphorical sense? Such a perspective on what is called the agency of tobacco turns it from a 'less-than-human' thing into an entity which is 'more-than-human', a conquering hero or villain with which we are all, to some extent, entangled and by which some are inextricably entrapped.[8]

But how is this 'more-than-human' entity constituted, linguistically and practically? The word 'tobacco' comes from 16th century Carib or Taíno origins. For some South American tribes it is *petun*, a term which came north around the time of the French exploration in the 17th century when, so industrious were the Tionontati people of Canada in their cultivation of the plant, the French gave them the epithet 'Petun' or 'Tobacco Nation' for a while. The Latin plant name *Nicotiana* reflects the reverence people have for its nicotine, named after the French ambassador to Portugal, Jean Nicot, who, in 1561, sent powdered leaves and seeds of the plant to delight the French court. Its origins are in lowland South America, which is where its story begins, but it is also now global in its spread; a case of tobacco world rather than tobacco nation.

There are at least 76 different *Nicotiana* species, 50 of them indigenous to North and South America, 25 to Australasia and one to Africa.[9] Tobacco is a member of the Solanaceae plant family, which includes tomatoes, potatoes, peppers, aubergines, petunias and deadly nightshade. Their transit from 'New World' to 'Old' from the start of the 16th century onwards was transformational in a number of ways. The Solonaceae "appear to have an almost in-built propensity for domestication and subsequent hybridisation".[10] Hybridization, as used here, refers to powerful genetic forces within the plants themselves, but the argument presented in this book is that tobacco has an equivalent ability to hybridize with people that has proved just as powerful as any genetic changes in its plant family. There is a story to this relationship and the half of it, to paraphrase a powerful study of slaves that laboured in American tobacco fields from the mid-17th century onwards to produce tobacco for an increasingly important global market, "ain't never been told".[11]

The march of tobacco has been the march of capitalism, the march of modernity and of a most peculiarly strong entanglement that has become increasingly recognized by the psychological term addiction. So 'taken for granted' is this situation that, until recently, in much of the world, tobacco was so common that the idea of its absence was, to all intents and purposes, laughable.[12] From its much longer evolutionary history in South America, with a shift into North America as a human domesticant around 2000 years ago (Chapter 1), the story I shall tell is of how, over the last 500 years or so, tobacco has become one of the most widespread psychotropic plants on the planet. There are no countries or regions in the world today where tobacco is not consumed in some form or other, and it is widely cultivated, thanks to its adaptability and resourcefulness in exploiting different environmental conditions. As with the other Solanaceae, tobacco's "association with people has proved a supremely successful evolutionary trajectory".[13]

Tobacco, as Fig. 0.1 shows, is a striking plant. But while some may cultivate it for its appearance, it is the nicotine present in its leaves and roots that is the basis for its overwhelming success in human entanglement. The two plants with the highest nicotine content are *Nicotiana tabacum* and *Nicotiana rustica* and these (particularly *Nicotiana tabacum*) have become the chief commercial species, "grown extensively for use for smoking, chewing and snuff manufacture".[14] Humans absorb nicotine via their lungs (in the case of cigarette smoke), oral mucosa (in the case – usually – of cigars, pipes or chewing tobacco), and nasal mucosa (in the case of snuff). Its addictive properties make it "one of the most popular but harmful plants in the world".[15] Chemically, its structure is similar to the neurotransmitter acetylcholine, which bridges the synapses between nerve endings. For this reason, tobacco acts primarily as a cognitive stimulant, with its popularity only partly explained by its physiologically addictive qualities.[16] Also important is its role as a vehicle giving some users focus and creative access to other worlds, or a 'time out' from this one. Its dual nature – as both poison and remedy – is at the crux of this book.[17]

Anthropological perspectives on the non-human

Until recently, the overriding – but not ubiquitous – tendency in anthropology, as in large swathes of the social and the natural sciences, has been to treat the non-

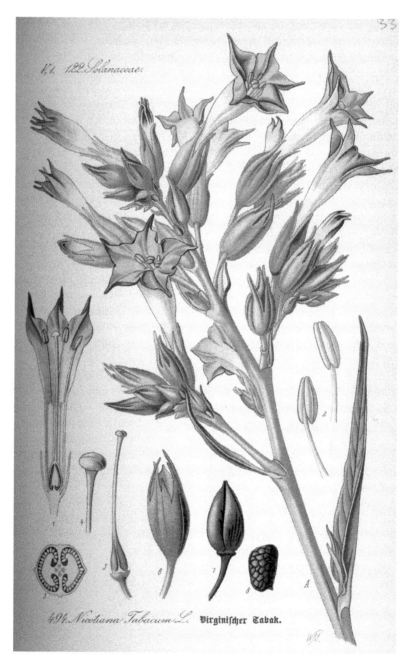

Fig. 0.1 'Nicotiana tabacum'
Source: Illustration from Thomé, 1885

human – plants, animals, minerals, concepts and ideas – as props for all things human, "to regard the world of things as inert and mute, set in motion and animated, indeed knowable, only by persons and their words".[18] For Malinowski, father of the 'fieldwork revolution' in anthropology, an object such as a canoe "is made for a certain use, and with a definitive purpose; it is a means to an end, and we, who study native life, must not reverse this relationship, and make a fetish of the object itself".[19] Thus, while objects could be "illustrative or representative of social orders, ideas, and imaginings" they remained "in our service, and we should take care not to think otherwise, no matter what the folk conceptions of our interlocutors were about the power of things".[20]

Julian Steward offers an example of a counter-tendency in anthropology that accords greater importance to aspects of the non-human. Steward became convinced that every culture had a limited range of possibilities hinged around sets of bounding environmental factors that he called the 'culture core'.[21] Marvin Harris, a self-styled 'cultural materialist', used non-human cultural features such as pigs and sacred cows to argue for the importance of material life more generally in explaining the ways of the world.[22] Such approaches are eternally damned, in some areas of anthropology at least, by the withering epithet 'environmental determinism'. But what if 'the environment' is more than an externality offering outer limits on people's lives, as per Steward, or more than a series of discrete explanations for phenomena that others have accounted for in purely social terms, as per Harris? Subsequent authors have argued for relationships between human and non-human that are much more interesting, more fundamental, and more profound than that. These have significant implications for the anthropology of tobacco.

Much more recently anthropologist Danny Miller has written about 'stuff' and the rich and meaningful relationships people often have with the material world, and has criticized our tendency to ignore or dismiss the importance of such connections.[23] Miller talks about "the humility of things", their tendency to remain "hidden in plain sight" with an uncanny ability "to fade out of focus and remain peripheral to our vision and yet determinant of our behaviour and identity". Miller attributes an almost homeopathic quality to this relationship; "the less we are aware of them, the more powerfully they can determine our expectations...They determine what takes place to the extent that we are unconscious of their capacity to do so".[24]

The idea of being 'hidden in plain sight' applies to how we perceive the world as well as how we engage more directly with it. Fig. 0.2 was used on the cover of a popular anthropological journal issue.[25] It references an article about khat, the exotic leaf stimulant and commodity found in north-east Africa and Yemen.[26] However, it is easy for a casual viewer of the photograph to overlook the fact that the Yemeni seller has another commodity in his hand, all the more powerful because it goes unacknowledged – a cigarette.

Miller criticizes the tendency for what remains hidden in plain sight to become, very often, the forgotten, overlooked or secreted. Why bother with

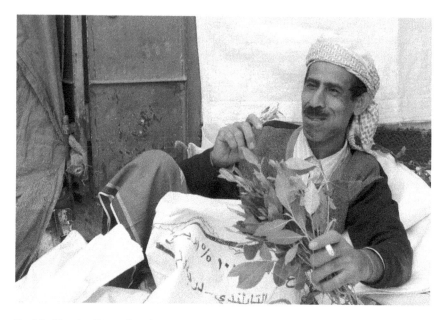

Fig. 0.2 Chewing *khat* in Sana'a, Yemen ("I love my *khat*")
Source: Ferdinand Reus, Arnhem, Holland, 2009 (Creative Commons license BY-SA 2.0)

nature when such deeply human topics as kinship, religion, politics and economics can appear almost without reference to a non-human realm at all? From such a standpoint, nature tends to be regarded as of peripheral significance, if it is regarded at all. Sometimes there may be non-human elements, biotic (plant/animal) or abiotic (matter, technologies, spirits) which have to be taken into, and occasionally called to, account.[27] But most of the time anthropologists have laboured in the productive seam of humanist knowledge in which people are the central focus and the non-human is generally only a backdrop, belittled or ignored. Such easy assumptions of dominance are coming to be challenged, however. Irrespective of the reactive effects of the Anthropocene when nature bites back,[28] tobacco is an excellent example of a non-human agent whose role in human life has been far from passive. The notion of 'agency' provides a way into understanding its dynamism.

Agency and the non-human

From one perspective, agency is all the ways in which one entity affects another. Tobacco, for example, gets people to do things – cultivate it, process and distribute it, use it, worship it, attempt to control it. There are also even people (such as myself) who are drawn to research it – not bad going for a humble plant! Taking the notion of non-human agency seriously turns the non-human from mere object, whether animate or inanimate, into something more akin to a co-producer of experience. For Miller "the things people make, make people".[29] Alfred Gell is similarly intrigued by the potential of artefacts to have agency. We frequently anthropomorphize things (i.e. attribute human characteristics to them), whether this is reflected in swearing at a car that won't start in the morning or praying to an effigy as if it were a person.[30] There are frequent examples of tobacco being accorded not just human but sometimes divine status in the pages that follow. However while both Miller and Gell argue that 'things' are more than mere objects in the service of humanity, people remain primary: the meanings that objects have are dependent on human sociality; without people, one cannot have agency. As Geismar puts it, "objects may have *impact* (like falling meteorites), but in order to have *agency* they must be entangled within social relations and indeed within our own humanity". She admires Gell for the care he takes "not to conflate the effects of inanimate objects with agency, which must itself be understood as a product of social relations".[31] What if, though, meaning and object were not necessarily dependent on human mediation? Some anthropologists have suggested that "things might be treated as *sui generis* meanings",[32] and others have been prepared to join them in taking a more straightforwardly ontological view on the notion of non-human agency.

Bruno Latour is an anthropologist who made his name as a researcher in science and technology studies, an area in which 'things' such as microbes, widgets and other technologies are often of supreme significance. Perhaps as a consequence of this, Latour insists on treating humans and non-humans symmetrically, as equally important 'actants' on a flattened plane of shared relationships, a 'network'.[33] Agency is the product of this interactive, hybrid network, and it is constituted by the diversity of elements – human and non-human – found within it.[34] Latour is assiduous in maintaining that neither side has priority over the other in his analyses.

One of the many examples Latour uses to illustrate his theory is the heated debate about gun control in the USA.[35] For representatives of the gun-control lobby, it is guns that kill people. For opponents in the National Rifle Association, it is people who kill through their misuse of guns. Neither are correct, in Latour's terms, since the agency resides in two together (what he calls a "hybrid assemblage" of person-with-gun, or gun-person). Similar, competing assertions are frequently made about tobacco. 'Tobacco kills people' argue those in tobacco control. 'Tobacco doesn't kill people, people kill themselves through misuse of tobacco', the industry might try, failingly, to reply. There is no such thing as misuse – 'every cigarette is doing you damage' (tobacco control).[36] 'You have the freedom, the right to choose' (industry). Whichever direction one pulls the trigger of causation, however, tobacco (like guns) is clearly a significant player in the tobacco-person bond.[37]

Latour's work offers exciting new ways of bringing the richly significant non-human world back into the frame and the 'hidden in plain sight' nature of something like tobacco back into focus. It can accommodate the changing status of tobacco as it shifts from animate plant to inanimate thing and moves through different contexts. It can also incorporate all the paraphernalia associated with tobacco-human hybridity, some of which will be presented in this book.[38] However, other theorists of non-human agency and hybrid relationships take more radical views about non-human powers. They see at least parts of the non-human in terms that include purpose, consciousness, and cognition. From such a position, it is not too much of a leap to see tobacco as having agency that is independent of its human entanglements, and is more than just impact in Geismar's meteoric sense.

Tobacco's hybridity: challenging the species divide

One early champion of a more radical philosophy of non-human agency is Spinoza (1632-1677). For him, "nature…is a place wherein bodies strive to enhance their power of activity by forging alliances with other bodies in their vicinity".[39] Spinoza would have been comfortable with Latour's notion of the hybrid assemblage, in our case the hybrid 'person-with-tobacco'. Indeed, Spinoza is himself an example of the many early modern thinkers who took "pleasure in smoking a pipe of tobacco".[40] The term I use in this book – 'tobacco-person' – reflects the way in which, with regular use, tobacco and persons become profoundly entangled; part of each other. Although, if we take Spinoza's view of nature seriously, one might prefer to see tobacco as enhancing its 'power of activity' through a Faustian alliance with its human host. However, for Latour the assemblage is more than dyadic. As well as the effect of tobacco itself on the human individual, its processing into a range of consumable items – cigarettes, roll-ups, cigars, pipe tobacco, snuff, chewing tobacco, tobacco paste, etc. – creates products (things) which in turn regularly make each other as well as people (tobacco-persons).[41] Another important hybrid that will be introduced in Chapter 8 is the 'tobacco corporation', reflecting the hybridity inherent in the profit-driven relationship of tobacco and late global capitalism. The hybridity of tobacco and humans, whether individual or corporate, permits them to perform the same, hybrid actions, even to the extent of speaking.[42] But they do so less as independent contractors in the relationship with tobacco and more as mutually constituted beings.

Another way of thinking about the associations between people and tobacco is Haraway's use of the term 'cyborg', half organism, half machine (or, more accurately, a hybrid of both). It is a concept appropriated from the technohumanist fantasies deriving from the research and policy era of the space race and Cold War. However, a cyborg is not only a creature of fiction, but a social reality.[43] It is a fitting way of conceptualizing the relationship between people and the paraphernalia surrounding tobacco, although terms like 'artefact', 'technology' or 'tool' probably work better than 'machine' for our purposes.[44] Haraway has broadened her interest from cyborgs to more general human/non-human relationships. She writes about the 'companion species'[45] with whom many humans share their lives and who play a part in making us what we are.[46] Horses, dogs, rats, birds, fish, fleas and intestinal parasites are amongst the many animal species which have influenced the course of history and contemporary societies worldwide, and a thriving literature has developed to chart some of these engagements.[47]

Plants generally receive less extensive attention in the interspecies literature, perhaps because they have fewer of the supposedly human attributes that make relationships with some (but not all) animal companion species so rewarding. Despite the fact that "in the majority of places that are inhabited by people...plants dominate the natural world",[48] people are "generally poorly acquainted with plants, looking down on them or simply ignoring them".[49] This may be due to a human 'plant blindness' that derives not only from ignorance but also the general similarity of plants' surfaces and textures, their relative lack of mobility and the fact that, unlike some animals, plants do not prey on humans.[50] Human interest, such as it is, often focuses only on the so-called 'economic crops'. Naturalist Richard Mabey, chides that despite understanding the importance of plants like never before, this is only insofar as this knowledge serves our human needs. "Plants have come to be seen as the furniture of the planet, necessary, useful, attractive, but 'just there', passively vegetating".[51] Although they both beautify our landscapes and help us breathe, we have lost any sense of wonder and respect owed them as active agents in their own life stories.

Plant behaviour: brains and intelligence

Recent work in botany has challenged such zoocentric notions of animal (and human) superiority. Charles Darwin himself conducted experiments on the highly reactive leaves of *Mimosa pudica*, the so-called 'sensitive plant', in order to challenge the assumption that plants were passive, insensitive beings. Plant behaviour is rarely as clearly or quickly displayed as it is in the case of *M. pudica*, though, since it normally occurs on a timescale quite outside everyday human perception. There is also the question of how plant behaviour is organized. Darwin considered it "hardly an exaggeration to say that the tip of the radicle [root]...acts like the brain of one of the lower animals; the brain being seated within the anterior end of the body, receiving impressions from the sense-organs, and directing the several movements".[52] The notion of some kind of nerve centre of 'root brain' has been revived recently, despite the reservations some express at the idea of 'plant neurobiology' or a plant brain.[53]

Whether or not they have a brain, there is ample evidence of plants responding to signals in their environment, both above and below ground.

Plant signalling takes place within and between plants, as well as between plants and other living beings. According to one expert, "territoriality, self and alien recognition and competition. . .predictive assessments, decisions and trade-offs are all involved, as well as countering the threat of herbivores and disease".[54] Some aspects of this behaviour, therefore, can accurately be described as 'intelligent',[55] while some go so far as to talk of cognition and consciousness.[56] "Plant behaviour", argue Trewavas and Baluška, "is active, purpose-driven and intentional. In its capability for self-recognition and problem-solving. . .it is thus adaptive, intelligent and cognitive".[57]

If plant behaviour does indeed demonstrate intelligence, then tobacco has it in abundance. The tobacco species *N. attenuata*, for example, is vulnerable to predation by the voracious larvae of the tobacco hawkmoth (*Manduca sexta*). Studies have shown how hairs on the tobacco plant secrete sugars that the larvae eat but which then give their bodies and excrement a distinctive odour that is attractive to other predatory insects and lizards.[58] The nicotine in *N. tabacum* evolved as a form of insecticide, an attempt by the plant to defend itself against caterpillar feeding.[59] An example of signalling between plant species can be found in a controlled experiment looking at the relationship between *N. attenuata* and sagebrush (*Artemisia tridentata*). Tobacco growing close to mechanically clipped sagebrush showed increased production of anti-herbivore defences compared to tobacco near unclipped plants.[60] Researchers were unable to demonstrate similar forms of 'eavesdropping' (as they called it) in any of the other broad-leaved plants that were subject to the same herbivorous predators as sagebrush and tobacco, [61] which raises the intriguing speculation that tobacco has higher levels of plant intelligence than most other species.[62]

Of course plants, animals, and people are different both individually and between groups. A potential criticism of Latour's work is that flattening the differences between the actant categories, or emphasizing their similarities, can lead to the distinctive elements of each being ignored simply because of their lack of symmetry with the qualities of others. "Unlike animals, which can escape or move to a more suitable place, or food or water, when under attack by other animals or from environmental stresses, higher plants cannot change site after germination, because their roots are anchored in the soil, and hence plants have to adjust to [any] biotic or abiotic stress factor they are exposed to".[63] People additionally have language, as do some animals in rudimentary form. Moreover where does morality, identity, motivation, feeling and emotion fit into Latour's approach? As we have seen above, scientists are starting to include entities such as these within the 'thing' domain.[64] In such ways entities previously regarded as uniquely and differentially human are now seen as symmetrical actants. Martin Holbraad calls this "the possibility – and in so many instances the fact – that the things we call 'things' might not ethnographically speaking be things as all".[65] All is not what it seems in the field of non-human agency.

Ambivalent agent of Enlightenment

To say "things are not what they seem" is to subscribe to the argument that tobacco is both non-human and more-than-human. Its ambivalent status and the tensions thus created are central to this book. Just like Odradek, the mysterious creature that lives under the stairs in Kafka's tale 'The Cares of a Family Man', tobacco is simultaneously visible and invisible, inanimate and alive, "verbal yet vegetal".[66] Anthropological hybridity challenges these polarities of contemporary life. In other cases, more marked, rigid and definable disjunctures between 'humans' and 'non-humans' or, in our case, 'people' and 'tobacco', are to be seen. Tags such as 'verbal but vegetal', or 'spirit and commodity', reflect tobacco's ambiguity, not only intrinsically but in relation to other human and non-human forms. Amongst some Amerindian peoples, for example, tobacco is a 'master plant', a divine gift that commands utmost respect,[67] a blessing from the gods that can facilitate entry into the spirit world or can be consulted for purposes of divination. For some it is also an herbal remedy that purifies through its smoke or relieves symptoms through its pharmacological effects; for others it is a product used for cementing intra- and inter-group bonds of conviviality and sociality.

With its passage across the Atlantic and rapid dispersal around the world from the end of the 15th century onwards, tobacco quickly turned into a commodity that could be bought and sold for profit like any other. Commodification has its own animacy, as we shall see in Chapter 6, and commodities develop their own agency. The fact they can do this, I shall suggest, is in no small part due to the development of increasingly strong boundaries around erstwhile fluid things, a process generated by the philosophical developments known as the Enlightenment. It seems to be a more-than-human coincidence that the growing popularity of tobacco in Europe coincided with the onset of a period of surging creative, critical and empirical enquiry in the late 17th and 18th centuries that has come to be known collectively as 'the Enlightenment'. Tobacco was a particularly significant actant in prefiguring and helping to shape the changes we associate with Enlightenment life and thought.

The Enlightenment had consequences for much of the natural world that were less than salutary. For Hall, "largely because it is depicted as devoid of the attributes which require human attention – such as mentality, agency, and volition – nature is left out of the sphere of human moral consideration".[68] Nor were all humans necessarily included in such a moral domain. Slaves, some of whom were required to work on the North American tobacco plantations, were a benighted corollary to the growth in economic prosperity that accompanied the increasing sense of human dominion over nature. With nature conquered and held to be passive, humanity in the Enlightenment paradigm becomes self-referential, a hall of mirrors in which the social can be explained purely in terms of the social.[69] The result, in Hall's view, are human actions which assault the very integrity of the biosphere.[70]

Challenging such dualisms is thus of more than academic importance. Doing so shifts our perspective from one of assumed human dominion, in which the non-human is merely a commodity ripe for exploitation, to one that more fruitfully regards people and nature as mutually interdependent. Tobacco has certainly benefitted from the many forms of dependency it has engendered with the rest of humanity in the 500 years since its escape from the confines of the Americas.

Another of the interesting ramifications of the renewed interest in human/non-human relations is the new ways the non-human 'other' can be talked about. The notion of the 'more-than-human' is reflected in books with titles such as *Plants as Persons*[71] or *How Forests Think*.[72] Titles such as these challenge our conventional sense of ontology (the nature of being) as well as how we conceive of the relations between species. They require us to take a lot on trust, though. "We are colonized by certain ways of thinking about relationality", Eduardo Kohn writes in defence of the notion that forests think. "Forests are good to think because they themselves think. Forests think...the fact that we can make the claim that forests think is in a strange way a product of the fact that forests think".[73] He accepts that such arguments require of the reader "a modicum of goodwill, patience, and the willingness to struggle".[74] However, forests' cognitive credentials require a lot more than trust. It demands what to many will seem like a theological leap of faith or, at the very least, a willing diversion into make-believe.

I expect no such leap of faith from readers of this book. I am quite happy to accept that, in a normal world, agency depends on a human/non-human hybridity to have efficacy in the non-human case. However, I do not want to exclude the potential for different perspectives on things that a more radical essentialism throws up. One of these is the possibility that, as Geismar phrases it, "instead of multiple *meanings* that stand in relief to a singular, objective reality, there are multiple *ontologies* – or worlds – which each stand apart from one another".[75] I take tobacco, through its linkages with people, to be 'more-than-human' in ways that owe much to ideas of plant intelligence (above) and the many tobacco-person, tobacco corporation and tobacco control relationships to be articulated in the following pages.

My arguments are supported by philosophical trends in the study of ontologies and material cultures. In the field of ontological studies 'correlationism', based on the premise that 'thinking' and 'being' can never be considered apart from each other,[76] is giving way to speculative realism, the notion that a life of objects exists (or, we can only speculate, may exist) outside of the humanly known world. Since we humans cannot know what these other worlds are really like, it is better (or at least permissible) to think of tobacco in an 'as if' sort of a way,[77] to explore the fanciful, superhuman and, sometimes, downright eerie dimensions of whatever, like Odradek, tobacco may or may not be.[78] Fiction has a part to play here as well as fact. There are many challenging ways to consider tobacco's hybrid agency 'as if' it were more-than-human, and many ethnographic adventures are promised in the attempt to represent tobacco's non-human worlds. I shall go on to introduce some of these in a thematic way, followed by a summary of their redaction within the contents of this book.

Constructing a non-human ethnography of tobacco

Ethnography is a research methodology with its roots in the study of people. If we accept the proviso that tobacco is in some respects 'more', rather than 'less than' human, then we have the makings of a method that can take its more-than-plant qualities seriously. Whether we accept Geismar's common-sense view of agency as only inhering in human relations, or a more 'radical essentialist' one in which non-human agency takes us in more speculative directions, ethnographic methods offer exciting new perspectives and the possibility for extensive story-making in the realms of non-human entities.[79] One such way of doing this has been termed 'follow the thing',[80] in this case, tobacco and its accoutrements, wherever they – and serendipity[81] – lead us. This calls not only for research across space (what the anthropologist George Marcus calls "multi-sited ethnography") but time as well; to follow the 'thing' wherever it goes, charting its relationships within and between the hybrid worlds with which it is mutually constituted. Marcus' approach is reminiscent of Latour's ant-like methods,[82] tirelessly investigating as many human and non-human components of the networks, their associations and connections, as we can.[83] The terms 'tobacco-person', 'tobacco corporation' and 'tobacco control' are useful in this context as representing three central sets of knots in the network to be investigated.

There are limitations, of course, to how comprehensively any 'thing' can be followed in time and space. We lack the possibility of being taken back into direct experience of the past and must resort to documents, archaeological and archival sources to follow tobacco's travels through time. Literature and the creative arts can sometimes provide additional 'existential' evidence of tobacco's power,[84] revealing "those dimensions of personal and social life we may have little access to when using other research strategies".[85] This book complements historical and ethnographic research with the analysis of literary and other artistic representations to explore the experience of tobacco-persons past and present. Unlike many a public health research project, literature offers access to people's inner lives as well as reflections on the external world. These representations may be based on personal experience or be the product of a purely literary imagination. While such accounts open up ground similar to that promised by qualitative researchers, literary accounts have the advantage of being able to reflect those aspects of the tobacco-person that may otherwise be missed – the life lived imaginatively, sensually, joyfully, motivated and influenced by tactile pleasures, beliefs (that may be irrational), enchantment and desire. In literary contexts, tobacco and its meanings can be portrayed in vivid ways that are sometimes inaccessible to purely scientific or social scientific analysis. Of course, such accounts cannot function as 'evidence' in the same way as empirical work. They cannot be read as representing experience in the way ethnography does, but they certainly enrich that account. Thus, I shall use both literary and ethnographic work in this book.

The research which has become the basis for this ethnography took place over an extended period, from 2005 onwards. During this time, I have been involved with or have led a number of projects researching tobacco in different forms and guises.[86] This period has been marked by the development of an increasingly confident and knowledge-based movement that has slowly shifted its position from tobacco control to envisaging a smoke-free future.

My involvement with this movement began when a colleague asked if I was interested in joining the 'intelligence sub-committee' for a new initiative that was being formed in the North East of England. Plans were afoot to develop a tobacco control office (Fresh North East) that would bring together smoking cessation, health education and lobbying work under one umbrella organization.[87] Unique within the UK at the time, after a few months we were able to take advantage of a funding opportunity to run a 'natural experiment' to see whether, and if so, how, the office had an effect on smoking prevalence rates in the region compared to the rest of the country. This offered a fascinating anthropological opportunity to investigate the interactions within and between the various categories of person – users and controllers – linked through the mediation of tobacco.[88] We went on to explore other aspects of tobacco's place in communities – a study exploring young people's views on smoking, for example, and the organization of criminal and public health activities around the movement of illicit (as opposed to legal) tobacco.[89] At the same time, I was able to supervise research taking place amongst tobacco-persons and tobacco corporations elsewhere in the UK and beyond. I also became interested in the path-breaking efforts to control tobacco at the global level through the World Health Organization (WHO)'s Framework Convention on Tobacco Control (FCTC).[90]

Working with people who live, breathe and sleep tobacco control, one quickly becomes impressed with the momentous facts and figures that drive their vocation. Smoking, for example, is "the world's greatest cause of preventable death";[91] "one in every two life-long smokers is killed by tobacco and most smokers lose many years of active life".[92] It is the only product which, in at least 50 per cent of cases, kills its consumer when used as directed. Tobacco, the cause of 100 million deaths in the 20th century, offers the prospect of causing one billion more in the 21st century; 70-80 per cent of these will be in low and middle-income countries. As an anthropologist, however, I had a growing awareness of the very different role tobacco assumes in some other parts of the world. Contemporary *curanderos* (traditional healers) in Peru, for example, describe tobacco as a plant with the "energy to clean and cure", an approach somewhat at odds with its villainous status in global public health. I met a colleague, Elizabeth Rahman, who had been doing doctoral research in Brazil amongst an indigenous group, the Xié. The Xié attitude towards tobacco smoke, she said, was one of great respect for its healing and purifying powers. In fact, so common was tobacco use amongst the Xié that she had almost taken it for granted in her DPhil thesis. For many researchers working in lowland South America, Miller's remark about things becoming 'hidden in plain sight' rang very true. Anthropologists working in the region tended to take more interest in indigenous cosmologies and exotic substances like the hallucinogen *ayahuasca* (rather like the *khat* example above) than they did in common or garden tobacco.[93]

Some scholars, in a rather blinkered fashion, devote their energies to frequently strident critiques of the agencies and individuals intent on following and supporting a public health view on tobacco. They bemoan a barrier of the "if you're not with us, you're against us"[94] variety which, they argue, stands in the way of anthropological research that doesn't follow such an instrumental format. 'With us' involves anthropology for tobacco control; 'against us' is broader-based anthropology of tobacco more generally, which may or may not include its control. Much of what takes place under the rubric of this 'critical public health' is valuable in addressing some of the 'hidden in plain sight' issues that those involved in tobacco control work day to day may overlook or ignore.

This book, then, is the result of trying to square a number of different perspectives on tobacco, its global spread, and its current situation. My research combines an ethnographic commitment to historical and cross-cultural specifics while at the same time recognizing and respecting tobacco as a global phenomenon. For tobacco is one of the most distinctive (some would say disastrous) commodity complexes to have arisen out of the process known as globalization; in so doing, it has become one of the most widespread and popular, as well as harmful, things on the planet. I intend neither to adjudicate the medical, social or policy evidence about its production and use, nor to replicate existing political criticisms of the structures and organizations that keep tobacco at the height of national and international health agendas. Instead, through restating and re-storying the different perspectives in what has become an increasingly politicized and polarized field, I intend to bring familiar and unusual perspectives together in ways that foment new understandings of this complex and extraordinary non-human entity. Doing so opens up new ways of looking at the insinuating relationship between plant and people.

Re-storying tobacco

The book divides naturally into two main parts. Part 1 (Life) focuses on the different worlds tobacco has created and occupied through history. We look first at the indigenous peoples of lowland South America for many of whom it is the 'other worldly' nature of tobacco which is of fundamental interest (Chapter 1). In the five centuries since its colonial discovery (recounted in Chapter 2) and rapid transport to other parts of the world, *Nicotiana tabacum*'s position has shifted, from being a 'master plant' in the reverential sense of the term amongst indigenous peoples of the Americas, to mastery of a different sort as one of the world's most heavily used and traded commodities. Chapter 3 looks at what happened in the 17th century as tobacco's influence in Europe took hold and reached further. Amongst the significant outcomes, Chapter 4 will propose, is the development of Enlightenment thought, in which I argue tobacco had a deeply implicated but largely unrecognized role. I shall then go on to look at some of the shape-shifting and diversification that took place from the 18th century onwards – into snuff (Chapter 5), cigars (Chapter 6) and cigarettes (Chapters 7 and 8).

Part 2 (Times) looks at tobacco's shaping of contemporary worlds through four chapters that look at the current situation of tobacco in the 21st century. Chapter 9 asks what it is like being a tobacco user in these times, when tobacco control is strong at both national levels (Chapter 10) and globally (Chapter 11). Chapter 12 considers the future and what needs to happen if, as current public health advocates would have it, we are seriously to imagine 'a world without tobacco'. From some perspectives, a plant which once held promise as a utopian panacea has become a dystopian health nightmare. I would like to move away from such polarities and put tobacco into a different category altogether, one that transcends even the dualism inherent in the notion of the *pharmakon*, the ancient Greek recognition that remedies can also be poisons, and vice versa.[95] We need to rethink tobacco's place in society and, conversely, our place in the social life of tobacco. The results may be somewhat surprising.

Some overarching themes come out of my analyses and reflect the value of taking a non-human agency approach to the story of tobacco. The first is that, while we might like to assume it is 20th century scientific evidence for its ill-effects that first challenged the production and marketing of tobacco, historical sources and literary and artistic outputs demonstrate that tobacco has been contentious ever since its first arrival on European shores. A second is that while it is easy to stress the disjuncture between the place of tobacco in Amerindian life and thought and its more recent rise as a global commodity, the concept of 'tobacco ideology', developed to explain some fundamental aspects of tobacco in lowland south America in Chapter 2, can be used to explain certain aspects of tobacco's human/non-human hybridity worldwide. I shall argue in Chapter 7 that despite a secular approach to policy making in the 20th century, a strange enchantment prevented scientists as well as other kinds of tobacco-persons from recognizing and accepting the serious human health implications of tobacco in general and cigarettes in particular. In Chapter 8 we shall see how many people had a stake in tobacco being readily available, affordable and desirable, and how tobacco corporations were involved in a conspiracy about the health risks associated with their product – except that, in the last decade of the 20th century, and unlike most conspiracies, theirs turned out to be true.

The fourth point arising from a non-human agency approach to tobacco is how tobacco control has been forced to expedite an increasingly global effort to solve what has become a significantly global problem. This raises issues about how we are to extract ourselves from the insinuating presence of tobacco in our lives – to 'imagine a world without tobacco', as the final chapter is titled. Fifty years ago, such a statement would have seemed unthinkable, at least in many parts of the western world. My argument is that the power of the imagination – detached, partly, by the machinations of tobacco in the first place – can be harnessed to counter the powerful agency of tobacco and encourage us towards thinking about different potential futures: how things could be, as opposed to how things are.[96] Various countries have developed policies – or policy intentions – for smoke- or tobacco-free futures. At the same time, tobacco itself is shape-shifting – from 'real' to 'electronic' cigarettes, for example, or from public health enemy to public health saviour. Such shifts raise new questions about what is the subject/object that is the focus of these attempts at control. In conclusion, the book argues that an ontological approach complements the predominantly epistemological approaches that have tended to dismiss, or make light of, the power of the non-human.

Follow that plant!

In the 21st century, tobacco, in not only its '-person' and 'corporate' but also 'control' forms of hybridity, is becoming increasingly uncommon in Salmond's terms. Tobacco in its hybrid forms responds to control attempts both by resisting denormalization and shape-shifting into other, more 'unusual' products – local home-grown, or e-cigarettes, for example. Tobacco control aims to tip tobacco into the domain of the unsettling and, as we shall see in Chapter 12, potentially almost inconceivable.

A book of this nature can only present a partial story of tobacco's rise to world domination and the increasingly complex practices its production, distribution, use, and regulation have occasioned worldwide. More important is the change in perspective that this book invites you, the reader, to undertake. To imagine a world without tobacco requires the re-imagination of what the world today – with tobacco in it – is like. This needs a re-assessment of the diversity of tobacco's 'thingly' properties: as a hybrid, a companion species, an assemblage, a spirit, a cyborg, commodity, non-human agent. This book extends the time and space across which tobacco is normally depicted and analysed by journeying into deep history, across cultures and through cognitive zones, and by considering the spaces of its production and manufacture as well as consumption. In looking to the future and considering the possibility of a tobacco-free world we need to look to the past and reconvene our present. To the extent that we have all in some way been touched by tobacco and its philosophical, cultural and historical legacies, we are all tobacco-people now.

Setting off

From the comfort of his armchair Sir James Frazer, eminent Victorian anthropologist, finishes the opening chapter of his classic *The Golden Bough* with an invocation to move from the antiquities of Italy to address a "wider survey". Although long and laborious, it "may possess something of the interest and charm of a voyage of discovery, in which we shall visit many strange foreign lands, with strange foreign peoples, and still stranger customs". He goes on "the wind is in the shrouds: we shake out our sails to it, and leave the coast of Italy behind us for a time".[97] Thus Frazer escapes into mythology and travellers' tales, leaving the fieldworker Malinowski to introduce us to our destination. "Imagine yourself suddenly set down surrounded by all your gear, alone on a tropical beach close to a native village, while the launch or dinghy which has brought you sails away out of sight". Later, Malinowski remarks, "some natives flock around you, especially if they smell tobacco".[98] What a powerful precursor to the role of the anthropologist is this – no sooner have we arrived than there is tobacco, hidden in plain sight yet ubiquitous, powerful, desirable. But what is the tale of tobacco to add to the tales of anthropological derring-do?

My intention is not to reconcile the competing viewpoints of people and plant – assuming a plant is what we take tobacco to be. Given the variety of contexts and concerns tobacco embodies, and sometimes even talks about in this book (either as a voice itself or speaking through some other kind of technological mediator), it is tempting to suggest that all human life adheres to this remarkable substance. Life but also, sadly, death. Given the heinous crimes by which it stands charged, one way to start our journey could be as a detective on a murder enquiry. Many witness statements will need collecting in the course of our work – from shamans in lowland South America, the English Elizabethan (and other) literati and musicians, a medical practitioner in the Sydney suburbs, the CEO of a transnational tobacco corporation, a former New Zealand tobacco picker and Booker prize-winner, a mother in the North East of England in the final stages of lung cancer. The outcome of these different perspectives[99] will be a non-human, global ethnography that encourages us to re-imagine what a world with tobacco is like. Many barriers, dead ends and subterfuges, real and metaphorical, will arise as we swerve and dodge oncoming traffic in our quest. Yet succeed we must, so, in the style of detective pursuits around the world, let us jump into a passing taxi (an 'unmarked vehicle' is probably the one most likely to succeed), and with all the breath that is left in our bodies, once tobacco has had its share, shout 'follow that plant'!

Notes

1   Fisher (2009) is a good exponent of some of these, although his work is never particularly material in nature.
2   Salmond (2017: 252), her emphasis.
3   Ibid.
4   Holbraad (2011) implies that all rather than some 'things' should be analysed together, through his thing=concept analogy.
5   Many authors provide such (essentially passive) commodity histories, however powerful the impact of the commodity in question on the human – e.g. Abbott (2010); Adshead (1992); Allen (2001); Cowan (2005); Dash (2000); Foust (1992); Gately (2001); Harvey et al. (2002); Kurlansky (1999; 2003); Mintz (1985); Pavord (1999) Pendergrast (2010); Reader (2009); Salaman (1949); Warman (2003); Wild (2010). Some write more generally about transformative relationships, positive and negative – e.g. Hobhouse (1999); Singer and Baer (2009). In this book I attempt to take a more "plant's eye view of the world" (Pollan 2002).
6   Ortiz ([1947] 1995).
7   Furst (1991: 319).
8   On the issue of entanglement vs. entrapment, see Hodder (2014); on the 'more-than-human', Tsing (2014).
9   For a recent authoritative list and indication of natural distribution, see Oyuela-Caycedo and Kawa (2015: 28-31).
10 Harvey et al. (2002: 25).
11 Cf. Baptist (2014).
12 In similar vein Fisher (2009: 1) suggests it is "easier to imagine the end of the world than the end of capitalism".
13 Harvey et al. (2002: 25).
14 Heywood (1993: 229).
15 Ibid.
16 Some have discussed tobacco's supposedly 'biphasic' attributes, meaning a substance which can both stimulate and relax, either simultaneously or consecutively. But such is the addiction which regular use of tobacco occasions in many people, it is likely that any relaxing effect is the result of the amelioration of the withdrawal symptoms that lack of tobacco causes rather than any intrinsic relaxing properties of the plant itself.
17 Martin (2006), after Derrida (1981), talks of the ambivalent nature of the Ancient Greek *pharmakon* – a word that meant both poison and remedy.
18 Appadurai (1986: 4).
19 Malinowksi ([1922] 2002: 80).
20 Geismar (2011: 212).
21 See Steward (1955).
22 Harris (1974) provides some examples. However Harris has won rather few champions for an approach that seems dismissive of ideological and symbolic systems (such as language and political beliefs) in shaping human experience.
23 Miller (2009).
24 Miller (2009: 50).
25 The picture relates to an article by McGonigle (2013) in the magazine.
26 Cassanelli (1986).
27 In my own sub-discipline medical anthropology, for example, Hunter (2010) reflects on the HIV/AIDS virus in South Africa, Garcia (2010) looks at heroin in the Rio Grande, and Petryna (2003) the effects of the radiation cloud from the Chernobyl nuclear reactor on inhabitants living nearby, to pick but three influential monographs that take the non-human seriously.

28 On anthropology and the Anthropocene, see a conversation involving Haraway et al. (2016); Latour et al. (2018) talk more generally about the effects of capitalism.
29 Miller (2005: 38).
30 Gell (1998).
31 Geismar (2011: 213), her emphasis.
32 Henare et al. (2007: 3).
33 Latour uses 'actants' in favour of 'actors' to help stress the equivalence of people and things, since the term 'actor' has distinctly human associations in many languages. His theory, however, which he argues is not really a theory at all, is known as Actor-Network-Theory (Latour 2005: 9).
34 This very much accords with Geismar's view (above).
35 Latour (1999: 147).
36 "Just one cigarette each day increases risk of heart disease and stroke" beams a front cover of the *British Medical Journal*, referring to an article by Hackshaw et al. (2018), based on a meta-analysis of 141 cohort studies in 55 reports.
37 Latour (1999: 180).
38 To make a list as long as Salmond's, they include pipes, cigars, curing sheds, tobacco fields, the safety match, lighters, cigarettes, cigarette-making machines, snuff grinders, cigarette packets, tobacco pouches, advertisements, health warnings and scientific literature.
39 Bennett (2004: 353).
40 Pollock (1880: 421).
41 In a similar fashion to the human relationship with another plant product similarly prominent around the time that tobacco erupted on the European scene, 'orange-persons' have been described as those who give themselves over "to the principle of connection that is 'orange'" (Yates 2006: 1007).
42 For more on this see Russell (2018). Holbraad (2011) stimulated my interest in the potential of things to speak.
43 Haraway ([1985] 1991: 149).
44 Black (2014: 41) distinguishes between tools – artefacts directly employed by the hand, and machines – artefacts designed to achieve a particular purpose. He admits, though, that the two categories overlap and the differences between them are becoming increasingly blurred in the 21st century world of handheld devices.
45 Haraway (2003).
46 "I love the fact that human genomes can be found in only about 10 percent of all the cells that occupy the mundane space I call my body", Haraway writes, "the other 90 percent of the cells are filled with the genomes of bacteria, fungi, protists, and such, some of which play in a symphony necessary to my being alive at all, and some of which are hitching a ride and doing the rest of me, of us, no harm" (2008: 3-4). In embracing the non-human elements in her being so enthusiastically, Haraway could be accused of an unnecessary zoocentrism. Tobacco's relationship with humanity, long term, is more complicated – it cannot be claimed as necessary for human life (despite the claims some users might make on its behalf); nor can it be regarded as doing no harm.
47 See, for example, Crosby (2003, 2004); Diamond (1997). For an example of the two-way interchange between people and animals, see Lien (2015) *Becoming Salmon*.
48 Hall (2011: 3).
49 Hallé (2002) quoted in Hall (2011: 5).
50 Wandersee and Schussler (1999).

51 Mabey (2015: 4).
52 Darwin (1880).
53 Baluška et al. (2009).
54 Trewavas (2012: 773).
55 See, for example, Trewavas (2014); Mancuso and Viola (2015).
56 E.g. Garzón and Keijzer (2011).
57 Trewavas and Baluška (2011: 1225).
58 Stork et al. (2011).
59 Steppuhn et al. (2004). It is fascinating to note other experiments, in which mechanical rather than caterpillar wounding triggered a more nicotine-rich response (Delphia et al., 2006). This has led scientists to conclude that the insect predators' saliva may have evolved to produce a counter-compound that suppresses the plant's nicotine response (Musser et al., 2002).
60 Karban et al. (2000).
61 Karban et al. (2004).
62 Trewavas (2014).
63 Li et al. (2007: 280).
64 Some commentators treat intangible 'things' like morality as kinds of 'quasi-actant' (Krarup and Blok 2011); others are more explicit in how they objectify abstract concepts and, conversely, abstract material objects.
65 Holbraad (2011: 12).
66 The Odradek story is recounted in Bennett (2010: 8). Bennett uses the story to argue for "the vibrancy of things" or "thing power". I am grateful to Arthur Rose for his more extensive exegesis of the tale during a 'Life of Breath' project meeting.
67 Russell and Rahman (2015).
68 Hall (2011: 1).
69 Latour (2005: 108) makes a related point when he says the social "is to be explained rather than providing the explanation".
70 Hall (2011: 1).
71 Hall (2011).
72 Kohn (2013).
73 Ibid. (21-2).
74 Ibid. (14).
75 Geismar (2011: 215). Emphasis on "meanings" original; emphasis added to "ontologies".
76 Meillassoux (2006: 5) defines correlationism as "the idea according to which we only ever have access to the correlation between thinking and being, and never to either term considered apart from the other". This is not dissimilar to Descartes' famous maxim "I think, therefore I am".
77 Ziser (2013: 185, fn.16) takes as an example the title of one book, seeking ways of living 'as if' nature mattered, which implies that, ultimately, it does not (Devall and Sessions (1985).
78 Fisher (2016) encourages us to consider the different dimensions of the eerie; see also Macfarlane (2015).
79 Raffles et al. (2015) offer one example of anthropologists who have followed such a trajectory.
80 Marcus (1998: 91-2).
81 Rivoal and Salazar (2013: 178) write "in anthropology, serendipity, together with reflexivity and openness, is widely accepted as a key characteristic (and strength) of the ethnographic method". They define serendipity as a quality involving 'chance' (good fortune) and 'sagacity' (recognizing the significance of one's findings).

82 Not only appropriate due to the acronym of Actor-Network-Theory.
83 Appropriately enough the term he uses for this painstaking work – tracing and tracking – is the expression used for the new technologies which follow the path of 'legal' versus 'illegal' cigarettes electronically across global trade routes; see Chapter 8.
84 Cf. Macnaughton et al. (2012: 457).
85 Van De Poel-Knottnerus and Knottnerus (1994: 67)
86 See, for example, Russell et al. (2009); Heckler and Russell (2008b); Lewis and Russell (2013); McNeill, Iringe-Koko et al. (2014).
87 For more information, see Russell et al. (2009) and Chapter 10.
88 See, for example, Heckler and Russell (2008b) and Lewis and Russell (2011).
89 Lewis and Russell (2013), McNeill, Iringe-Koko et al. (2014).
90 See Chapter 11.
91 Kohrman and Benson (2011: 329).
92 ASH (2008: 1).
93 The result of my discussions with Elizabeth was an edited volume deriving from a workshop held in 2013 to which we invited fellow anthropologists who had worked extensively in lowland South America and who had fascinating things to say about tobacco production and use amongst the indigenous peoples with whom they had worked there. See Russell and Rahman (2015).
94 Bell and Dennis (2013: 12)
95 Derrida (1981)
96 This distinction is made by Holbraad et al. (2014)
97 Frazer (1920: 43). I have been unable to find out whether Frazer smoked a pipe or other object while he was in his armchair.
98 Malinowski (1922: 5)
99 Using 'perspective' in the sense Viveiros de Castro (1998) uses it – see Chapter 1 and subsequent chapters.

Part I

Life

Shamanic dreaming

For someone working in the field of public health, discovering the importance of tobacco in what is almost certainly its source region, Amazonia, is rather like going through Lewis Carroll's looking glass. Suddenly what was once familiar seems strange, what was strange, familiar. Far from the source of a 'golden holocaust', as one book describes the western experience of tobacco without hint of hyperbole,[1] in lowland South America, the region where tobacco's relationship with humanity has been longest, the plant is widely and variously regarded as a blessing from the gods, a 'master plant', a spirit in its own right, a food for the spirits, and a plant with the energy to cleanse and cure. In this chapter I look at the relationship between people and tobacco in lowland South America in order to understand the place of tobacco in this particular world, and its implications for a non-human ethnography of tobacco worldwide.

Of the 50 *Nicotiana* species indigenous to the Americas, 41 are specifically from South America. Species diversity of this kind can occur for a number of different reasons, but the disproportionate representation of tobacco species in those parts lends support to the argument that tobacco has a long evolutionary history in the Americas.[2] The tobacco species with the highest concentration of nicotine are *Nicotiana tabacum* and *Nicotiana rustica*, at 1.23 per cent and 2.47 per cent respectively. Received wisdom has it that such high levels of nicotine are the result of human domestication, but recent DNA evidence suggests that much of this evolution took place prior to any human involvement.[3] For example, an ancestral parent of *Nicotiana tabacum, Nicotiana sylvestris*, is found in north-west Argentina and Bolivia, from where genetic evidence suggests it hybridized and moved eastwards into lowland Peru, Brazil, Paraguay and the humid Amazon forests some 200,000 years ago, long before the entry of humans into the Americas. *Nicotiana rustica* likewise hails from the arid landscapes of Peru, Ecuador, and the Bolivian lowlands where it evolved prior to the arrival of people.

North and South America were the last continents to be settled by humans. Genetic and archaeological evidence is mixed, but one strongly argued suggestion is that this peopling took place quite rapidly from a relatively small pool of migrants, known as the Clovis people, who split off from a central Asian population in the Palaeolithic period and settled in a land bridge area called Beringia, between Russia and Alaska, where the Baring Straits now flow. They stayed in this area for anything up to 20,000 years until about 11,500 years ago, when the retreat of the Wisconsin ice sheet permitted movement down an 'ice-free corridor', along which bands of no more than 8,000 to 12,000 persons transited rapidly from North to South (Fig. 1.1).[4]

Imagine the experience of the first people to make the transit from Beringia down the coast of what is now Alaska and British Columbia, into the warmer climes to the south. This, unlike the misguided claims made by European colonialists who came thousands of years later, really was untamed wilderness. It was not the presence of other people, their accessories and legacies that was surprising – there were none. Rather it was the diversity of plant and animal life that was a source of amazement. Instead of 'culture shock', as they proceeded from the permafrost terrain of Beringia into warmer, more benign and biodiverse environments, the overriding feeling the wandering bands most likely had was one of 'nature shock' from an abundance of beneficent nature. They preyed on mastodons and other large mammals, cumbersome creatures that were easy prey for the fleet-footed, proto-Amerindians and some of which were eventually hunted to extinction. As the first peoples came south, across the Isthmus of Panama and into the Amazon region, the range of flora and fauna became even greater.

Amongst the cornucopia of new plants and animals surrounding the early migrants arriving in South America were the impressively large and florally colourful examples of the *Nicotiana* species which, after millennia of waiting, "simply benefitted from...dispersion by humans beyond their original range".[5] *N. rustica* probably dispersed northwards into Central and North America with the help of hunter-gatherer groups before the advent of agriculture: the earliest *N. rustica* seeds identified in North America are from around 2,000 years ago. The archaeological record in South America is sorely lacking, but estimates here are for a much longer period – some 8,000–10,000 years – of *N. tabacum* domestication and use.

During this time, tobacco became strongly entwined with human life and thought. The deep history of the plant in North and, particularly, South America is reflected in the extensive range of contemporary indigenous terms for tobacco, the many myths and stories surrounding it, the diversity of ways in which it is used, and what it is used for. Chewing the leaf, drinking tobacco juice, licking its paste, using it as an enema, snuffing its powder and smoking its leaf – all can be found in different parts of North and South America, along with the paraphernalia associated with each.[6] Across the Americas we find many people using tobacco smoke, spit or poultices for purification and healing purposes – amongst them its decoction and use as an embrocation for sprains and bruises, and the use of its crushed leaves as a poultice applied to wounds. However, anthropologists have tended to over-look these everyday uses in favour of more dramatic ways tobacco can be

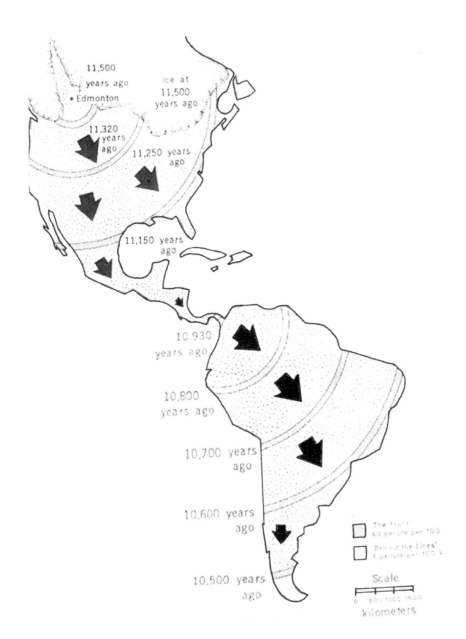

Fig. 1.1 The peopling of the Americas

Source: Martin, 1973

used – often in hallucinatory quantities[7] – in shamanic practices, and how these practices interdigitate with indigenous perceptions and cosmologies.

Tobacco and shamanism

Shamanism is the blanket term given to a range of activities that involve certain people (shamans) moving between spiritual and physical worlds in order to effect change. To do this, practitioners must enter into an altered state of consciousness that enables them to make this transition.[8] Of the at least 130 plants with hallucinogenic properties in South America that are put to use in this way,[9] the one used by shamans more than any other is tobacco.[10] The Matsigenka people of Eastern Peru are typical of the many groups where a shaman is "the one intoxicated by tobacco",[11] and amongst whom tobacco is "the hallmark of shamanic activity".[12] Wilbert defines the tobacco shaman as "the religious practitioner who uses tobacco, whether exclusively or not, to be ordained, to officiate, and to achieve altered states of consciousness".[13] Sometimes, tobacco is the means of creating communication with parallel, spirit worlds. Sometimes it is used as an offering to attract the spirits residing in those worlds.[14] Sometimes it transports the shaman directly, its analgesic properties rendering the shaman's body insensitive to heat and pain. However, it is its intoxicating and hallucinatory properties that make it such a central feature of shamanic healing and sorcery.

Here is an account by Gertrude Dole of the experience of a Kuikuru shaman, Metsé, imbibing tobacco in a ritual séance. It raises several themes concerning tobacco shamanism that will be returned to later in the chapter:

> Metsé inhaled deeply, and as he finished one cigarette an attending shaman handed him another lighted one. Metsé inhaled all the smoke, and soon began to evince considerable physical distress. After about ten minutes his right leg began to tremble. Later his left arm began to twitch. He swallowed smoke as well as inhaling it, and soon was groaning in pain. His respiration became labored, and he groaned with every exhalation. By this time the smoke in his stomach was causing him to retch...The more he inhaled the more nervous he became...He took another cigarette and continued to inhale until he was near to collapse...Suddenly he 'died', flinging his arms outward and straightening his legs stiffly...He remained in this state of collapse nearly fifteen minutes...When Metsé had revived himself two attendant shamans rubbed his arms. One of the shamans drew on a cigarette and blew smoke gently on his chest and legs, especially on places that he indicated by stroking himself.[15]

The anthropologist Johannes Wilbert is insistent that shamanism must have come first, and envisions hunter and gatherer groups originally relying "on endogenous and ascetic techniques of mystic ecstasy rather than on drug-induced trance".[16] Siberian shamans are a good example, although Wilbert remarks how quickly the Siberians adopted tobacco into their later 16th century shamanic rituals, "thus recapturing for it the religious meaning that it has always had for the American Indians",[17] but which had been lost in its habitual and addictive use amongst Europeans. For Wilbert, the distinctive physiological and psychological effects of tobacco provide empirical, experiential support for shamanic practices, including initiations, near- and actual death experiences such as Metsé's (above), shape-shifting and other experiences. However, his argument is that tobacco's effects served to confirm rather than shape the "basic tenets of shamanic ideology".[18]

Of course, tobacco shamanism is not ubiquitous in South America. Some groups practice forms of shamanism in ways that are 'drug-free'.[19] The anthropologist Claude Lévi-Strauss was likewise aware that in tropical America "some tribes smoke tobacco, while adjoining tribes are unacquainted with or prohibit its use. The Nambirwara are confirmed smokers, and are hardly ever seen without a cigarette in their mouths. …Yet their neighbours, the Tupi-Kawahi, have such a violent dislike for tobacco that they look disapprovingly at any visitors who dare to smoke in their presence, and even on occasions come to blows with them. Such differences are not infrequent in South America, where the use of tobacco was no doubt even more sporadic in the past".[20]

Yet there are similarities as well as differences. Wilbert argues for the "strikingly similar tobacco ideology of American Indians that coincides with the limits of tobacco distribution in the New World",[21] going on to describe expansively what such an ideology might be through demonstrating "the extraordinary power of this agent of diffusion".[22] Lévi-Strauss was similarly preoccupied with commonalities across the whole American landmass. In his masterwork, the four-volume study, *Mythologiques*, he follows a single mythic form from the southern tip of South America up through Central America and eventually into the Arctic Circle, tracing its cultural evolution and variations from group to group. He professes interest in the underlying structure of relationships amongst the different elements of the stories rather than their content, seeing them as evidence of immutable structures of the human mind. Both Wilbert and Lévi-Strauss put shamanic practices and human mental structures as primary, and tobacco as secondary. Yet in lowland South America, the part of the world where people's relationship with tobacco has been longest, we may find aspects of shamanic ideology that have been shaped by tobacco, rather than simply confirmed by it. After all, Volume 2 of *Mythologiques* (*From Honey to Ashes*) presents a mythic system which "revolves round the central theme of tobacco".[23] In the rest of this chapter, I shall look at the stories about tobacco in lowland South America, and the commonalities that can be identified, based on numerous ethnographic examples, with a view to better understanding Wilbert's 'tobacco ideology' and its possible influence in shaping, rather than just confirming, certain cultural tropes in human life and thought in Amazonia.

Untangling 'tobacco ideology'

The long history of tobacco use in lowland South America and the respect it is accorded by many indigenous peoples gives us further clues about what Wilbert intended the term 'tobacco ideology' to encapsulate. The Yanomami are one of many Venezuelan groups in whose lives tobacco plays a central role. Here is the story of how tobacco was originally acquired through two Yanomami culture heroes, Haxo-riwë and Tomï-riwë:

> The old Yanomamo did not have tobacco. Instead they used to chew *taratara*, an elongated leaf that is rather harmful because it intoxicates. Haxo-riwë was sad, and he cried because he could not chew *taratara*. Seeing him weeping, Tomï-riwë took pity on him. He knew of another leaf which was less powerful than the *taratara* and which did not intoxicate. It was tobacco. So he called Haxo-riwë, took a few tobacco seeds that he had, wrapped them in a banana leaf, put everything inside a tube container, and gave it to him, saying: "Take this. Go home, and then to your plantation and plant these".

There follow some quite detailed instructions about how to sow, cultivate and process tobacco into a small roll which is placed between the gum and lower lip, because "when you're sucking tobacco like that you'll have the strength to work and won't feel so hungry". The story continues as follows:

> Haxo-riwë did everything that Tomï-riwë had told him. The plants that he had sown grew. Then he went to the plantation, picked a few leaves, returned home, and made a roll. When he began to suck, he felt such great pleasure that he went crazy with happiness. Running off to the forest in big leaps, he turned into a *kinkajou*. Afterward Tomï-riwë went into the forest where he was transformed into an *agouti*. To this day we Yanomamo cultivate tobacco the way Tomï-riwë showed Haxo-riwë. We call on them to make the seeds fruitful. If it rains a lot we harvest only a little tobacco, but if there is a drought we get an abundant harvest".

The *kinkajou* is a small nocturnal member of the racoon family[24] and is seen by the Yanomami as the animal-person responsible for the discovery and celebration of tobacco. But it was another folk hero, Nosiriwë, who was responsible for its spread. In the contemporary myth world he wanders through the forest, driven mad by a desire he cannot express. "*Peshiyë, peshiyë, peshiyë!*" he cries.[25] After a series of frustrating encounters with different forest beings, each of which tries to offer him some kind of wild fruit to assuage his desire, he meets Kinkajou. Kinkajou first gives Nosiriwë some *pahi* fruits, but when these fail to satisfy his desire he points him towards his stone axe where a wad of tobacco is lying on the handle. Nosiriwë puts a large cut of tobacco under his lip and goes off crying with satisfaction. The tale concludes: "In the places where Nosiriwë spat as he walked, tobacco plants sprouted in his wake. It was Nosiriwë who caused tobacco to spread everywhere, but it was Kinkajou who discovered it".[26] In this myth the Yanomami not only recognize the intense desire tobacco can engender but how this can mobilize journeys for consumption and exchange.[27] Such feelings will strike a chord with any regular tobacco user who has gone without their expected intake. Less familiar, but explored further below, is the idea that these cravings are common to animals and humans, indeed that one can shift from one category to the other at will and see how easy it is to see things from the other's point of view.

The Warao of the Orinoco Delta are another group for whom "tobacco is of utmost cultural significance despite the fact that they cannot grow it in their swampy habitat but rely on its importation from the island of Trinidad and from regions adjacent to the Orinoco Delta".[28] In one Warao myth explaining the origin and importance of tobacco, the longing for tobacco transmutes into the grief of a man at the loss of his son, Kurusiwari, and a longing to see him once more. Kurusiwari was the product of a second marriage, as the man's first wife could not bear him a child. The first wife was, however, very good at weaving hammocks, and Kurusiwari was good at distracting her from her work. One day she pushed him aside roughly, the child cried and left the house unnoticed by his parents as they made love in one of the hammocks. By the time his parents caught up with him, the boy was with two companions and the three of them had grown up. His parents begged Kurusiwari to return home, but he would only agree to appear if they built him a Spirit house to which they would 'call' him with tobacco. In those days, people knew nothing about tobacco, as it grew only on an island in the sea, guarded by women. Of the birds used to attempt to fetch some of the tobacco seeds, only a crane and humming bird, in partnership, were able to bring back some seeds for planting. The father became a shaman, singing to the accompaniment of a rattle. His son and the two companions were now the three tobacco spirits and always came in answer to the rattle's call.[29]

This myth alludes to the importance of tobacco in the exchange economy in lowland South America, particularly for groups who lack ready access to it and hence must outsource it from elsewhere. Meanwhile the neglect of Kurusiwari (dismissed by his non-biological mother and ignored by his biological parents due to their sexual desire for each other) is redeemed only by the parents agreeing to provide the child (now a spirit) with tobacco, and by the father becoming a shaman, using tobacco as both the bridge between himself and his spirit son, and the lure to ensure his return. In another Warao

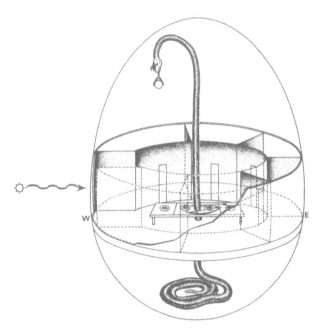

Fig. 1.2 The Zenithal house of the tobacco spirit

Source: drawing by Noel Diaz, from Wilbert, 2004: 26, reproduced with the kind permission of Johannes Wilbert and Utah University Press.

myth, also quoted by Wilbert, the tobacco spirit lives in an egg-shaped house, the cosmic centre of the Warao light shamans (Fig. 1.2). Everything in the house – its contents and residents – is made of the thickened smoke of flowering tobacco plants. These plants stand on both sides of a rope bridge also made of smoke and which links the house to the apex of the world. A shaman lives in the Tobacco Spirit's house. His wife, once a bee, now a frigate bird, is a white female shaman who specializes in curing nicotinic seizures. Four insects live in the house. From time to time they "gather around a gambling table on which they move specific counters to invade each other's spaces according to a dice arrow cast by the Spirit of Tobacco...Depending on which gambler wins, someone will live or die on earth".[30]

These extraordinarily complex metaphysical accounts are frequently presented as intriguing folk tales, yet they are certainly more than 'myths' in the western sense of fiction or fable. For indigenous peoples in lowland South America such myths are an important part of contemporary life. One anthropologist working amongst the Yanomami heard the Haxo-riwë myth related above used by Yanomami cultivators in the form of a propitiatory spell when planting their tobacco crop, for example.[31] We can also see them as presenting a more directly sensorial account of people's relationship to and experience of tobacco – the raw desire for tobacco expressed in the Nosiriwë myth, for example, or the loss of a son as a result of similar, more carnal desires such that only tobacco could woo him back in the Kurusiwari myth. It is also tempting to see the insect gambling game in the Warao house of the Tobacco Spirit as an allegory for the dual nature of tobacco as a plant with the ability to deliver both life and death. In all cases, there appears to be what Barbira Freedman calls "the collusion of the empirical and symbolic properties of tobacco".[32] Could the imbibing of tobacco in the hallucinatory quantities associated with shamanic practices have had pharmacological consequences reflected in the dream-like quality of the myths presented here? Is shape-shifting, body transformation and seeing things from the perspective of other beings likewise facilitated by tobacco? If so, how very convenient for the long-term success of tobacco.

All these stories demonstrate the extraordinarily rich mythologies surrounding tobacco in lowland South America. By drawing out some of their common characteristics, we can perhaps come to a better understanding of the possible parameters of Wilbert's 'tobacco ideology'. The three aspects I would like to focus on in what follows are the notion that tobacco constitutes and helps to strengthen the body, the contribution tobacco makes to understanding a multiperspectival universe, and the way tobacco may be associated with the generation of cognitive dualisms.[33]

Tobacco constitutes persons

The Baniwa of north west Brazil have a story about Dzuliferi, the 'owner of tobacco', who gave fresh, green tobacco to culture hero Nhiaperikuli at the beginning of time, long before the first ancestral humans were created. Each lineage has its particular kind of ancestral, sacred tobacco which was given to the souls of their ancestors, along with sacred pepper, when they emerged. For them, tobacco is an important part of all healing rituals because the sweet smell of its smoke coaxes the soul of the sick person back to life. Robin Wright, the anthropologist who has worked with the Baniwa, describes the processes involved as follows:

> Smoking freshly grown green tobacco makes the soul 'content' and the body 'strong'. Passing a fresh cigar around a circle of people is a mark of harmonious sociality in the sacred stories and in real life. '*Alira*,' the Baniwa say, as the tobacco cigar goes around, leaving each person with a strong and contented heart-soul. The evangelical missionaries, who condemned tobacco smoking as being 'of the devil', in reality were condemning Baniwa souls.[34]

The interconnectedness of people and tobacco is strongly marked in this passage. Tobacco plays an important role in creating, shaping and transforming people of all sorts, including shamans, throughout North[35] and South America.[36] For many Amerindian populations the body is chronically unstable, nothing but a superficial and ephemeral cloak to a single, meta-'soul'. The Achuar, another Amazonian group, are described as refusing to divide their world into the cultural world of human society and the natural world of animals. Instead, their cultural realm contains animals, plants and spirits which some (including members of other Amerindian societies) might be inclined to put in the realm of nature. In the latter realm are consigned those living species which lack a soul [wakan] and hence the ability to communicate – this category includes "most insects and fish, poultry, and numerous plants, which thus lead a mechanical, inconsequential existence".[37] The soul is shared with other living species and gives them the ability to communicate. Tobacco is a master plant with 'soul' in abundance. In a familiar shamanic healing gesture throughout South America, a shaman blows smoke over the patient's clasped hands and the crown of the patient's head (as well as the heads of fellow shamans). This is seen as strengthening and protecting both the body and the soul, concentrating the life force within it.

The fluidity and vulnerability of bodies[38] and the use of tobacco to firm these up is used to good effect in child rearing as well as adulthood. During childbirth, tobacco smoke is sometimes used as a shield to distract potentially harmful spirits from attacking the vulnerable mother and new-born. Tobacco smoke is also used in order to cool, dry out, and firm up or harden the neonate. The Xié, for example, regard the newborn as a 'little fish': a creature in need of forming into a fully-fledged human being.[39] Indeed for the Muinane, Witoto and Andoke peoples living along the Brazilian/Colombian border, tobacco is seen as actively constituting persons. "We all have the same hearts, made from the same tobacco" say the elders of these different language groups, collectively called 'the People of the Centre'. In other contexts, the differences between people that westerners might attribute to cultural differences are accredited to differences between their tobaccos.[40]

The mutually constitutive relationship between people and tobacco has resonance with statements attributed to the Yanomami about the environment not being separate from the people: "We are inside it, and it is inside us. We make it, and it makes us". The parallel with the notion of non-human agency espoused by Miller (Introduction), "the things people make, make people", is obvious. The Yanomami spokesperson most renowned for his espousal of environmental values, although he rejects use of the term environment as something separate from humanity, is the shaman Davi Kopenawa. Tobacco is an important element in his life, although his shamanic journeys take place through the medium of a different hallucinogenic substance.[41]

Tobacco changes perspectives

In contrast to western notions of the 'natural body', regarded as a stable substrate for the range and diversity of human cultures, the Xié example (above) reflects the commonly held view amongst many Amazonian peoples that it is the soul which is the stable constant, underpinning a multiplicity of natural forms of which humans are only one. This notion – of one shared soul and many natures – has been glossed as 'multinaturalism'. In a 'multi-natural' world such as that inhabited by the Achuar (above), it is unstable bodies (rather than cultures) which can alter and transform, a tendency known as shape-shifting.[42] A jaguar, for example, may be a shaman in disguise; shamans are particularly renowned for their shape-shifting abilities. This is not an easy matter for Amerindians to contend with. In McCallum's words, for the Amazonians, "the world is riddled with misinformation and lies, truth a matter of dispute".[43] According to one anthropologist who worked with the Wari', a group living in the Rodonia region of Brazil, "it is always best to distrust one's own eyes...metamorphosis is something that haunts the native imagination".[44] The following Wari' story is typical:

> A child is invited by her mother to take a trip to the forest. Many days go by as they walk around and pick fruit. The child is treated normally by her mother until one day, realizing just how long they have spent away from home, the child starts to grow suspicious. Looking carefully, she sees a tail discreetly hidden between her mother's legs. Struck by fear, she cries for help, summoning her true kin and causing the jaguar to flee, leaving a trail of paw-prints in its wake. One woman, telling me about this event, said that, after finding her, the girl's true mother warned her to always distrust other people. Whenever she went far from home, either with her mother or father, she should take along a brother or sister as company (in order, I assume, to secure her point of view).[45]

As well as multinatural shape-shifting, this story features the need to secure a point of view, which is predicated on it being possible to see things from the point of view of another. This other does not have to be human. Anthropologist Eduardo Viveiros de Castro talks of "the conception, common to many peoples of the continent, according to which the world is inhabited by different sorts of subjects or persons, human and non-human, which apprehend reality from different points of view".[46] So marked is this propensity that Viveiros de Castro coined the term 'cosmological perspectivism' to encapsulate it.

This ability to put oneself in the place of another being is reflected in a pattern of speech common to many lowland South American groups. Here is one anthropologist writing about the Juruna of Brazil:

One of the first phenomena to catch my attention during my fieldwork were the indelible, though elusive, marks left by the notion of point of view. Certain phrases spoken to me in Portuguese, such as "this is beautiful to me", "for him, the animal turned into a jaguar", "to us, there appeared prey while we were making the canoe" seemed to refer exclusively to the grammatical structure of a language which I did not master but which nonetheless became transparent through the Juruna's Portuguese. Even after I began to put together one or two phrases, the constructions which invited these types of translation never ceased to sound strange: without doubt, I would classify them as the most difficult Juruna practice to assimilate. "*Amana ube wi*" – it is not easy to utter these words without becoming disconcerted, unpleasantly or otherwise. I felt I was saying "to me, it rained" and not "it was raining there, where I was". This way of relating even the most independent and alien phenomena to the self leaves its mark on Juruna cosmology, yet I neither presume that all grammatical categories play the same role in a culture, nor do I believe that there is even a remote possibility that one of us could put ourselves in the skin of one of the Juruna in order to capture the sense which human life would assume in a situation in which, for us, suddenly, it became acceptable, or at least perfectly valid, to say "it's raining for me". At most, this sense would relate to a virtuality which is within us, thereby turning us inside-out.[47]

The point being made about relating what might otherwise be seen as phenomena independent to the self is interesting. To say "it rained to me", rather than just "it rained", paradoxically enhances the sense of 'self' while emphasizing its relationship to other human and non-human beings; a constant linguistic reminder that, while this is how it was for me (or us), others might see things differently. This could be something as apparently mundane as the weather, but extends into all aspects of life such as a sense of beauty, the idea that an animal or person might have turned into a jaguar, or that prey appeared while making a canoe. In other words, there is a strong sense of appreciating the relativity of one's own, and the reality of others', points of view. This extends not simply to humans but to the range of non-human animals, plants and objects that share the common 'soul essence'. It is a foundational claim of cosmological perspectivism that indigenous Amazonian animals, "the archetypal 'natural' creatures, subjectively identify themselves as humans, the archetypal cultural beings".[48] Thus peccaries are a favourite prey amongst Juruna hunters, but the peccaries see themselves as humans engaged in warfare, not animals at the receiving end of a hunter's dart.

It would be wrong to attribute the development of such perspectival thinking exclusively to the effects of tobacco, although contemplation of the shamanic uses of tobacco makes such a possibility quite likely. McCallum mentions *nixi pae* (the word for the hallucinogen *ayahuasca* amongst the Amerindian group she studies) as another perspective-changing compound that turns visible what is normally unseen.[49] For her, it is "the controlling presence of language" which is fundamental in making sense of hallucinogenic experiences. Yet its ubiquity and frequently prodigious use in shamanic rituals, it seems to me, makes tobacco similarly strongly implicated in these transformations and, we might surmise, cosmological perspectivism more generally. There is a danger in ignoring the material substances (tobacco included) which underpin such 'out of body' or shape-shifting experiences. After all, prodigious tobacco ingestion frequently leads to such interpretations, rather than simply confirming them.

Tobacco generates dualisms

Lévi-Strauss' structuralism, while regularly taught, is now perhaps regarded as a little *passé* by many anthropologists. Fashions have changed, and many are wary of assuming unverifiable structures for the human mind, while others feel his theories do not attend to issues such as power, political-economic relationships such as colonialism, and the question of human and non-human agency and practice (as opposed to abstract mindsets). There is also a distaste amongst many anthropologists for the idea of binary opposites on which much of Lévi-Strauss' theorizing is based. Yet such dualisms, as Lévi-Strauss demonstrates so magisterially in *Mythologiques*, are alive and well, embedded in indigenous thought processes throughout North and South America. Indeed, Lévi-Strauss's fundamental premise – the categorical opposition of nature and culture, whatever the contents of these two poles are taken to be in specific circumstances – has been described as a core Amerindian cosmological concern.[50] Little wonder, given his fieldwork location, that Lévi-Strauss was able to develop structuralist theory where and when he did.

Anthropologists following in the wake of Lévi-Strauss, however, seem strangely reticent about discussing such dualities, tending to underplay or deny the binary pairings on which structuralism is founded.[51] Tim Ingold, for example, applauds the idea of a "paradigm of embodiment" because of its "promise to collapse the Cartesian dualities between mind and body, subject and object". This, he suggests "holds a certain appeal for many anthropologists whose familiarity with indigenous, non-Western understandings – which are not generally concordant with such dualities – predisposes them to adopt a critical attitude towards the foundational assumptions of Western thought and science".[52] Stolze Lima similarly writes of "a binary system [in Juruma cosmology]…all these categories being the object of a dispute between humans and another category of alterity" (i.e. non-human others).[53] But she goes on to mask the significance of this binary thinking by the use of semantically distracting words such as 'duplicity' (rather than 'dualism'), as when she writes:

duplicity is the law of every being and every event. Let us take human experience as an example. It never presents a single dimension; it is double by definition. One dimension is that of sensible reality....the other is that of the soul. The latter develops in dreams and its rules are not necessarily the same as those active in sensible reality.[54]

The word 'dialectical' is sometimes used in a similar (might we say duplicitous?) fashion. Yet despite the efforts of some anthropologists to avoid acknowledging the binary thinking which is its bedrock, it is interesting to note how often structural theory seems to fit the ethnographic data in North and South America. Is it a complete coincidence that this is precisely the same hemisphere marked by Wilbert's ubiquitous 'tobacco ideology'? Could it be that the sense of such binary oppositions has something to do with the presence of tobacco and its influence (both subtle and not-so-subtle) in people's lives and thoughts?

Cosmological perspectivism is sometimes called 'post-structuralist' theory in South American studies; the binary oppositions it contains sometimes appear as rather an embarrassment. For example, in one passage emphasizing the fluidity between the 'human' and 'non-human' in Amazonia and the 'multinaturalism' of Amazonian societies, Viveiros de Castro relegates "the syncretic master opposition between nature and culture" found in them to a mere footnote.[55] Yet this dualism, for him, is marked by particular config-urations of dyadic pairs such as "universal and particular, objective and subjective, physical and social, fact and value, the given and the instituted, necessity and spontaneity, immanence and transcendence, body and mind, animality and humanity, among many more".[56]

From Honey to Ashes is based on commonly recurring symbolic oppositions in Amerindian mythologies. Lévi-Strauss, like Viveiros de Castro, interprets these as being fundamentally between nature and culture. Nature is represented by honey; a natural, moist, raw and pre-processed product. Tobacco, by contrast, is culture; a refined product that is dry and cooked (or rather, burnt, which, in Lévi-Strauss's eyes, makes it 'meta-culinary', compared to honey, which, as a raw material, is 'infra-culinary').[57] He presents tobacco as establishing the dominance of culture, a product which "unites properties that are normally incompatible",[58] such as the natural and the supernatural, and the physical and metaphysical. Tobacco and honey both occupy "an ambiguous and equivocal position between food and poison" in the myths he analyses.[59] Tobacco's good and bad forms are based on their mode of consumption: exhaled tobacco smoke establishes a beneficent relationship with the spirit world, but inhaled smoke is likely to lead to the transformation of the inhaler into an animal.[60] Lévi-Strauss sees the act of smoking as the quintessential transformation of nature into culture, an act "essentially social; while at the same time it establishes communication between mankind and the supernatural world".[61]

Another dualism we could add to Viveiros de Castro's list is that between male and female. Barbira Freedman has written about tobacco's contribution to gendering of the South American cosmos. Amongst the Lamista Quechua shamans, "tobacco is considered to be the male catalyst that enhances the effects of all other shamanic plants".[62] Certain plants are recognized in both the Amazon and the Andes as 'plants who have mothers'. "Those that do are regarded as 'powerful plants', whose subjectivities can be enlisted to prevail over those of less powerful beings which may encroach upon or attack humans in the cosmos, and even rob their souls, de-substantialising them. All shamanic plants, unlike commonly used medicinal plants, are 'plants with mother spirits' with a connotation of psychotropic attributes".[63] Tobacco is the male consort for the female spirit of such plants and is therefore the catalyst necessary to ensure their effectiveness.[64] Given its significance, it is little wonder it is so commonly (but not inevitably) the hallmark of shamanic activity!

Anthropologists have tended to be reluctant to acknowledge the binary nature that appears to be the epistemological bedrock of lowland South America (as it is pretty much everywhere else in the world, according to structural theory). Yet it is but one of the ways in which tobacco can be seen to have contributed to the shaping of Amazonian life and thought. Others we have observed are the co-constitution of tobacco and persons, the fluidity of bodies and the shifting of perspectives. Structuralism does not always provide predictable answers or results, nor does it necessarily deal with the nitty-gritty of everyday life and experience. Likewise, anthropologists' interests in animism have sometimes been at odds with the more down-to-earth concerns of the people with whom they have been living. One anthropologist, reflecting on her fieldwork experiences in Amazonia, reports that

> while I often struggled to get someone to help me collect stories about shamanism or to transcribe myths and chants, I had no difficulty in finding people willing to show me how to prepare a banana plantation, or to explain the specific uses of a particular plant.[65]

There can also be exceptions to the structural binaries so deftly woven by Lévi-Strauss. Tobacco undermines its own binary (in Lévi-Strauss' mind) in failing to consider modes of production and consumption of tobacco that are not dependent on it being dried, burnt and inhaled. Amongst the Witoto and other groups known collectively as People of the Centre, for example, the most common form of tobacco use is as a licked or sucked paste – indeed, this is a defining feature of the groups concerned. Juan Alvaro Echeverri has lived and worked closely with the Witoto. The paste that men, women and children consume extensively is "a thick decoction of tobacco juice mixed with vegetable salt".[66] This doesn't fit the raw/cooked, burnt/moist, supra-culinary/infra-culinary oppositions that characterize the relationship Lévi-Strauss charted between tobacco and honey. Instead, Alvaro Echeverri suggests, tobacco paste and honey co-exist on the same side of a binary of which vegetable salt (which is burnt) and coca powder (which is roasted) are the opposites. The people to the south, whom Lévi-Strauss used as his exemplars, smoke tobacco leaves rather than licking tobacco paste. They love honey and make it a feature of special festivals. Amongst the Witoto, by contrast, honey is never consumed raw, because it is considered to be blood. Tobacco paste, seasoned with vegetable salt, occupies the same semantic pole that honey does further south. Tobacco paste *is* the Witoto honey, argues Echeverri, and "plays a central role in the ceremonial life of the People of the Centre".[67] The Matsigenka use *opatsa-seri*, a paste mixed with *ayahuasca*, to create a form of 'dream tobacco'.[68] As well as its shamanic connotations, there are "the less explicitly 'mystical' everyday functions of the plant" to consider.[69] Think, for example, of the everyday cultivation practices of smallholder farmers of Borba in Amazonas, whose tobacco cultivation on black *terra preta* soils is "the product of long-term indigenous settlement and management during the pre-Columbian era".[70]

It seems to me we need to supplement the ways in which scholars have considered tobacco cognitively, by acknowledging and exploring the physical, physiological experiences of the plant itself, both its production and consumption. We need to consider tobacco as an entity – plant, spirit, voice – with a 'social life',[71] a life concerned not only with people but also in combination to or opposition with paraphernalia ('things') and other ambivalent substances such as coca and *ayahuasca* (South America), alcohol or marijuana. Such connections form the subject matter of the rest of the book.

Conclusion: then and now, here and there

It is nighttime, and in the communal house of the Xié river dwellers in the north-western headwaters of the Brazilian Amazon the men sit together enjoying a smoke after supper. Visitors are invited to roll themselves a cigarette from the pouch of commercial tobacco sitting on the table. The Brazilian *Fumo Extra Forte Coringa* ['Extra Strong Coringa Smoke'] is the preferred brand; the Portuguese catchphrase on the packet is *'vamos a pitar'* ['Let's smoke!']. The pages of old school exercise books, obtained from the local school teacher, become rolling papers.[72] Such a vignette shows Amazonian peoples are far from immune to corporate tobacco and the forces of global capitalism. Contemporary anthropologists have observed many examples of change and adaptation in indigenous practices as commercially manufactured tobacco products are brought back into these communities. For the Ashaninka people, recovering from a brutal civil war, tobacco offers ways of becoming Peruvian. In such ways, tobacco changes its relationship to the people living the myth of its origins, extending its reach even wider, engaging with and shaping hitherto undreamt of material and spiritual shores.

'Indigenous' is a relative term, and so too is 'traditional'. It is wrong to suggest that what we see in the contemporary practices described in this chapter are 'traditional' practices surrounding tobacco which have been passed down since times immemorial. Tradition has a habit of getting its feet under the cultural table very quickly. In fact, practices considered traditional are often quite recent inventions.[73] Sometimes the word is invoked, either unconsciously or deliberately, to serve particular ideological or commercial ends. The use of hallucinogenic *ayahuasca* for shamanic purposes in south-western Amazonia is a case in point. *Ayahuasca* shamanism might be assumed to be a traditional practice lost in the mists of time, and certainly this is how it is presented to numerous (gullible?) westerners who come to South America on a 'shamanic tourism' trail, as well as to followers of various Brazilian, *ayahuasca*-based religions such as 'Santo Daime' and 'União do Vegetal', which now have followers worldwide. However, contemporary *ayahuasca* use has now, with some certainty, been connected to the expansion of the rubber industry in the late 19th century, having been brought by workers moving to the area from further north.[74] It is currently enjoying a resurgence through the development of '*ayahuasca* tourism', largely targeted at westerners and feeding into a desire for individual, commoditized, sacred experiences.[75] While tobacco use clearly has a much longer history in the region, the *ayahuasca* example should warn us to guard against assuming the ways in which tobacco has been used – or indeed whether it has been used at all – have been stable through time.[76]

Anthropologists tend to back off from grand statements concerning particular things (such as tobacco) and their role in the development of modes of thought, preferring to think of people in general – or, more often, particular people – as having the upper hand in terms of agency. Yet the power of tobacco – generative in the contexts we have been exploring it of sociality, purification, healing and shamanic vision – makes it a strong contender for equality with, if not mastery of, indigenous life, thought and experience in the Americas. While we can accept Wilbert's contention that shamanism came first, and tobacco use later, given the intoxicating quantities consumed, at least in shamanic rituals, and the commonalities of metaphysics across the region where tobacco was used, we can assume that tobacco has also helped shape its own ideology. In other words, it has engaged with, shaped and transformed at least some of the metaphysical structures of which it was a part. Cosmological perspectivism, its associated view of 'many natures', and a sense of the fluidity of bodily forms are all aspects of lowland South American thought processes which feed an anthropological fascination with exotic metaphysics. Less commonly celebrated is the strong sense of binary dualisms as another key organizing principle in indigenous American thought. Tobacco, I argue, has played an active role in shaping all aspects of Amerindian cosmology. To use Juruna perspectivalism, "to me, tobacco has been an active partner in shaping Amerindian perspectives".

Tobacco has tended to be taken for granted by anthropologists working in lowland South America. Its ubiquity has led to it being 'hidden in plain sight'; a passing reference in ethnographic accounts of life in the region if it is referred to at all. The "everyday blessings"[77] of tobacco in Amazonia are in stark contrast to the 'banal evil' of tobacco use from the perspective of public health (Chapters 10-12). Yet there may also be common ground that exists between these two poles, and this is what the rest of this book will investigate, under the common rubric of tobacco's agency. Are there similarities, as opposed to contrasts, between the tobacco ideology here briefly charted in the Amazonian context, and the hybrid tobacco-human experiences elsewhere in the world once the plant escaped its continental origins, approximately 500 years ago? Are there certain elements of this transit that are ill-apparent to modern sensibilities and that have remained unacknowledged in consequence? Why is such a distinction (between 'modern' and 'traditional') made in the first place?[78] Did tobacco, perhaps, have a role generating it? The three Amazonian elements of tobacco-human relations that I have identified in this chapter – making up persons, changing perspectives and the generation of dualisms – are dimensions of tobacco's presence that will recur in later chapters, as the master plant sets out to conquer the rest of the world.

Notes

1 Proctor (2011).
2 Feinhandler et al. (1979) claim that tobacco is also native to Australia and the south-west Pacific, but it is likely that lowland South America is the progenitor of tobacco worldwide.
3 Indeed recent research has indicated that the Solanaceae in general evolved much earlier than previously thought – see Wilf et al. (2017).
4 Martin (1973); Tamm et al. (2007); Mulligan et al. (2008); Meltzer (2015). Kinoshita et al. (2014) present new evidence from north-east Brazil that suggests human transit south may have been much earlier, possibly by boat.
5 Oyuela-Caycedo and Kawa (2015: 32).
6 Wilbert (1987) provides what remains the definitive account of the different modes of consumption in South America. For North America, see Winter (2000).
7 The prodigious amounts reportedly consumed are extraordinary. Amongst the striking observations made by Johannes Wilbert is that of a male Yaruro shaman who "in the course of an all-night performance…was observed to have consumed forty-two industrial cigarettes and about one hundred native cigars".
8 I am focusing on South America here, although von Gernet concludes "there is abundant evidence to reject any opinion that the use of tobacco to produce major dissociative states was confined to South America" (2000: 74).
9 Some of the most well-known are datura, mescal, peyote, coca, and *ayahuasca* (or *yagé*, produced from the vine *Banisteriopsis caapi*) and *pariká*. "Pariká is a crystalline powder made from the blood-red exudates of the inner bark of *Virola theidora* and *Ananenanthera peregrine* trees found in the north-west Amazon region. Its active chemical principle is DMT (dymethyltriptamine)" (Wright 2013: 26).
10 Goodman (1993: 24). This is something conveniently overlooked by travellers to South America who come in search of *ayahuasca*-based spiritual experiences rather than the much older, but less romantic in western terms, tobacco-based shamanic practices (Brabec de Mori 2015).
11 Baer (1992). On tobacco use in the Matsigenka context, see also Shepard (1998; 2004).
12 Fausto (2004: 158).

13 Wilbert (1987: 150 fn1).
14 See for example Sarmiento-Barletti (2015).
15 Dole ([1964] 1973: 300-301).
16 Wilbert (1987: 149).
17 Wasson (1968: 332) in Wilbert 1972: 56n.
18 Wilbert (1987: 148). His assumption that tobacco was assimilated into a pre-existing set of practices and metaphysical beliefs is highly reminiscent of Sahlins' theory of commodity indigenization, which we shall meet in Chapter 2.
19 The social anthropologist Signe Howell reports that Chewong hunter-gatherers in central Malaysia similarly conduct shamanic séances which involve practices such as shape-shifting (the ritual transformation of a human into an animal or vice versa) simply through the use of drumming.
20 Lévi-Strauss (1973: 59-60).
21 Wilbert (1987: 202).
22 Ibid.
23 Lévi-Strauss (1973: 29).
24 The Latin name of the *kinkajou* is *Potus flavus* (Wilbert and Simoneau 1990: fn 362 p. 335). *Agouti* designates at least 11 species of forest rodents in the genus *Dasyprocta*.
25 *Peshiyë* derives from *pëshi*, a verb that usually expresses sexual desire, but also tobacco craving. Indeed, in another version of this tale, the protagonist is told by the inhabitants of a communal longhouse to go and have sex with the women and make them pregnant.
26 Wilbert and Simoneau (1990: 168).
27 Reig (2015).
28 Wilbert (1987: 83).
29 This is a summary of the Warao myth "The origin of tobacco and of the first medicine-man" in Lévi-Strauss (1973: 423-5).
30 Wilbert (2004: 26).
31 Cited in Reig (2015: 178).
32 Barbira Freedman (2015: 78).
33 Londoño Sulkin proposes an "Amazonian package" amongst the heavily tobacco-using "People of the Centre", viz. "that human bodies are fabricated socially, that this occurs in the context of a perspectival cosmos, and that relations with dangerous outside Others are necessary to the process" (2012: 24). This has resonance with all three elements identified here.
34 Wright (2013: 176).
35 In North America, "tobacco is so important in the [Eastern] woodlands that the Seneca, Cayuga, Onondaga, Oneida, and Mohawk...or Iroquois Nation, depend upon it for their very spiritual and cultural survival, as do their linguistic relatives the Huron, Neurtral, and Khionontaternon (the Petun or Tobacco Nation)" (Winter 2000: 16).
36 Hugh-Jones (2009: 34, 42).
37 Descola ([1986] 1993: 325).
38 For Vilaça (2005), Amazonian bodies are "chronically unstable".
39 Rahman (2015).
40 Londoño Sulkin (2012: 102-3).
41 Kopenawa and Albert (2013). Tobacco is fundamental to Kopenawa's account of Yanomami lore.
42 This invites comparison with a multicultural world. Viveiros de Castro is quick to suggest, however, that such a polarity is "perhaps too symmetrical to be more than a speculative fiction" (2012b: 46). Viveiros de Castro has been criticized by Ramos (2012: 482) for the false impression cosmological perspectivism gives of

cultural homogeneity, with each new publication taking "his generalizing imagination a little further away from the nitty-gritty of indigenous real life".

43 McCallum (2014: 512).
44 Vilaça (2005: 451, 458).
45 Vilaça (2005: 451).
46 Viveiros de Castro (1998: 469).
47 Stolze Lima (1999: 116).
48 Turner (2009: 11).
49 McCallum (2014: 511).
50 Turner (2009: 11).
51 Ingold (2000: 170). A similar point was made in the explication of the Human
Nature strand of the decennial conference of the Association of Social Anthropologists in 2014, which made the claim that "anthropologists have followed the
example of many of the peoples among whom they have worked in rejecting any a
priori division between nature and humanity in favour of an understanding of forms
of life as emergent within fields of mutually conditioning relations, by no means
confined to the human" (Association of Social Anthropologists, 2014). At the same
time, however, "they have continued to assert the ontological autonomy of the
social and cultural domain from its biological 'base', and with it, the distinctiveness
of sociocultural anthropology vis-à-vis the science of human nature".
52 Ingold (1996: 116).
53 Stolze Lima (1999: 120).
54 Ibid. (121).
55 Viveiros de Castro (2012b: 46 fn1).
56 Viveiros de Castro (2012b: 46-7).
57 Lévi-Strauss (1973: 20).
58 Lévi-Strauss (1973: 29).
59 Lévi-Strauss (1973: 66).
60 Lévi-Strauss (1973: 65). Honey similarly has both good and bad (poisonous)
forms, the latter produced by certain species of wasps or from bees which have
fed from poisonous flowers, tree saps or bird droppings (Lévi-Strauss, 1973: 51-2).
61 Lévi-Strauss (1992: 105).
62 Barbira Freedman (2010: 151).
63 Barbira Freedman, (2015: 70-71).
64 Barbira Freedman (2010: 151).
65 Rival (2014: 226).
66 Echeverri (2015: 108).
67 Echeverri (2015: 114).
68 Shepard (1998).
69 Sarmiento-Barletti (2015).
70 Oyuela-Caycedo and Kawa (2015: 40).
71 Appadurai (1986).
72 This description is based on Rahman (2015).
73 Hobsbawn and Ranger (1992).
74 Gow (1994); Brabec de Mori (2011).
75 Anderson et al. (2012); Fotiou (2014).
76 For more on this topic, and how anthropological methods can be deepen our
knowledge of the ethnohistorical past, see Gow (2015).
77 Rahman (2015).
78 After all, Latour (1993) insists, *We Have Never Been Modern*.

Chapter 2

First contact

O metaphysical tobacco.[1]

Michael East, 1606

Dried leaves

At first tobacco was relatively insignificant, just one of a panoply of herbal products that the Iberian conquest of the Americas yielded to explorers and colonialists from Christopher Columbus onwards.

In his diary of October 15th, 1492, Columbus wrote:

> Being at sea, about midway between Santa Maria and the large island, which I name Fernandina, we met a man in a canoe going from Santa Maria to Fernandina; he had with him a piece of the bread which the natives make, as big as one's fist, a calabash of water, a quantity of reddish earth, pulverized and afterwards kneaded up, and some dried leaves which are in high value among them, for a quantity of it was brought to me at San Salvador.

The author was writing his diary with a sense of disappointment. Having failed in his quest to find a westward passage, Columbus was motivated less by an interest in plants than in the possibility of finding gold and gemstones. This explains his casual approach to the first exposure of any European to the plant, one of several from the so-called 'New World', which was to become so significant in global affairs later on. Some weeks later, members of his crew encountered Taíno Indians smoking rolled tobacco in the woods near Cuba's Bahia Bariay harbour: "The Spaniards upon their journey met with great multitudes of people, men and women with firebrands in their hands and herbs to smoke after their custom".[2] These herbs, like the leaves on the canoe, were almost certainly tobacco.

It is hard to underestimate the impact that contact between Europe and the New World had on both sides of the Atlantic from the end of the 15th century. The first transit of the Atlantic brought in its train mayhem that was both human and non-human in its origins. For the historian Alfred Crosby, it was germs rather than guns that enabled Europeans to colonize the world's temperate zones, thus putting non-human agency – specifically microbial agency – in the driving seat of world history. However, such a viewpoint has been criticized for inadvertently or intentionally serving to absolve Europeans of responsibility for some of the terrible things which took place at their hands.[3] "For how is it possible to speak of the fate of American Indians in terms of holocaust or genocide when accidental factors such as microbes were so critical?", asks one commentator.[4]

Bartolomé de las Casas was a Dominican priest who came to the island of Hispaniola (now Haiti/Dominican Republic) in 1502 with a view to learn more about native peoples in order to convert them to Christianity. So horrified was he by Spanish behaviour against the Indians, he decided to devote the rest of his life to condemning Spanish atrocities and advocating and extolling the virtues and accomplishments of indigenous cultures.[5] He was critical of Spanish settlers he met on the island who had developed a strong dependence on tobacco and were finding it hard to give up, and he was mystified as to what pleasure or advantage they might be taking from the habit.[6] Spanish colonists began cultivating tobacco in Santo Domingo in 1531. Gonzalo Fernández de Oviedo y Valdés noted that his fellow Spaniards were turned into drunks by tobacco. In his *Historia*, published in 1535, he wrote that "among other evil practices, the Indians have one that is especially harmful, the inhaling of a certain kind of smoke which they call tobacco, in order to produce a state of stupor". Like de las Casas' comments on the Spanish settlers, the author of *Historia* was unable to imagine what pleasure they might have been deriving from the practice, "unless it be the drinking which invariably precedes smoking...It seems to me that here we have a bad and pernicious custom".[7] The development of colonial settlements based on cultivars such as tobacco continued, however. The Caribbean island of Trinidad, also held by the Spanish, became eponymous with the esteemed tobacco ('Trinidado') that came from there.

The Milanese explorer Girolamo Benzoni was similarly stupefied (intellectually, not experientially) by tobacco. In the account of his travels over a 14 year period in the "newly discovered islands and seas" on the other side of the Atlantic, he described the island of Hispaniola thus:

> In this island, as also in other provinces of these new countries, there are some bushes, not very large, like reeds, that produce a leaf in shape like that of the walnut, though rather larger, which (where it is used) is held in great esteem by the natives, and very much prized by the slaves whom the Spaniards have brought from Ethiopia.
>
> When these leaves are in season, they pick them, tie them up in bundles, and suspend them near their fire-place till they are very dry; and when they wish to use them, they take a leaf of their grain [maize] and putting one of

the others into it, they roll them round tight together; then they set fire to one end, and putting the other end into the mouth, they draw their breath up through it, wherefore the smoke goes into the mouth, the throat, the head, and they retain it as long as they can, for they find a pleasure in it, and so much do they fill themselves with this cruel smoke, that they lose their reason. And there are some who take so much of it, that they fall down as if they were dead, and remain the greater part of the day or night stupefied...See what a pestiferous and wicked poison from the devil this must be. It has happened to me several times that, going through the provinces of *Guatemala* and *Nicaragua*, I have entered the house of an Indian who had taken this herb, which in the Mexican language is called *tabacco*.[8]

The first European to write about the effects of tobacco smoking based on his own use of it, rather than relating what it looked like or its observable effects on others, was a Breton sailor, Jacques Cartier. He went on three voyages to what is now eastern Canada between 1534 and 1541, sailing up the St Lawrence River and being offered a pipe of tobacco by an Iroquois chief on arrival. He describes the process of pipe smoking in some detail, ending with the comment that his hosts "say that this does keep them warm and in health. We ourselves have tried the same smoke, and having put it in our mouths, it seemed that they had filled it with pepper dust it is so hot".[9]

A Jesuit missionary reporting about the Montagnais Indians of Quebec in 1634 found:

The fondness they have for this herb is beyond all belief. They go to sleep with their reed pipes in their mouths, they sometimes get up in the night to smoke; they often stop on their journeys for the same purpose, and it is the first thing they do when they re-enter their cabins.[10]

Tobacco enthralled the French in Canada as it had their Spanish counterparts in Santo Domingo. Writing about a Montagnais convert to Christianity who had forsaken the plant, the Jesuit priest comments: "Those who know what a mania the Savages and some Frenchmen have for smoking tobacco, will admire this abstinence. Intemperate drinkers are not so fond of wine as the Savages are of tobacco".[11]

These initial reactions to tobacco and the people who used it are epitomized in the (imagined) image provided by De Bry of Europeans stumbling upon a Tupinamba ritual in which tobacco was clearly playing a central part (Fig. 2.1). The visitors gaze astonished from the edge of the scene.

Going global

Tobacco's transit around the world between the middle of the 16th and 17th centuries was extraordinarily rapid considering the speed of the ocean-going

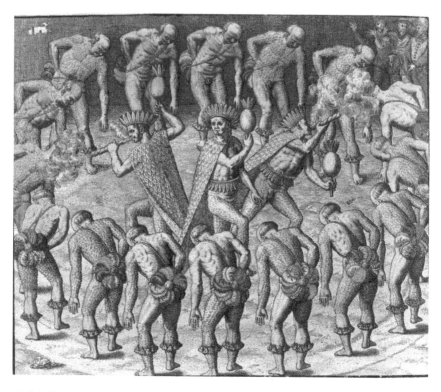

Fig. 2.1 Tupinamba Indians, observed by Hans Staden during his voyage to Brazil
Source: De Bry 1592, courtesy of the John Carter Brown Library at Brown University.

galleons and the hazards they faced from uncharted and frequently treacherous waters. With their colonies in Brazil, Mexico, and Peru, Portugal and Spain were able to include tobacco in the exotic substances their fleets took with them back across the Atlantic and onwards around the globe.

One of the most astonishing trade routes developed by the Spanish was the 'Manila galleons', journeying from their colony on Cebu in the Philippines (established in 1565), across the Pacific to Acapulco in Mexico. Tobacco arrived in the Philippines from here in 1575, and proved a productive cash crop, one able to exploit the well-established, sophisticated trading networks maintained by Arab and Chinese merchants throughout Southeast Asia, where the Japanese also had significant settlements. Fujianese traders probably first introduced it to southern China.[12]

When a decree by the Chinese emperor lifted restrictions on trade with Southeast Asia in 1567, it was something the Portuguese, with their trading base in Macao on the Chinese mainland, doubtless used to their advantage.[13]

Domestic tobacco cultivation and use was well established in China by the time the Chongzhen emperor ascended to the throne in 1628, particularly around Zhangzhou in the province of Fujian.[14] A Fujian poet, Yao Lü, writing during the Wanli period (1573-1620) commented:

> There is a plant called *tan-pa-ku*, produced in Luzon [Philippines]...You take fire and light one end and put the other in your mouth. The smoke goes down your throat through the pipe. It can make one tipsy but it can...keep one clear of malaria. People have brought it to Changchou [Fujian] and planted it, and now there is more there than in Luzon, and it is exported and sold to that country...It is commonly called gold-silk-smoke. Its leaves are like those of the lichee. After these are pounded, the juice...can kill off lice on the scalp. The leaves make the tobacco.[15]

By 1600, the Portuguese had introduced tobacco to Iran, India, Java, the Moluccas and Japan.[16] They may well have introduced it to coastal African societies en route, although the kind of pipes that remain characteristic of Senegal and Gambia are curiously similar to a native American style from Louisiana and suggest that the French may also have played a part in the introduction of tobacco to these countries.[17] Moluccan (Indonesian) traders carried tobacco from what is now eastern Indonesia to New Guinea, while Macassan traders came from Celebes to the coast of northern Australia.[18]

Tobacco also colonized China from the north-east, via Manchuria, where imports from Japan probably started concurrently with its introduction into Korea.[19] Once established, tobacco's domestic cultivation increased rapidly. A Beijing official wrote sometime in the early 1640s, "within the last twenty years, many people in the Beijing area are growing it. What they make from planting one *mu* of tobacco is equal to what they can make from planting ten *mu* of grain fields. It has got to the point that there is no one who doesn't use it".[20]

Another noteworthy route taken by tobacco was to arctic North America. The Siberian Inuit brought it across the Bering Sea to the extreme western peninsula of Alaska, and from there it was traded with the Norton Sound Inuit. Tobacco then followed a tortuous route through various other Inuit and some native American groups further inland, such as the Gwich'in.

> Pewter and wood pipes patterned after Japanese and Chinese opium pipes also circulated throughout the Arctic trade system, with the western Inuit carving ivory pipes that they traded to whalers for English and American tobacco....The Eastern Inuit also obtained their tobacco through trade with the Greenland colonists...Many colonists from Denmark married Inuit women who acquired the tobacco habit and then passed it on to their families. Today the Inuit are avid tobacco users, purchasing it in stores, cooperatives, and trading posts scattered throughout the Arctic.[21]

Because of its relatively late arrival (rather like tobacco in Europe), however, "there is no mention of the plant in Inuit mythology, and none of the rich symbolism, tobacco shamanism, and tobacco deities that are found to the south".[22] Likewise, unlike their Siberian counterparts, Inuit shamans appear not to have picked up the habit of using tobacco to help themselves enter trances, communicate with spirits, or heal the sick.

Tobacco's indigenization and transculturation in Europe: from accommodation to transformation

The term 'commodity indigenization' refers to the process whereby different cultures respond to and absorb new commodities.[23] Commodities brought by Europeans to other cultures are accommodated within the life ways of that culture, while commodities from non-European cultures may be similarly accommodated by Europeans. However, commodities don't simply 'fit in' to existing cultural formats; they can radically change them. Fernando Ortiz, who claimed that Havana tobacco had conquered the world (Introduction) discusses transculturation as "the process by which habits and things move from one culture to another so thoroughly that they become part of it and in turn change the culture into which they have moved".[24] Both commodity indigenization and transculturation can be seen in the case of tobacco, a product whose transit, I shall argue, has involved not simply absorption but socio-economic, political and cognitive transformations as well. The commodity in question has also generated new and changed objects for its storage, transport, consumption, and disposal, as well as novel human behaviours, such as smoking, required by these new commodity-object assemblages. Responses to such commodity complexes are unlikely to be uniform or unequivocal, however. This is clear when considering how tobacco spread within Europe. Certain features of European life and thought appear to have been accommodating of tobacco's spread after 1492; however there were significant changes wrought by the herb that can be found depicted in poems and songs of the period.

The first reason for tobacco's easy incorporation into 16th and 17th century life in Europe was the significance attributed to breath and breathing. The Greek word *pneuma* was seen, in variously interconnected ways, as breath and spirit/soul. For Plato, whose *Timaeus* was probably the most influential Greek text in early modern Europe, the soul both suffused the universe and was contained in innate form within every individual. The innate *pneuma* increased in volume during the growth of an individual by means of respiration. Aristotle rejected the idea that the soul could be a separate entity existing independently of the body, and considered *pneuma* the physical instrument of the soul. The physician Galen, whose influence came into Medieval Europe during the 12th century through Arabic texts, had incorporated Aristotelean logic, and considered the soul to be maintained through the work of both blood and air, with the latter drawn into the body through the windpipe. With Christian theological notions linking breath, life and the holy spirit ('inspiration'), and the ecclesiastical penchant for using incense to purify, bless and symbolically link Earth with the more ephemeral (but sweet-smelling) Heaven, smoking was a novel behaviour that entered a domain pregnant with powerful semiotic connections. It made breath, literally, incarnate.

Another reason for tobacco's successful indigenization was the manner of its entry, and who brought it. Soldiers and sailors returning from voyages of exploration and conquest across the Atlantic were probably the first to introduce the herb to an incredulous public, although most examples of them doing so, since no written or artistic records remain, are lost.[25] One of the first reports in England of a sailor causing a sensation from his novel behaviour, smoking in the street, dates from 1556.[26] Because of its wide distribution across the Americas, tobacco entered through a range of different European ports concurrently.[27] Sailors coming ashore in Seville after voyages to the New World were probably typical of their counterparts elsewhere in bringing tobacco to supplement their pitiful wages by petty trading on the dockside or in the taverns, inns and workers' neighbourhoods of the city.[28] Goods for 'personal use' were exempt from customs duties, hence small amounts coming in pockets and pouches in this way would have gone unrecorded. In his *Commissio pro Tobacco* (see Chapter 3), King James I of England bemoaned the arrival of tobacco "from foreign Partes in small quantitie' into this Realm" by "Merchants, as well Denizens [citizens] as Strangers".

So unusual was the new arrival, and so strange the behaviour surrounding it, that the word for 'smoke' in the transitive sense of smoking *something* did not become established in English until around 1600.[29] Nor was this form of smoking (as opposed to fumigation or preservation) known in other parts of Europe.[30] Instead, the act of inhaling the burning leaves of the tobacco plant was termed 'eating' or, more usually, 'drinking' (Fig. 2.2). This should not surprise us unduly: anatomy as a subject of organized, empirical enquiry rather than occasional opportunistic insight was still in its infancy, and the idea that the lungs could take in liquid as well as breath had a long pedigree.[31]

Tobacco was also a poor man's drug, at least at first. Its physiological ability to suppress appetite and reduce hunger helps explain not only its spread but why it might have been regarded as a form of food, or 'drug food', in many parts of the world. One Castilian poem, 'In praise of tobacco' published in 1644, includes the lines "a few balls of tobacco are enough/carrying them in the mouth/stays thirst and hunger".[32] The privations of peasant life in Spain were mirrored in England's capital, where the way of life

> was brutal, coarse, inured to physical suffering and endurance. The pillory and the scaffold provided constant excitement and thrills; the heads impaled on London Bridge, the procession of a traitor to his fearful

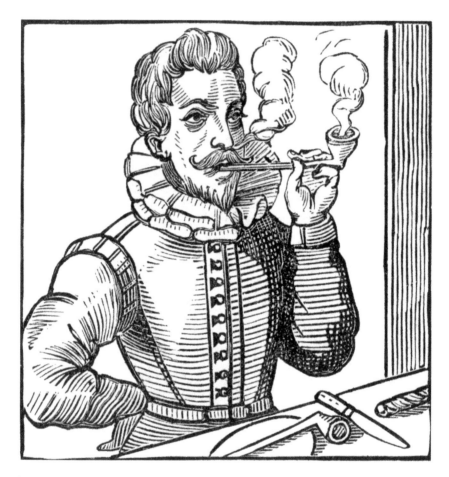

Fig. 2.2 'A tobacco drinker, 1623'
Source: Penn, 1902

> end, the bear-baiting and bull-baiting – these and many other things
> remind us that a tough fibre was necessary to live at ease of mind in
> Elizabethan London.[33]

So too was a strong constitution. Another reason for the ready acceptance of
tobacco was the biotic environment it was entering. Across the continent,
bubonic plague continued its frequent outbreaks. During the 16th and 17th
centuries, syphilis, probably first introduced into Europe from the Americas
by Columbus' returning seamen, also became rife.[34] Effective treatments were
limited – leaving the path clear for claims to be made for a substance like
tobacco on medical grounds alone.

Another reason for tobacco's ready uptake around Europe was the increasing availability of books and other forms of print media in conjunction with the growing rates of literacy, at least amongst the wealthier classes. Over time, more translators and translations of popular works appeared, and books started to appear simultaneously in English, French, German and Latin editions.[35] The quality of illustrations also improved. These developments increased the rapidity with which knowledge about the new plants could be disseminated, even ahead of people actually coming into direct contact with them. It is worth looking at some of these artistic representations of tobacco – in books, pamphlets and song – in order to gain a richer impression of the responses triggered by tobacco, as well as how it was being used and to what effect.

Tobacco as herbal panacea

In 1574, the Sevillian physician Nicolas Monardes' history of the medicinal plants of the Western hemisphere was published in Spain, translated and printed in English as *Joyfull Newes from the New Found World*.[36] Monardes wrote of tobacco's "marvellous medicinable virtues" including in particular "to heale griefes of the head, and in especially coming to colde causes, and so it cureth the headake when it commeth of a cold humor, or of a windy cause". Given the challenging bacterial environment, the arrival of an exotic new pharmacopoeia offering the potential for hitherto unimaginable cures was potentially joyful news indeed. However, Monardes was scandalized by what he had gleaned from travellers' reports about the religious use of tobacco by its Indian users – how Indian priests, before divining the future, would become so dazed by tobacco smoke that they would fall to the ground as if dead. On returning to their senses, they would respond to queries put to them, interpreting what they had seen while in their cataleptic state "in their own way, or following the inspiration of the Devil". In Monardes' view, it was the trickery of the Devil and his knowledge of the power of the herbs who had "taught the Indians the virtue of tobacco: and leads them into deceit through visions and apparitions which the tobacco procures".

Matthias de l'Obel (1538-1616) was an herbalist and author whose life reflects the growing cosmopolitanism of the time. Born in Lille, France, he studied in Montpelier before moving to England where he published *Stirpium adversaria nova*, dedicated to Queen Elizabeth, in 1571. He was the first herbalist to include a description of tobacco as a separate plant. His respect (not to say reverence) for the plant is reflected in this passage, translated from the Latin:

> This [plant], if it could speak, would reproach the more reckless detractors of botany for their inactivity, but it would congratulate intelligent investigators for their zeal, because of which, a few years ago, it from the West Indies, became a dweller in Portugal, France, Belgium and England.[37]

After his herbal was published, de l'Obel moved to Antwerp where he practiced medicine for several years before returning to England to manage an herb garden in Hackney; he became botanist to James I. However, none of his writings were published in English during his lifetime.

John Gerard's 1597 book *The Herball or Generall Historie of Plantes* was a popular English publication of the period. Much of it is based on the work of the Flemish botanist Rembert Doedens, who produced the first representation of a tobacco plant (misnamed *Hyoscyamus luteus* or yellow henbane) in his herbal published in Antwerp in 1553.[38] Gerard maintained a confusion which had developed between *Nicotiana rustica* and yellow henbane although, given the rapidly spreading smoking habit and the willingness of some sections of the medical profession to suggest it was a panacea or cure-all, Gerard spent some time describing the two kinds of plant, stating:

> [Tobacco] being now planted in the gardens of Europe, it prospereth very well, and commeth from seede in one yeere to beare both flowers and seede. The which I take to be better for the constitution of our bodies, than that which is brought from India [by which he meant the West Indies]; and that growing in the Indies better for the people of the same country; notwithstanding it is not so thought nor received of our Tabackians; for according to the English proverbe; Far fetcht and deare bought is better for Ladies.

While he had found compounds including tobacco successful as cures for some diseases, Gerard cautioned against drinking [i.e. smoking] it for fear of "wantonnesse" and did not hold this "fume or smokie medicine" in high regard when smoked in a pipe, only recommending doing so once a day, before breakfast.[39] For William Vaughan, however, whose *Naturall and Artificiall Directions for Health* was first published in 1600 but enlarged and reprinted seven times during the next three decades, "Tobacco, well dryed and taken in a silver pipe fasting in the morning cures the migraine, the toothache, obstructions proceeding of cold, and helps the fits of the mother". He cautioned, though, that "after meales it doth much hurt, for it infecteth the braine and the liver".[40] By the 6th edition, in 1626, however, he condemned smoking as a pastime for being a "wasteful and vicious" habit.

These are somewhat equivocal accounts. Other New World plants appear to have been valued more highly than tobacco for their assumed curative powers. Guaiacum (*Zygophyllaceae*), sarsaparilla (*Smilax spp.*) and sassafras all received far more champions, largely because of their hoped-for ability to cure syphilis. Indigenous people used tobacco symptomatically against the effects of syphilis, but Hispaniola's military governor, Gonzalo Fernández de Oviedo y Valdés, pitied settlers who did likewise "for they say that in the state of ecstasy caused by the smoke they no longer feel their pain". In his opinion, the man who acts thus merely passes while still alive into a deathly stupor. It seems to me that it would be better to suffer the pain, which they make their excuse, for it is certain that smoking will never cure the disease.[41]

Thus, regardless of the claims made for its health benefits by Monardes and others, it may be that the medicinal qualities of tobacco were not so much a reason as an excuse for people to seek out this new-found commodity.

The new pharmacopoeia was not without its critics. Most European societies were still enthralled by the myth of a 'golden age', the era of classical antiquity deemed far superior to the miseries of the present. In terms of herbalism, the classical lodestone was Dioscorides' *De Materia Medica*, a five-volume pharmacopoeia written around A.D. 70 based on his observations of plant and other medicinal materials gathered while working as a military surgeon with the Roman Army. Many botanists tried to fit the thousands of new plants identified in the Americas to the 600 or so included in Dioscorides' work, rather than recognizing them as completely new species to the European world. The Galenic, humoral theory of medicine – that health was the product of the balance of the four bodily humors with their associated qualities – phlegm (cold and moist), blood (hot and moist), black bile (cold and dry) and yellow bile (hot and dry) – also acted against tobacco. Tobacco was regarded as a 'hot' substance, but there were already many remedies that were 'hot', leading some to argue there was little to be gained by adding more from the New World to them. On the other hand, the dampness of the northern European climate, and the humoral effects this was reputed to cause, made the prospect of an additional warming and drying addition to the pharmacopoeia quite appealing.

There was also a belief, persistent in theories of macrobiotics to this day, that plants grown in specific localities were best for the treatment of illnesses in those localities, and that their curative potency would decline with travel. We saw echoes of this in Gerard's suggestion that tobacco grown in the Indies was better for the inhabitants of that country. Timothy Bright's tract 'wherein is Declared the Sufficiencie of English Medicines for the Cure of All Diseases', published in 1580, takes a stronger tack in suggesting that all non-English medicines were unnecessary.[42] His contemporary Ralph Holinshead likewise suggested that every region had abundance of whatsoever was needed and most convenient for the people that lived within its borders, suggesting it might be "repugnancie in the constitution" of the English or a quality of the soil that might explain why tobacco was not as efficacious as might be expected. Edmund Gardiner, a physician who supported the medicinal use of tobacco, however, wrote a counter argument in 1610 that it was "nature gave it, and nature doth nothing in vaine".[43]

What we see in these conflicting accounts is a more complex picture of tobacco than that of "panacea or precious bane".[44] Monardes and l'Obel both spoke for the virtues of tobacco whereas, as time went on, other influential physicians such as Vaughan became sceptical about its properties. Tobacco's lack of anything other than symptomatic success against syphilis also suggested the need for caution, as did the difficulty of placing tobacco in any traditional pharmacopoeia or of making it stand out against other plants with similarly hot, dry humoral properties. Finally, the differences of opinion about whether a plant grown in a certain part of the world could be used to treat ailments elsewhere added to the confusion. It was for its exotic associations and narcotic effects, rather than for its medicinal properties, I suggest in the following sections, that tobacco really came into its own, both on paper and in practice.[45]

Tobacco as Algonquian exotic

The 60 herbals printed in Europe in the 15th and 16th centuries contrast numerically with the roughly 4,000 books on the "New Found Land" of the western hemisphere printed during the same time period.[46] With more than 60 of these books saying at least something about tobacco, it is likely that these publications were at least as important as the herbals in explaining tobacco's rapid integration into Europe.[47] A noteworthy example of these early published reports is Thomas Hariot's *Briefe and True Report of the New Found Land of Virginia*, published in multiple translations in 1590. Hariot had been a leader of an English attempt to settle Roanoke Island in 1585.[48] Unlike most colonizers, he had some respect for the indigenous people already living in the vicinity. He bothered to learn the language of the area from two Algonquians, Manteo and Wanchese, brought to England by Sir Walter Raleigh on an earlier voyage. As well as being one of the first Englishmen to see tobacco being grown, he describes how the natives:

> Use to take the fume or smoke thereof by sucking it through pipes made of claie into their stomacke and heade, from whence it purgeth super-fluous fleame & other grosse humors, openeth all the pores & passages of the body: by which meanes the use thereof, not only preserveth the body from obstructions; but also if any be...[assuming] that they have not beene of too long continuance, in short time breaketh them.

For Hariot, its use to prevent as well as treat short-term 'obstructions' helps explain why the Algonquian's "bodies are notably preserved in health, and know not many greevous diseases wherewithal wee in England are oftentimes afflicted".[49]

Hariot reports how the Algonquians also used tobacco to communicate with metaphysical beings. For example, if they are "in a storme upon the waters, to pacifie their gods, they cast some up into the aire and into the water". Tobacco was "of so precious estimation amongst the[m], that they thinke their gods are marvelously delighted therwith". Hariot, like De Bry's depiction of the

Tupinamba (above), found Algonquian rituals bizarre ("all done with strange gestures, stamping, sometime dauncing, clapping of hands, holding up of hands, & staring up into the heavens, uttering therewithal and chattering strange words & noises"). But, unusually for most colonists of the time, Hariot acknowledged some positive aspects of the Algonquian's way of life, such as their abstemious diet whereby they avoided sickness. He went on:

> I would to god we would follow their example. For we should be free from many kinds of diseases which we fall into by sumptuous and unseasonable banquets, continually devising new sauces, and provocation of gluttony to satisfy our unsatiable appetite.[50]

Hariot himself followed the Algonquian example and began a smoking habit. It was probably the unusual manner of smoke exhalation learned from the Algonquians that caused him to die of a nasal cancer in 1621. It was a sorry commentary on the 'tobacco for health' arguments he and some of some of his compatriots had been so quick to expound. On the other hand, Thomas Hobbes (1588-1679) is said to have been a regular pipe user when thinking and writing, and he lived to the age of 92.

Poetic insinuations of divinity

Tobacco first appeared in English poetry in as insignificant a way as its passing mention in Columbus's journal 100 years before. In Spenser's *The Faerie Queene* (1590), the fairy Belphoebe seeks herbs for King Arthur's wounded squire Timias. "Divine *Tobacco*" is one of the three she picks and applies, Amerindian style, in a poultice to staunch the flow of his "hart-bloud". "What could be more fleeting a reference?" asks the literary critic Jeffrey Knapp. "A plant growing in not only distant but fairy woods, and then only one of three alternatives for the herb Belphoebe actually does fetch...Spenser's poetry never mentions the word, the novelty, again". Yet, he points out, "no epithet for tobacco comes close to being as standard in later Elizabethan literature as Spenser's 'divine'".[51]

John Donne had actually referred to tobacco in seven Latin epigrams written as juvenilia five years earlier.[52] The depiction of tobacco in these verses is very different to Belphoebe's fairy-like ministrations. 'Upon a Pipe of Tobacco Mistaken by the Author for the Tooth-ach' relates Donne's first reaction to it:

> Outlandish Weed! whilst I thy vertues tell.
> Assist me Bedlam, Muses come from Hell.

The second continues:

> An Hearb thou art, but useless; for made fire,
> From hot mouths puft, thou dost in fumes expire.

After this:

> Lothings, stincks, thirst, rhumes, aches, and catarrh,
> Base weed, thy vertues, that's thy poysons are.

> I love thee not, nor thou me having tri'd
> How thy scorcht Takers are but Takers fry'd.

The tobacco seller is likewise rebuked:

> Merchant of smoke, when next thou makes a feast
> Invite some starv'd *Chamelion* to be guest.

The chameleon reference is to an animal believed to live on nothing but air. Donne's confusion over taking a tobacco pipe for "tooth-ach" (when some kind of tincture of the sort Belphoebe used on Timias, or the use of a small ball of tobacco leaf, would have been more appropriate) reflects how the epigrams' composition, before pipe smoking – particularly the smoking of pipes for pleasure – was generally known about.[53] Unlike Spenser, tobacco for Donne was far from 'divine'. One author suggests the tobacco epigrams were written at or around the siege of Antwerp in 1585, when Donne would have been 13; Donne was quite precocious, matriculating at Oxford University at the age of 12, and it is quite likely that he spent time in Europe after that point and was initiated into tobacco smoking there.[54] Like most people's unpleasant first experiences of tobacco, it is hardly surprising that he averred "I love you not" after his initial acquaintance with it.

The other mention of tobacco in Donne's poetry is similarly disparaging. In his First Satire, he and a companion meet a number of "guls" in the street, including one "which did excel/Th'Indians in drinking his tobacco well". "Guls", an early incarnation of the dandy or man about town, were well-known tobacco users and followers of fashion.[55] Donne's reaction to this encounter is to whisper to his friend "Let us go,/'T may be you smell him not; truly I do".[56]

Detracting statements about the olfactory experience of smoking do not mean Donne was averse to partaking of the weed later in his life, however. He was probably one of the first secret smokers (Chapter 9). He was an ally of the courtier Sir Edward Hoby, himself in an early and vitriolic "pamphlet war" with the Jesuit writer John Floyd. Floyd referred to Donne as one of Hoby's "fellow Tobaccaean writers".[57] "Was Donne himself a smoker?" asks Donne scholar Alison Shell, in response to Hoby's remarks. She concludes equivocally that such a notion "is a pleasurable idea, and it may even be true".[58] Given the company he kept and – as we shall see in Chapter 3 – the company he joined, as well as some of the later poetry he wrote, Donne would appear to have been "Tobaccaean" through and through. It is interesting that 'Metaphysical' - the term applied to the poetry of Donne and a loose circle of his contemporaries – was, like 'divine', commonly used as an adjective to describe tobacco, as in the title of Michael East's madrigal at the start of this chapter.

A "Smoakie Society"

From 1595 onwards, treatises started appearing that focused on tobacco in its own right, rather than it being mentioned in herbals or travellers' reports. There was a subtle change in tone in these accounts, based as they often were on the author's own experience of the plant. While the panegyrics about tobacco tended to repeat the medicinal benefits claimed by Monardes, English publications based on closer, direct experience were starting to emerge. The first of these, in 1595, was Anthony Chute's *Tabaco. The distinct and severall opinions of the late and best Phisitions that have written of the divers natures and qualities thereof.* As was becoming increasingly common with a growing number of publications, his book owed much to other works, such as Monardes, and he in turn was borrowed by William Vaughan in his *Naturall and Artificiall Directions for Health*, mentioned above. However, Chute also comments on how the authors from which his own work derives say little about "receiving it in pipes, as we now use".[59] The work is dedicated to one Humphrey King, "What your experience is in this divine hearbe, al men do know; and acknowledge you to bee *The Sovereign of Tobacco*". There is also allusion to a 'smoakie Society' of which this Sovereign of Tobacco was head. Chute expounded on the virtues of tobacco. "For my selfe in few, I think that there is nothing that harmes a man inwardly from his girdle upward, but may be taken away with a moderate use of *Tabacco*".[60] He also comments on its excellent "preservative against the late dangerous infection",[61] by which he meant the rampant curse of syphilis. Finally he describes taking "sixe or seven pipes full" to ensure a profound sleep:

> The next day, I did perceive my wearinesse almost utterly gone, although not quite, which perhaps might be for wante of custome, or because my sicknesse before was apt to make me feele that longer than I should have done being well.[62]

His "sicknesse" was the dropsy. Barclay (1614) observed that "the Hydropisie [dropsy] is one of the ordinaries customers that commeth to crave health at the shop of *Tobacco*". Chute unfortunately died of it before his treatise was published.

John Beaumont's rhyming couplet poem *The Metamorphosis of Tobacco*, published in 1602, invites the reader to

> Take up these lines Tabacco-like unto thy braine,
> And that divinely toucht, puff out the smoke againe

Beaumont celebrates the muse-like nature of tobacco ("By whom the Indian priests inspired be") seeking it to "infume" his brain and make his "soule's powers subtile". "Inspire me with thy flame, which doth excel/The purest streams of the Castalian well".[63] This is a 'devil may care', light invocation of both the power and pleasures of tobacco.

According to Knutson, everyone – dramatists and poets alike – was talking about tobacco by 1599.[64] Various songs were likewise fulsome in its praise. Its narcotic effects are represented in the sixth of Thomas Weelkes' *Ayeres or Phantasticke Spirites for Three Voices*, "Come, sirrah Jack, ho! Fill some tobacco", published in 1608. "Bring a wire [presumably to cut the tobacco plug] and some fire...I drank none good to-day". In the next stanza Weelkes' request has been satisfied. "I swear that this tobacco, it's perfect Trinidado...for the blood it is very very good". Then "fill the pipe once more, my brains dance trenchmore. It is heady, I am giddy. Head and brains, back and reins, joints and veins from all pains it doth well purge and make clean".[65] Here we have tobacco taken for its stimulating cognitive effects as much as for its alleged health-giving benefits - the trenchmore being danced by Weelkes' brains was a lively contemporary folk dance. A change in time signature reflects the changing timbre and possibly the narcotic effects of tobacco. Weelkes' song ends by mocking those who condemn or fail to appreciate tobacco. "Let them go pluck a crow, and not know as I do the sweet of Trinidado".

Another example of madrigal verse from the period that presents tobacco in a positive light is that of Scottish mercenary-cum-musician Tobias Hume. His song, "Sing sweetly for tobacco", is reminiscent of the way the Yano-mami crave tobacco, or at least describe an aching desire for it, in their myths (Chapter 1). For Hume "tobacco is like love, O love it, for you see I will prove it". Tobacco, like love, "maketh lean the fat men's tumour".

> Love still dries up the wanton humour
> Love makes men sail from shore to shore
> 'Tis fond love often makes men poor
> Love makes men scorn all coward fears
> Love often sets men by the ears.[66]

Thomas Ravenscroft meanwhile praises both the medicinal and pleasurable qualities of the herb in his madrigal "Tobacco fumes/Away all nasty rheums". He also compares the conjoined effects of tobacco and alcohol (in this case, ale). "Nappy" (foaming, strong) ale "makes mirth". Tobacco "clears the brain" while ale "glads the heart". But taken to excess tobacco makes the will "giddy", while ale turns good cheer into headiness. Music – in the form of "crotchet rules" – furthers these effects, swelling "low" brains and encouraging participants to feed further on ale and tobacco until they become "heady giddy fools".[67] Others made similar connections between tobacco and alcohol. In his book of instruction for London "young gallants" in how to behave, Thomas Dekker suggests: "After the sound of pottle-pots is out of your eares, and that the spirit of Wine and Tobacco walkes in your braine, the Taverne door being shut uppon your backe, cast about to passe through the widest and goodliest streetes in the Cittie".

Pieces like these acknowledge and celebrate the various narcotic effects produced by tobacco "walking in your braine". While lip service was paid to the medicinal properties discussed above (as in Ravenscroft's example), it is the pleasurable aspects of tobacco which feature most as justification for using the plant.

Tobacco speaks

De l'Obel (above), tongue in cheek, suggested that tobacco might speak to challenge its detractors. In the 1607 play *Lingua*, by Thomas Tomkis,[68] tobacco gets that chance. The subtitle to the play is *The Combat of the Tongue and the Five Senses for Superiority: a Pleasant Comoedy*, and in it we find Lingua (the tongue), "an idle, prating dame", campaigning to become the sixth sense in what until then has been the exclusively male domain of *Microcosme*. In Act 4, Scene 4, tobacco is brought on stage by Olfactus (smell) to champion his claim to be the superior sense. The elaborate stage directions describe an apparition which must have been a sight indeed.[69]

"Foh, Foh, what a smell is heare?" asks one of the judges. "What fiery fellowe is that, which smoakes so much in the mouth?" asks another. "It is the great and puissant [powerful] God of Tobacco", Olfactus replies. And tobacco speaks, except that the language it uses is incomprehensible to its audience:

> Ladoch guevarroh pusuer shelvaro baggon,
> Olsia di quanon, Indi cortilo vraggon.

One of the judges considers it the "tongue of the Antipodes". For another "it was the language the Arcadians spake, that lived long before the Moone". Fortunately Olfactus is able to offer a translation. "This is the mighty emperor Tobacco, king of Trinidado, that in being conquered, conquered all Europe, in making them pay tribute for their smoake..." He goes on to translate some of the other nonsense utterances, describing tobacco as "expeller of Catarhes, banisher of all agues [fevers]", and "son to the god Vulcan". Finally, tobacco's speech is translated as

> Genius of all swaggerers, profes't enemy to physicians, sweet ointment for sower teeth, firme knot of good fellowship, Adamant of Company, swift winde, to spread the wings of Time, hated of none, but those that know him not, and of so great deserts, that who so is acquainted with him, can hardly forsake him.

This fascinating scene reveals much about sensibilities and understandings accorded tobacco at the time, while the master stroke of tobacco speaking an unintelligible language reflects its exoticism and alien status. Olfactus provides a sophisticated analysis of the qualities of 'the great and puissant God' that were recognized at the time. Medical claims are recognized in Tomkis' references to tobacco as "profes't enemy to physicians" and "sweet ointment for sower [sour] teeth". There is also an interesting observation on the "firme knot of good fellowship" it provides, something which was to come to the fore in the coffee houses that were starting to appear in the capital and elsewhere. Here those "adamant of company" met for the discussions and where, through (and perhaps because of) a fug of tobacco smoke, the ideas and ideals of the Enlightenment came to be forged (Chapter 4). The "swift winde, to spread the wings of Time" is an allusion to the narcotic properties of tobacco and its place in punctuating and stalling the rhythms of daily life. Finally Tomkis alludes to how, once tobacco's pleasures are known, one so acquainted "can hardly forsake him". It is interesting to note how even then the addictive properties of tobacco were becoming recognized, even if the term 'addiction' was not used as such.[70]

Another 17th century play that gave a walk-on, speaking part to tobacco was *Wine, Beere, Ale and Tobacco: Contending for Superiority*. This time, tobacco spoke contemporary English, although the first edition, published in 1629 following its translation from a Dutch original, omitted tobacco. The play follows a tradition in European literature of personifying beverages in competition with one another. Wine, Beer and Ale are supported respectively by Sugar (a page to Wine), Nutmeg (an apprentice to Beere), Toast ("tost" – servant of Ale) and Water, a parson who oversees all the others. Tobacco, described as "a swaggering gentleman", tries to assert his authority early on by claiming "I am your Sovereign, the sovereign drink, Tobacco". Wine, Beer and Ale are unimpressed by this assertion, however. They see their intoxicating qualities as making them alike, and equal, despite tobacco arrogantly championing his "divine breath" that "doth distill eloquence and oracle upon the tongue".[71] Wine questions his strength (as opposed to his eloquence) to which Tobacco retorts "Whose brain hath not felt the effects of my mightiness? He that opposes me shall find me march like a tempest, waited upon with lightning and black clouds".

Ale then takes a different tack, mocking the 24 "postures" required to smoke a pipe, which one has to do repeatedly "till you stink, defile the room, offend your friends, destroy your Liver and Lungs, and bid adieu to the world with a scowring flux". Tobacco dismisses these concerns as "childish inventions", but Wine considers them "most proper to illustrate your magnificence", since "howsoever you pretend that you converse with men, it is apparant, that you make men children again, for they that use you most familiarly, do but smoke all the day long". The three drinks agree with Wine's suggestion, however, that they should "admit him [Tobacco] to our

society...least he seduce men to forsake us". After all, "he is a dry companion, and you may observe how he hath insinuated already with the greatest". The four 'drinks' (because "Tobacco is a drink too") thus end up settling
their differences and joining in a dance together.

Despite the jocular intentions in tobacco gaining the power of speech (and
hence a profoundly human aspect), disquiet about tobacco, its power and
ambivalent effects on people's lives and actions is expressed in both plays.
Lingua raises the 'who has conquered who?' question, while in *Wine, Beere,
Ale and Tobacco* the suggestion is made that tobacco infantilizes men by
making them unable to control their desire for it, in the process destroying
their vital organs. Tobacco scoffs at these "childish inventions", after which
he is grudgingly but interestingly admitted to the company of other drinks –
an early indigenization that turned to transculturation with the invention of
the term 'to smoke'.

Satirical reflections

As well as the comic dramas discussed above, Ben Jonson's *Every Man in His
Humor* (1598) includes mildly satirizing vignettes that similarly represent the
ambivalent status of tobacco. When he revised the play in 1616, Jonson
transferred its setting from Italy to England. In this later version, Captain
Bobadill seeks to initiate Stephen into a tobacco habit. Speaking in a style
which "would have done decently in a tobacco trader's mouth", Bob argues
for tobacco's divine status, claiming that men have lived nearly half a year on
nothing but its "fume":

> I have been in the Indies, where this herb grows, where neither myself,
> nor a dozen gentlemen more of my knowledge, have received the taste
> of any other nutriment in the world, for the space of one and twenty
> weeks, but the fume of this simple only: therefore, it cannot be, but 'tis
> most divine.[72]

He then goes on to argue for its qualities as an emetic and cleansing antidote
to the deadliest of plants, concluding: "By Hercules, I do hold it, and will
affirm it before any prince in Europe, to be the most sovereign and precious
weed that ever the earth tendered to the use of man".

A water bearer, Oliver Cob, however, can't understand what pleasure men
get from "taking this roguish tobacco":

> It's good for nothing but to choke a man, and fill him full of smoke and
> embers: there were four died out of one house last week with taking of
> it, and two more the bell went for yesternight; one of them, they say,
> will never 'scape it; he voided a bushel of soot yesterday, upward and
> downward. By the stocks, an there were no wiser men than I, I'd have it

present whipping, man or woman, that should but deal with a tobacco
pipe: why, it will stifle them all in the end, as many as use it; it's little
better than ratsbane.[73]

This was before serious medical arguments against tobacco had been
published; but post-mortems were starting to query the safety of tobacco,
and some poor individuals may well have had some kind of unexpected
reaction to it. Alternatively, it is possible that the "pure Trinidado" people
thought they were smoking had been adulterated with other products. The
possibility of adulterated tobacco is taken up by Jonson in his more famous
play, *The Alchemist*. Speaking about a tobacconist,

> He lets me have good tabacco, and he do's not
> Sophiſticate it, with ſack-lees, or oyle,
> Nor waſhes it in muſcadell, and graines,
> Nor buries it, in gravell, under ground,
> Wrap'd up in greaſie leather, or piſs'd clouts:
> But keeps it in fine lilly-pots, that open'd,
> Smell like conferue of roſes, or french beanes.
> He has his maple block, his ſilver tongs,
> Wincheſler pipes, and fire of iuniper.
> A neate, ſpruce-honeſt-fellow, and no gold-ſmith.[74]

Tobacco is celebrated in the above works, rather as in John Beaumont's
couplets (above), with a certain 'devil may care' attitude. Not all musicians,
poets and playwrights felt able to write so freely about tobacco, however,
unless they adopted a critical tone about it like John Donne. Even Ben
Jonson's presentation of it has an equivocal, satirical air. For the reaction to
tobacco in some circles was a reaction to something regarded as more than
just a pleasant narcotic. The larger associations of the plant – with paganism,
popery and religious radicalism more generally – could lead to serious
problems for its consumers, particularly those who sought to explore its
'divine' virtues in a more literal sense. Some of these dangers will be apparent
in the next chapter.

Conclusion

This chapter has described the first contact phases between tobacco
encountered by Europeans in the Americas and the effects of its spread
from 'New World' to 'Old', largely through perusal of the poetic, dramatic
and musical representations of tobacco in England at that time. We have
considered those elements in the global assemblage – the chaotic mix of
biota, people and publications – which contributed to tobacco's rapid and
frequently successful traverse across these worlds. It has demonstrated that

while responses to tobacco often fit a 'commodity indigenization' model, some aspects of its transit were more transformational of the cultures into which it came. Given the strong association of tobacco with what were then regarded as heathen and barbarous rituals, and the dominant role played by the Church in 15th and 16th century European society, the adoption of tobacco across Europe with such alacrity is in many ways remarkable and needs explanation, both in terms of what were the alluring aspects of tobacco's agency (this Chapter) and what were some of the responses that attempted to resist it (Chapter 3).

In the 16th and early 17th centuries, tobacco as panacea was an important aspect of the 'commodity indigenization' process, but more so people's interest in the 'New World' as an intriguing, exotic curiosity. Yet neither medical, geographical nor economic accounts acknowledge some of the more phenomenological (and, quite frankly, phenomenal) aspects of tobacco's spread. Tobacco's presence in period plays and popular songs can give us insight into the pleasures people took in encountering a narcotic, intoxicating, and ultimately addictive substance that was exotic in its origins and, in many cases, required new sets of behaviours, materials and vocabulary for its administration. Such outputs were also the way, in England at least, that ordinary, frequently non-literate folk garnered their attitudes and ideas about tobacco's power. Only later in the 17th century did the continuing success of tobacco globally lead to its further promotion becoming "a deliberate, profit-driven process".[75] The historian Victoria Berridge commends an author for adopting a comparative approach that moves "away from a topic or substance-specific approach".[76] I argue for the need to move back to substance-specificity to understand the ways in which tobacco changed the world, its material agency reflected in this chapter by its role as a substance that speaks for itself in some early 17th century dramas.

As well as its habit-forming powers, summed up but not encapsulated by the term 'addiction', tobacco executed changes to the way society was or could be organized. Its effects contributed to a flowering of new recreational avenues for ordinary folk – as well as elites – in many Old World societies. While the precise manner in which tobacco was ingested and the social meanings it acquired varied from place to place, whether in Europe, the Middle East, or Asia, it has been argued that tobacco "helped to frame a distinctively early modern culture in which the pursuit of pleasure was thereafter more public, routine, and unfettered".[77] The author of this statement was talking about the Middle East specifically, but his comments could be applied pretty much anywhere in the world. However, tobacco's power was not to be exercised without resistance. The next chapter will look at how the more ambivalent dimensions of people's responses developed into a more negative set of arguments against tobacco, in England and elsewhere.

Notes

1 Concluding song of East's second set of madrigals. The complete text is "O metaphysical tobacco, fetched as far as from Morocco, thy searching fume, exhales the rheum, O metaphysical tobacco" (Fellowes, 1967: 91). The music accentuates the slightly narcotic, time-warping effect of tobacco in the way the initial 'O' is held.

2 Quoted in Mackay and Eriksen (2002: 18).

3 "The Americans were not conquered, they were infected" writes Blaut (1993: 186).

4 Coates (1998: 102).

5 He also advocated the use of West African rather than Indian slaves in West Indian plantations, a position he came to recant in subsequent writings.

6 Dickson (1954: 106).

7 Translation of de Oviedo y Valdés (1535).

8 Benzoni (1565).

9 Cartier ([1545] 1580).

10 Thwaites 1896-1901 recounted in von Gernet (2000: 76-77).

11 Thwaites 1896-1901 in von Gernet (2000: 77).

12 Marshall (2013: 10, 13).

13 According to Benedict "tobacco was already well established as a commercial crop in coastal Fujian and some districts of Guangdong by the early 1600s" (2011a: 19).

14 Brook (2004: 85).

15 Quoted in Dickson (1954: 166).

16 Courtwright, (2001: 15); on Japan, see Suzuki (2004). Screech (2004: 92) says tobacco was growing so well in the Japanese archipelago that in 1612 it was declared a drain on food production and banned.

17 Roberts (2004: 47).

18 Brady considers the distinctive design of the pipes they brought with them originates from opium rather than tobacco smoking, since the Macassans had no strong tradition of the latter (Brady, 2013).

19 Benedict (2011b) reports on a group of eight hapless Korean smugglers who tried smuggling tobacco and ginseng from Korea to Manchuria in 1638, during the time the Manchurian leader Hong Taiji was preparing a campaign to overthrow the Ming dynasty in China. Hong Taiji was also attempting to prohibit the growing, selling or smoking of tobacco, and the smugglers risked serious lashings and facial disfigurement if caught, as well as fines. In order to evade duties and restrictions on the Korean/Manchuria border, they decided to make a sea crossing over Korea Bay to the coast of Manchuria. Unfortunately, their craft encountered a typhoon which blew them to Chinese Ming island, where they were prosecuted instead for "consorting with the enemy".

20 Yang Shicong quoted in Brook (2004: 85).

21 Winter (2000: 11-12).

22 Winter (2000: 11).

23 Sahlins (1988).

24 Brook (2008: 126) summarizing Ortiz.

25 Norton (2008: 158) talks of the "plebeian Atlantic circuit" whereby tobacco spread via a cosmopolitan mix of white crewmen, black slaves and freedmen, and other sundry passengers.

26 There is a similarly apocryphal story of Sir Walter Raleigh (more correctly spelt Ralegh) smoking a pipe. His servant was so alarmed, thinking his master was on fire, he threw a bucket of water over him.

27 Goodman (1993: 49).

28 For an account of life for Spain's 'Men of the Sea', see Peréz-Mallaína (1998).
29 Long and Sedley (1987: 315).
30 According to Gately (2001: 23) "no one smoked anything in Europe. They burned things to produce sweet smells, to sniff, but not to inhale. Smoke was for dispersal, not consumption". There has been speculation that a 14th century French literary clique centred around the poet Eustace Deschamps (c.1346-c.1406) called the Society of Fumeurs ['Smokers'] may have had access to marijuana or opium. A curious three-part motet *Fumeux fume par fumée* lends weight to such an argument, although, as in English, there are no other indications of the verb *fumer* having been used transitively until the advent of tobacco (Lefferts, 1988; Unruh 1983). Were there any evidence of smoking in Europe prior to the 16th century, we might expect to see it represented somewhere in the corpus of pre-modern European art, but we don't. Yet the possibility of *fumer* meaning more than just 'fuming' in medieval French remains an intriguing one.
31 Plato's *Timaeus*, for example, saw the lungs as a coolant surrounding the heart – he argued that the lungs took in both breath and drink for this purpose.
32 Norton 2008: 157.
33 Bennett (1949: 49-50).
34 Cf. Harris (1998: 55) concerning the situation in London. The devastation wrought by European viruses travelling in the opposite direction across the Atlantic was far greater than that of syphilis in Europe.
35 Hariot (1590) was one such book – see Mancall (2004: 658).
36 Monardes (1577).
37 De l'Obel (1571) *Stirpium Adversaria Nova*, quoted in Dickson (1954: 44).
38 Henbanes are a member of the nightshade family. Dickson (1954: 34n14) suggests that this classification may have contributed to the belief that tobacco was evil.
39 In Gerard (1597).
40 Vaughan (1600: 26, 27).
41 Translation of de Oviedo y Valdés (1535).
42 Worth Estes (2000: 116).
43 Gardiner (1610) quoted by Cowan (2005: 37).
44 Dickson (1954).
45 Norton (2008) comes to a broadly similar conclusion.
46 Mancall (2004).
47 Ibid. (659).
48 Roanoke island was in what is now North Carolina.
49 Harriot (1590: 16).
50 Ibid. (60). Spellings modernized for clarity.
51 Knapp (1988: 27; 1992: 134).
52 Flynn (1995).
53 Ibid. (191-2); Whitlock (1962: 16-17).
54 Flynn (1995: 192).
55 See Dekker's manual (1609).
56 Sugg (2007: 44) describes the face at the window as a mistress. However, the sex of his "love" is unclear and given the preceding verses it could as well be male.
57 Pamphlet wars were a feature of literary life at the turn of the 17th century, reminiscent of 21st century internet 'flaming'. Tobacco was often invoked in contentious ways amongst the combatants in these disputes, but this was not necessarily to the disservice of tobacco. For example, two literary combatants, Thomas Nash and Gabriel Harvey, were both in their own ways favourably disposed towards tobacco, and their dispute fuelled the publicity it received.
58 Shell (2003: 132).

59 Chute (1595) quoted in Kane (1931: 158).
60 Chute (1595) quoted in Kane (1931: 159).
61 Ibid. Kane assumes this to be a reference to the plague of 1592-93. The fact that Chute does not recommend tobacco for any harmes "below the girdle" indicates he had no faith in its abilities to cure syphilis.
62 Chute (1595) quoted in Kane (1931: 159).
63 Beaumont (1602). The Castalian well was a spring at Delphi which was a source of poetic inspiration. For a fuller exposition of this poem, see Knapp (1992) Chapter 4, Part 5.
64 Knutson (2001: 81).
65 Fellowes (1967: 296-7).
66 Ibid. (252-3).
67 Ibid.
68 Authorship is disputed, with some claiming Anthony Brewer wrote the play. The quotes that follow are all taken from Tomkis (1607).
69 "Tobacco apparelled in a taffata mangle, his arms browne and naked, buskins made of the pilling of Osiers, his necke bare, hung with Indian leaves, his face browne painted with blue stripes, in his nose swines teeth, on his head a painted wicker crown, with tobacco pipes set in it, plumes of tobacco leaves, lead by two Indian boyes naked, with tapers in their hands, Tobacco-boxes and pipes lighted".
70 We should not leave the play without acknowledging Lingua's "unremittingly misogynist confirmation of Jacobean patriarchal ideology" (Harris 1998: 111). "The five senses' petition practically exhausts the inventory of misogynist Tudor and Stuart characterizations of women and their tongues. Lingua is branded variously as a liar, a witch, a whore, a back-biter, a scold, a gossip, a flattered and, 'worst' of all, 'a Woman in euery respect'" (ibid: 112).
71 Anon. (1630). For further consideration of the commonality with which tobacco and alcohol were regarded as intoxicants, see Withington (2011).
72 Jonson (1616: 61-2). Spellings modernized for clarity.
73 Ibid. (62-3).
74 Ibid. (16).
75 Courtwright (2001: 9).
76 Berridge (2013: 12) discussing Nathanson (1999).
77 Grehan (2006: 1377).

Chapter 3

Counterblastes and compromises

Tobacco as panacea and, more importantly, as part of the vast cornucopia of materials unleashed by the 'discovery' and subsequent colonization of the peoples and worlds of South and North America, were important tropes in tobacco's early European indigenization. However, tobacco was being hybridized or indigenized into and across societies in complex ways. In the process, its power stimulated various kinds of theological and monarchical opposition. On the theological side, strong countercurrents included the view that tobacco was the work of the devil ('Divell' in early modern English). Monarchically, tobacco's rapid dispersal around the world led to various attempts by jealous rulers to counteract its seductive powers. James I of England (and VI of Scotland) is a typical example and is the author of the *Counterblaste* (1604) that appears in the title of this chapter. I argue for the need to take James' arguments about tobacco on their own terms and seek to understand them according to the norms and values of their time. By doing so, I will show how much of what he says makes sense in terms of current ideas about 'lay epidemiology'.

Despite his antipathy, James, like many other leaders, very soon became as dependent on tobacco as were those 'gallants' or 'tobacconists' who became aficionados. The historian Jordan Goodman points out the multiple 'cultures of dependence' created by the arrival of tobacco in different parts of the world. "The history of tobacco is full of conflict, compromise, coercion and co-operation. It is through this historical process that tobacco has become a universal addiction for consumers, for growers and for governments".[1] Goodman identifies multiple forms of dependency – of people on their product, of governments on tobacco's revenues, of businessmen on their profits and of agricultural and manufacturing labour on the employment it provides. Even the field of tobacco control, a new social form in public health (Chapters 10-12) has elements of self-perpetuation within its fabric. But 'dependence' hardly captures the strength of tobacco's influence. There is a colonialism to tobacco which can be seen in both its effects on the individual user and its important role in the formation of the first European colonies in Virginia. These would have failed without the development of tobacco cultivation. The deep imbrication of tobacco with colonial and nascent capitalist enterprises such as the Virginia Company, and the effects of this hybridization, are themes that will recur not only in this chapter but throughout the rest of the book.

Tobacco as Divell's work

1602 saw the publication of what was probably the first pamphlet strongly opposed to tobacco ever published in England. The author of *Work for Chimny Sweepers*, Philaretes, was most likely a physician, "a very well-educated and probably prestigious one".[2] He argued that tobacco consumption was a "vulgar practise...hurtfull and pernitious to the life and health of man". Philaretes was critical of "our smoky gallants" (the period dandies or men about town) who have for a "long time glutted themselves with the fond fopperies and fashions of our neighbour Countries". As well as this xenophobic distaste for the habits of England's neighbours, he criticized the plant for its "venome and poison" and "heat and dryness". However, for Philaretes, tobacco was as importantly dismissed on religious grounds, because "the first author and finder [of tobacco] was the Divell". He reprised Monardes' comments about Indian priests drinking the tobacco fume to the extent that "with the vigour and strength werof, they fall sudently to the ground, as dead men, remaining so, according to the quantities of the smoake that they had taken". It was the Devil, according to Philarates, who showed them "the virtue of this hearbe, by meanes whereof they might see the imaginations and Visions that hee represented unto them, and by that meanes dooth deceive them".[3] Even Monardes, champion of tobacco's medicinal powers, averred that the visions induced by the heavy use of tobacco must have come from the devil.

The *Counterblaste to Tobacco*

It was the newly anointed English king, James I, however, who in 1604 authored the most polemical piece against tobacco perhaps ever penned. It was certainly the most influential, triggering what has become known as 'The Great Tobacco Controversy in England'.[4] However, to call it this implies a finite period of dispute after which the controversy was resolved. In fact, what James I did in his *Counterblaste to Tobacco* was bring together a set of arguments against both tobacco itself, and people's perceptions of it, that were mostly already in circulation; some of them have maintained their salience to this day. The *Counterblaste* was also a political document. In it, James rails at being head of a country which "though peaceable, though wealthy, though long flourishing in both...hath brought foorth a general sluggishnesse, which makes us wallow in all sorts of delights, and soft delicacies". He saw such habits as a breeding ground for sedition. His criticisms cross class lines – the clergy are singled out for being "negligent and lazy", the nobility and gentry for being "prodigall, and sold to their private delights". Lawyers, meanwhile, are "covetous" and commoners "prodigall and curious". In short, "all sorts of people [are] more carefull for their privat ends, then for their mother the Common-wealth". James argued it was his role as King to act as "the proper Physician of his Politicke-body...to purge it of all those diseases, by Medicines meete for the same". With an eye to tobacco, the subject of his diatribe, he comments that some kinds of abuses in "Common-wealths" can evade state sanctions of different kinds, being "too low for the Law to looke on", and too "meane for a King to his authoritie, or bend his eye upon". In the case of smoking tobacco, he would have liked the people to act as their own physicians, "by discovering and impugning the error, and by persuading reformation thereof". The pamphlet ends by describing tobacco smoking as "a custome lothesome to the eye, hateful to the nose, harmful to the brain, dangerous to the lungs, and in the black and stinking fume thereof, nearest resembling the horrible stygian smoke of the pit that is bottomless".

"The Deceivable Appearance of Reason"

Apart from theological allusions to Hell, one of the arguments against smoking in the *Counterblaste* is "The Deceivable Appearance of Reason". Tobacco, it had been argued, was "dry and hote" and hence good for the brain, which is "colde and wet". James could have followed those herbalists mentioned in Chapter 2, who argued that there were already plenty of "dry and hote" remedies for the problems caused by "colde and wet". Instead, the *Counterblaste* attempts to argue that the principles of humoral medicine have been misinterpreted. The body is a diverse "*Microcosme* or little world within our selves". In this world, the application of a thing of contrary nature to any part disrupts the "perfect harmonie" constituted by the whole body. Thus, the coldness and wetness of our brains, James I argued, is "the onely ordinarie means that procures our sleepe and rest". Tobacco smoking puts this rest in jeopardy. He also developed a convoluted argument that claims tobacco smoke cannot be drying anyway, because it is "neere to the nature of the air" and hence, he surmises, is more like water vapour than dry smoke.

"The Mistaken Practicke of General Experience"

We can make more sense of James' second set of arguments, those founded on "the mistaken Practicke of general Experience". The argument was abroad that "people would not have taken as general a good liking...[for tobacco] if they had not by experience found it verie soveraigne and good for them". However, James argues shrewdly that people are "drawn to the foolish affectation of any noveltie" and feel compelled to imitate the use of it. For "we imitate every thing that our fellowes doe, and so prove our selves capable of every thing whereof they are capable, like Apes, counterfeiting the manners of others, to our owne destruction".

James also challenges the health arguments being made at the time, that so many "by the taking of *Tobacco* divers and very many doe finde themselves cured of divers diseases...[and] no man ever received harme thereby". How could it be, he opines, that "it cures all sorts of diseases...in all persons, and at all times"? There had to be contradictions in such panacea claims. For example, "[i]t refreshes a weary man and yet makes a man hungry. Being taken when they goe to bed, it makes one sleepe soundly, and yet being taken when a man is sleepie and drowsie, it will, as they say, awake his braine, and quicken his understanding". "What greater abusurditie can there bee", James I went on, "then to say that one cure shall serve for divers, nay, contrarious sortes of diseases?"

Furthermore, many of the cures claimed seemed quite illogical to him in their attribution of causation. The "mistaken practice of general experience" meant that if a sick man took tobacco and got better, even if his illness had simply taken its natural course, he was likely to attribute his recovered health to the miracle of tobacco. By the same token, if someone smokes themselves to death with tobacco, as it was claimed many had done, some other disease might well be blamed for this misfortune. The prominent survival of certain individuals in apparently rude health who might have been expected to die is also significant. "So doe olde harlots thanke their harlotrie for their many yeeres, that custome being healthfull (say they)...but never have minde how many die of the Pockes in the flower of their youth". Similarly "olde drunkards thinke they prolong their dayes, by their swinelike diet, but never remember howe many die drowned in drinke before they be halfe olde".

"Habitum, alteram naturam"

The third explanation for people's behaviour, after those arguing for a misplaced faith in experience or reason, demonstrates King James' emergent appreciation of tobacco as an addictive substance or, as he put it, the 'bewitching qualitie' of the weed, which leads to the "great takers of *Tobacco*" having to take increasing amounts of it. "Many in this kingdom have had such a continuall use of taking this unsavorie smoke, as now they are not able to forbeare the same...for their continuall custome hath made to them, *habitum, alteram naturam* ['habit alters nature']", such that for "those that from their birth have bene continually nourished upon poison and things venomous, wholesome meats are onely poisonable".

However, it was not only bodily nature which was altered by the tobacco habit. Social mores were also changed. Tobacco, James I says, "has become in place of a cure, a point of good fellowship". "Is it not a great vanitie, that a man cannot heartily welcome his friend now, but straight they must bee in hand with *Tobacco*?" This, James felt, was leading to men "sound both in judgment, and complexion", feeling pressure to take it even when not wanting it, for fear of being "accounted peevish and no good company".

Becoming papist, heathen or barbarous

For James I, though, tobacco had symbolic associations as well as bodily consequences. He abhorred all things papist, heathen, or simply primitive, and asked his countrymen to consider "what honour or policie can move us to imitate the barbarous and beastly maners of the wilde, godlesse, and slavish *Indians*, especially in so vile and stinking a custome?" If disdaining French manners and the spirit of the Spaniards (whose king, he warned, had become "comparable in largenes of Dominions, to the great Emperor of Turkie"), James argued, why should his countrymen lower themselves to imitate the customs of the *Indians*, "slaves to the Spaniards, refuse [outcasts] to the world, and as yet aliens from the holy Couvnant of God?" If we are going to do that by smoking, James I went on, "[w]hy do we not as well imitate them in walking naked as they do? Preferring glasses, feathers, and such toys, to gold and precious stones, as they do? Yea why do we not deny God and adore the Devill, as they do?" It is in the Indians' preference for worthless trinkets and geegaws to the "gold and precious stones" that were the primary object of European forays which James finds perhaps their most damning criticism.[5]

Corrupting her "sweete breath"

Finally, James expressed concern for the way a husband's smoking habit might corrupt his wife's "sweete breath", thus leaving her with little choice but to "resolve to live in a perpetuall stinking torment".

Discussion: a text in its context

It is important to see the *Counterblaste* in the historical context of James I's kingship. James saw himself as the political father of his people, head of the 'microcosm' of the body of man. In a speech to the English parliament in 1610 he claimed that "Kings are justly called Gods, for that they exercise a manner or resemblance of Divine power on earth". He felt his 'divine right' threatened, however, by anything else making such a claim, whether divine or diabolical, tobacco or witchcraft (to name one of James' other preoccupations). It was hardly surprising, therefore, that God's lieutenant on earth felt threatened by, and attempted to counterattack, a substance people were calling the 'great god' or 'divine' (Chapter 2). However, using pamphlets for this purpose was perhaps not the most dignified thing a man claiming divinity could have done, and risked him becoming a subject of satire and ridicule (again in much the same way the 'great god' tobacco is ridiculed in Tomkis' *Lingua* – Chapter 2). We shall see in subsequent chapters that many rulers elsewhere in the world had a similar reaction to the arrival of tobacco in their polity – but then had reasons to rethink their position as, somewhat miraculously, did James I.

Berthold Laufer, curator of Asian anthropology at the Field Museum of Natural History, Chicago, in the 1920s, claimed James I's pamphlet "has met with almost universal condemnation".[6] Although from his perspective tobacco was "a great benefactor of mankind", in good anthropological style, he went on to argue that "to condemn [James I] is easier than to understand". In this vein, "while the royal diatribe is sizzling...with misstatements, exaggerations, and outbursts of gloomy pessimism and unrestrained animosity, it was a natural reaction against the many exorbitant claims made by the friends and defenders of the narcotic".[7] However, it is an oversimplification to say James I condemned the use of tobacco "primarily out of motives of racial and national pride", as Laufer suggests. James I's comments on experience being a dubious source of evidence remain as relevant today as they were in 1604 and raise interesting comparisons with contemporary interest in what has been called perception bias. Perception bias is clearly illustrated in a joke about why dolphins have the reputation for pushing swimmers in difficulties towards the shore. The answer is that we never hear back from the swimmers who are pushed in the other direction. Those swimmers are the same as James I's harlots and drunkards whose premature deaths preclude a negative story about their experiences.

Meanwhile, the living tend to be over-impressed by 'good news' stories about dolphins, or tobacco. In 1991, the anthropologist Charlie Davison led a project looking at people's perceptions of the causes of coronary heart disease (CHD) in South Wales.[8] One hundred and eighty people were interviewed to find out their views on who would be a likely candidate for CHD. What transpired was that although almost everyone knew the public health messages about the disease's likely causes (such as smoking or over-eating), just about everyone knew or had known someone in their social circle who gave the lie to these messages for reasons of fate, luck or destiny. This 'lay epidemiology', as it was termed, was based on people's experience of those who had flouted the normal rules of epidemiology. One was an 'Uncle Norman' figure who had reached a healthy old age, despite heavy smoking, eating, and drinking. Most people could identify such a figure in their lives, irrespective of their age, gender, or class. An obverse case, if less frequently observed, was provided by the individual we might call 'Fit Fred', a slim, clean-living "last person you'd expect to have a coronary...who is then unfortunate enough to succumb".[9] Both exemplify James' "mistaken practicke of general experience". Hughes identifies a tendency for rationalizations of smoking, and the arguments against it, to converge in the contemporary world, a process he calls "nihilist cynicism".[10] Some people, much to the exasperation of King James, seem only too willing to 'accept the exception' and ignore more problematic population-based, statistical evidence. This is that roughly half of those who smoke regularly over a long period of time (and a quarter of those who chew tobacco) will become the lost souls whom the dolphins push out to sea.

This is not the only way that perception bias can take hold, however. Those who succumb to a range of 'smoking-related' diseases have a tendency to become invisible. Such diseases either kill them prematurely or make it difficult for them to appear in public and for their presence to be witnessed or their voice (sometimes quite literally) to be adequately heard. Such difficulties are directly related to their health problems, but they can also be the result of the stigma they experience. For people in the latter stages of smoking-related lung diseases like Chronic Obstructive Pulmonary Disease (COPD), for example, the problems of breathing, walking, speaking, and avoiding exacerbations often make it easier to stay indoors than to appear in public. Lung cancer can cause similar difficulties. Heart disease, stroke and other circulatory problems associated with long-term tobacco use also serve to hide people from sight. This can make it difficult for the young and unafflicted to get a true sense of the effects of tobacco on long-term users. Furthermore, smoking is overwhelmingly portrayed in contemporary media as a subject performed by people who appear largely unaffected by their habit. We are not introduced so regularly to people who are terminally ill from smoking-related respiratory illnesses, and certainly not to those who have passed away.

James I had understood something quite profound in human experience and was using it in an early attempt to change the place of tobacco in the public imagination. Other perspectives on tobacco come from its place in religious, literary and gender politics during this time.

Religious politics of tobacco in the 16th and 17th centuries

Tobacco, Catholicism, and the 'School of Night'

Tobacco was also acquiring fairly unsavoury associations with dissenting religious voices and those who championed a questioning of the scriptures in the interests of rationalism. The playwright Christopher Marlowe (1564-1593), an inveterate 'tobacconist', was part of an intellectual circle known as the 'School of Night'. This 'School', a group rumoured to meet at Sir Walter Raleigh's London residence, included the Algonquian sympathist and tobacco champion Thomas Hariot.[11] Raleigh had many enemies at court and abroad who were only too happy to demonize his enterprise. A pamphlet published in 1592, for instance, disparaged 'Sir Walter Raleigh's school of atheism' and accused Hariot of being 'the conjurer that is master thereof'.[12] In the highly charged religious atmosphere of the time, it is hardly surprising that Hariot came in for accusations of necromancy because of his scripture-questioning rationalism. Marlowe likewise did himself no favours by suggesting, according to one informer, that the Eucharist would be "much better if administered in a Tobacco pipe". This, and the purported statement "all they that love not tobacco and boys are fools", were regarded as so blasphemous that both were deleted in an informer's account presented to Queen Elizabeth in 1593. A warrant was issued for Marlowe's arrest, and he was stabbed in mysterious circumstances some 12 days later. The writings of Hakluyt, Hariot and others, with their accounts of delirious heathen priests using tobacco for divinatory purposes, gave its detractors plenty of scope to associate it with religious deviance. One contemporary Protestant zealot accused Catholics of being overly affected by tobacco, and argued the Gunpowder Plotters acted as they did because their brains were befuddled by heavy smoking.[13] Guy Fawkes and his fellow conspirators are reported to have smoked prodigious amounts of tobacco as they awaited their execution in January 1606, "with a seeming carelessness of their crime".[14]

The association between tobacco and Catholicism gave other writers good reason to feel they should distance themselves from tobacco. "Tobaccaean" John Donne (Chapter 2) was one example. Donne's family was Catholic at a time when it was difficult being a Catholic family in England. His younger brother Henry, a university student, was arrested in 1593 and accused of harbouring William Harrington, a Catholic priest accused of sedition. Betrayed by his friend under torture, Harrington was himself racked and then hanged until not quite dead, after which he was disembowelled. Henry Donne subsequently died of bubonic plague in Newgate prison. After this time, we are told, Donne began to question his Catholic faith, and was probably quite wise to go 'underground' with his tobacco habit, particularly since – in an almost complete renunciation of his religious roots – he went on to become Dean of St Paul's Cathedral.

Catholic associations to one side, King James' attitude to tobacco did little to encourage writing in favour of the 'loathsome weed' particularly if, like Donne, you were an "awkward would-be courtier grovelling for James' favour".[15] Perhaps the "tobaccaean" epithet was an attempt by Floyd (Chapter 2) to flip the argument about tobacco and heresy back on his Protestant enemies, or a subtle reference to Donne's Catholic origins. Hoby's response in a *Counter-Snarle* (an allusion to the King's *Counterblaste*, perhaps?) sees Donne's ally somewhat on the back foot. Hoby writes: "I confesse in my time I have not been an enemy to that *Indian* weede...[but] if he [the informer] be as free from all his olde vices, and drunken conceites, as I am from this vanity [smoking], hee shall not neede any great penance".[16] Tobacco was clearly not being consumed in an unequivocally 'pro-tobacco' environment at this time.

Why is there no tobacco in Shakespeare?

Given the associations analysed above, it is perhaps no wonder that William Shakespeare was reluctant to be associated with or, indeed, use the word 'tobacco' at all in any of his known works. Yet given the innovative disruption tobacco's arrival on European shores caused, and Shakespeare's intense observation of and literary engagement with the lifeways of his time, its absence is all the more remarkable. Neither do the words 'smoke', 'smoking' or 'pipe' appear in his works, at least not with regard to tobacco.[17] Shakespeare was a member of the Lord Chamberlain's company which performed Ben Jonson's *Every Man in His Humor* in 1598 (see Chapter 2),[18] so must have been well aware of the dramatic potential offered by 'the weed'.

In fact, 'weed' is the only metonym that might, on just two occasions, refer to tobacco in Shakespeare. In Act 4 Scene 2 of *Othello: Moor of Venice*, Othello exclaims of Desdemona "O though blacke[19] weed, Who are so lovely fair and smell'st so sweet/That the sense aches at thee, would thou hadst never been born!"[20] And then in Sonnet 76, when berating himself for dullness and repetition in what he writes, Shakespeare asks:

> Why is my verse so barren of new pride?
> So far from variation or quick change?
> Why with the time do I not glance aside
> To new-found methods and to compounds strange?
> Why write I still all one, ever the same,
> And keep invention in a noted weed...

Assuming 'weed' in both cases refers to tobacco and not to clothing (as several commentators assume) or cannabis (as some etymologically challenged 20th century critics seem to think), Shakespeare could have been discretely acknowledging the 'inventive power' of tobacco while overtly disdaining its use.

Shakespeare's remarkable reticence about tobacco remains a conundrum, though. He may have been worried about falling out with James I, but this seems unlikely given the frequent appearance of tobacco in other literary and musical outpourings from the period (despite its heathen and Catholic associations). J.M. Barrie (an inveterate smoker himself, as we shall see in Chapter 6) refused to believe that Shakespeare lacked acquaintance with the Arcadia or similar mixture that was so close to Barrie's own heart. In his homage to tobacco in his collection *My Lady Nicotine*, Barrie ends his chapter about the Elizabethans, 'The Grandest Scene in History', with a picture of "the figure in the corner...He is smoking the Arcadia, and as he smokes the tragedy of Hamlet takes form in his brain...I know that there is no mention of tobacco in Shakespeare's plays, but those who smoke the Arcadia tell their secret to none, and of other mixtures they scorn to speak". Maybe Shakespeare did occasionally partake of 'the weed' but was ashamed to say. Certainly Sonnet 76, one of his 'Fair Youth' series, is reticent with regard to 'the love that dare not speak its name',[21] given what had happened to Christopher Marlowe. Such reticence may be mirrored in his refusal to acknowledge tobacco.

Tobacco and the Puritan radicals

As the 17th century progressed, tobacco became an equally important feature in the lives of those at the other end of the religious spectrum, the so-called

Puritan radicals opposed to 'state-sponsored' Protestantism. Some 50 years after Marlowe's death John Erbery, a representative of the shadowy world of 'Seekers' and 'Ranters', made similar proposals to those of Marlowe about enlivening Christian rituals through use of tobacco. The Ranters were a loose group of pantheist itinerants who believed, in the words of one of their following, that God is in "this dog, this tobacco pipe, he is me and I am him".[22] Erbery proposed making holy communion a full meal, with lots of drink. "Why do they not say their prayers before a pipe of tobacco?" he asked, adding "a good creature".[23] George Fox (1624-1691), founder of the Religious Society of Friends (Quakers), reported being accosted by "a forward, bold lad" at a Ranters' meeting who offered him a pipe saying "Come, all is ours". Fox disdained tobacco, but on this occasion he decided to take it "and put it to my mouth, and gave it to him again to stop him, lest his rude tongue should say I had not unity with the creation".[24] These were revolutionary times, the revolution in question being Thomas Cromwell's short-lived 'Long Parliament' and the English republic. In a time when "anything seemed possible",[25] Seeker and Ranter groups formed part of the revolt within this revolution. Many of the sects met in taverns and tobacco houses; Baptist services were an occasion for tobacco smoking. According to Hill, "the use of tobacco and alcohol was intended to heighten spiritual vision...the millenarian John Mason was excessively addicted to smoking and 'generally while he smoked he was in a kind of ecstasy'",[26] while across the Atlantic "in New England, Captain Underhill told Governor Winthrop 'the Spirit had sent into him the witness of free grace, while he was in the moderate enjoyment of the creature called tobacco'".[27]

Hill remarks "'Unity with creation', tobacco 'a good creature', parodying holy communion: we should never fail to look for symbolism in what appear the extravagant gestures of seventeenth century radicals. Ranter advocacy of blasphemy...was a symbolic expression of freedom from moral restraints".[28] We could add that their views − not to mention actions − would have found favour amongst the animist and perspectivist Amerindians in their tobacco heartlands.

Gender politics of tobacco

Gender politics has been a feature of tobacco ever since first contact, in literature as well as life. In the play *Antonio and Mellida* by John Marston, written in 1599, tobacco features heavily in the choices Mellida's cousin makes about marriage. One potential suitor, who looks "for all the world like an o'er-roasted pig", is "A great tobacco-taker too, that's flat,/For his eyes look as if they had been hung/In the smoke of his nose".[29] Another fancies himself as worthy because of a good head of hair and "I ha' not a red beard, take not tobacco much".[30] Mellida's cousin finally decides she will have none of them, saying she will marry "when men abandon jealousy, forsake taking of tobacco, and cease to wear their beards so rudely long. O, to have a husband with a mouth continually smoking...ah, 'tis more than most intolerable".[31]

In an altogether earthier pamphlet published in 1675, female antipathy towards tobacco extended beyond a distaste for 'smoking mouths' to concern for the effects tobacco might have on men's procreative abilities. In *The Women's Complaint Against Tobacco*, a woman at "Gossips' Hall" is reported as saying:

> I have been married to my Husband about fourteen years, this Man hath been all his time a great Smoaker, and to tell you the truth I was never got with child by him but once, and that was so feebly done, that I may boldly say it was not half gotten, though he is a Man as likely as any of his Neighbours, and as for my own part I am sure I am not in the least defective, but am as apt and fit for the work of generation as any of my Neighbours, nay I may say as likely to be got with child as any Woman in *England*, let the other be what she will, yet this Man cannot do the feat, and the reason why it is not done, I must clearly impute to his smoking that Infernal *Indian* Weed, which they call Tobacco.[32]

Tobacco's potential effect on procreative powers, and the resistance of women to tobacco more generally, is a thematic skein throughout the historical and contemporary life of tobacco.

Commissioning compromise

Only six months after his *Counterblaste*, James I published his *Commissio pro Tobacco*, intended to give legal 'teeth' to his views. The change in tone it signifies is quite remarkable. It commences with the warning that, in ten days' time, the:

> Treasurer ... Customers Comptrollers Searchers Surveyors, and all other Officers of our Portes ... shall demaunde and take to our use of all Merchauntes, as well Englishe as Strangers, and of all others whoe shall bringe in anye *Tabacco* into this Realme ... the Somme of *Six Shillinges and eighte Pence* upon everye Pound Waight thereof, over and above the Custome of *Twoo Pence* upon the Pounde Waighte usuallye paide heretofore.

A 4,000 per cent increase in revenue for importers of this "drugge" surely augured a significant change in the relationship between tobacco and the state. On the one hand disparaged, it suddenly had the makings of a financial opportunity. The *Commissio pro Tobacco* was necessary in order to ensure the "weale and prosperitie" of an expanding "common-wealth", argued James. Yet the duty paid did not go directly to the treasury, the collectors of duties paid the Crown £2,000 a year for the privilege.[33]

Perhaps it was to enable some revenue to be collected that a distinction was made in the *Commissio* between "persons of good Callinge and Qualitye" who used tobacco ostensibly on health grounds, and its use "by a number of ryotous and disordered Persons of meane and base Condition". Such people "doe spend most of there tyme in that idle Vanitie, to the evill example and corrupting of others". James notes the hardships faced by families where additional work is necessary to garner enough money to maintain a tobacco habit. He complained that by the

> great and immoderate takinge of *Tabacco* the Health of a great nomber of our People is impayred, and theire Bodies weakened and made unfit for Labor…a great part of the Treasure of our Lande is spent and exhausted by this onely Drugge so licentiously abused by the meaner sorte.

However, with these words James I stopped short of attempting to secure an all-out ban on tobacco. Instead he declared that the government would allow the import of tobacco "to serve for their necessarie use who are of the better sort, and have and will use the same with Moderation to preserve their Healthe".

What reasons could there be for James' seeming about-face in permitting the import of tobacco for medicinal purposes by those "of the better sort"? James had signed a treaty with the new King of Spain, Philip III, thus ending the hostilities between the two countries, which had been going on since 1585. He was keen to avoid further excuses for belligerence between the two nations, so the privateering which had been an important source of Trinidado, Orinoco and other tobaccos from the Americas had to stop. James had been poor as a Scottish monarch and was generous in his bestowal of honours when he ascended the English throne in 1603.[34] He had an urgent need to raise funds in order to avoid being financially beholden to an overly large array of nobles. As the Canute-like impossibility of countering the tide of tobacco became apparent, the impetus became one of ownership rather than conquest. James did in fact insist that all claims and rights to property were under his control, in accordance with his views on the divine right of kings.[35] Ratcheting up the tax on tobacco in the way he did gave him the opportunity to ensnare this devilish commodity – and make a substantial profit for the Crown in doing so.

Compromise as a global phenomenon

James I represents a pattern which was common worldwide almost anywhere tobacco came into contact with quasi-divine or autocratic leaders. Such leaders initially sought to protect themselves and their countrymen from what they saw as a powerful threat to their polity, usually by attempting to ban tobacco, but generally rethought this approach when the opportunity to raise revenues from tobacco became apparent. However, some other practical concerns were also raised. Attempts to grow tobacco by an Alsatian farmer in Strassburg (1620) were resisted by the city council, worried that tobacco growing would discourage the production of more worthy food crops.[36] The Archbishop of Cologne in 1649 preached that smoking corrupted youth and started fires. In China, in the final years of his reign, the last Ming emperor attempted to criminalize tobacco, although his ineffectual edicts were openly flouted by smokers, even in Beijing. The Qing dynasty emperor Hong Taiji also tried the criminalization approach but he, in common with the Indian Mughals, the Iranian Safavids and the Turkish Ottomans, found such attempts at regulation or prohibition failed; thus, their efforts shifted to attempting to boost their revenues through taxing tobacco, either at the point of its production, manufacture, import, or use.

In India, Shah Jahangir issued a decree against smoking in 1617, but such was the potential benefit to his treasury from its taxes that, within a few years, commercial tobacco production was taking place within his borders. Of course, the emerging colonial situation made his situation rather different to that of James I. The East India Company (EIC), described by one commentator as the first corporate multinational,[37] had started curing tobacco in its Indian factories in 1612 and was waiting for any opportunity it could to turn India into a hub for the export of tobacco across Asia.[38] In this way, as in Virginia (below), tobacco was at the forefront of the colonial and, subsequently, capitalist economy. The Iranian Shah Abbas, concerned about the amount his troops were spending on tobacco, attempted to prohibit its use by cutting off the lips and noses of people who smoked.[39] He tried further prohibitions in 1621 but then acquiesced to legalization while heavily taxing consumption; the EIC was able to start importing tobacco into Iran by 1628-29. By the middle of the century, however, tobacco had become a cash crop in Iran and the Iranians were able to export it to the Ottomans and India.[40]

Ottoman attempts at suppression went in two waves. The first was during the reign of Ahmed I, "a young and unusually pious sultan who seems to have given his personal backing to the cause".[41] However, despite its impact in some provinces (for example Egypt, where the incoming governor burnt large quantities of tobacco and declared it a contraband item), the campaign soon lapsed. Twenty years later, however, Sultan Murad IV, under the influence of a popular reformist preacher,[42] made smoking an offence punishable by death, citing the risk of fires.[43] However, there may also have been concern at what tobacco presaged in terms of its shared consumption and the breakdown of longstanding social hierarchies (as with the coffee shops then coming into vogue and which Murad IV also closed down in 1633).[44] Murad IV died in 1640, however, and by 1650 tobacco was legal again, becoming heavily taxed in 1691 to help pay for the costly campaigns of the Ottomans against the infidels in Austria and elsewhere.

Only in Muscovy (Russia) did the tsars, starting with Ivan the Terrible, hold out against this pernicious habit. Ivan the Terrible shared the Orthodox

Church's antipathy towards tobacco. The English Muscovy Company (EMC), established on the same lines as the EIC and preceding the latter by about 50 years,[45] was hopeful it could follow the EIC's example by breaking into the lucrative Russian market. But the situation in Russia was very different to that in India. The Russians were concerned with non-Russian and non-Orthodox populations within their borders and the 'evil customs' and 'lawlessness' to be found in the countries beyond them – categories that were both covered by the same Russian word *inozemsty* ('foreigner'). A prohibition passed by Tsar Mikhail Fedorovich in 1627, prohibiting the sale of tobacco in Siberia, was extended to all Russian territories in 1633/34 "on pain of death". A traveller in Muscovy reported seeing eight men and one woman being flogged with a knout (a potentially fatal 'cat-o-ninetails' instrument) for selling tobacco and vodka in 1634.

Since environmental conditions in Muscovy, unlike India or Iran, were not conducive to growing tobacco, there was no incentive to legalize production in order to save on the loss of revenue through imports. While several smuggling routes opened up through Sweden and Moldova, the English were unable to expand their official tobacco trade as the EMC was only allowed to operate in a direct line between Arkhangelsk (their northern entry point) and Moscow. When the English started trying to smuggle tobacco directly along this route (in order to circumvent the Swedish middlemen) two Englishmen were arrested and imprisoned by the Russian authorities, and King Charles I was forced to intercede on their behalf. The English were strong advocates of 'free trade', which in their terms, according to one writer, meant "their right to unrestricted trade with foreign countries, with severe restrictions on any competitors".[46] Increasing production in Virginia (see below) was leading to a fall in prices and Virginia plantation owners petitioned the Crown to break into the Russian market. The Russians, however, preferred establishing export monopolies, and the one for tobacco had already been secured with the Dutch. A Dutch emissary to Moscow in the early years of the 17th century did nothing for Anglo-Russian relations through blaming the English ambassador for a "great conflagration which caused much damage" with his tobacco smoking.[47]

All hail the Virginia Company

Another influence on James I's decision to tax tobacco to the heavens rather than attempt to ban it altogether might have been lobbying by members of the fledgling Virginia Company (initially called the London Company). The Roanoke settlement Thomas Hariot had been involved in establishing was abandoned a year later. It was part of what became increasingly desperate efforts by England to emulate the "golden successe",[48] in colonial terms, of its European rivals. A subsequent attempt to establish a colony, in what became called Virginia in honour of Queen Elizabeth I, also failed due to the ongoing naval hostilities between England and Spain and the consequent difficulties in supplying the settlers with adequate provisions. What subsequently happened to these Roanoke settlers is something of a mystery.[49]

The kings of Spain, Portugal, and France established royal tobacco monopolies, making it a crime for anyone other than sanctioned leaseholders to trade in tobacco grown in their territories. In England, contrary to its continental neighbours, the colonial enterprise was largely financed by merchants creating joint stock companies. The Virginia Company came into existence by royal charter in 1606. In 1607, a further group of colonists attempted to found a settlement. One hundred and forty-four men set out, of whom 105 reached Virginia alive. They established a settlement in the tidewater area of the Chesapeake Bay, at a site they called Jamestown.

George Percy, one of the 38 noblemen in this party, described their experiences in his *Discourse of the Plantation of the Southern Colony in Virginia by the English*. There were some initial skirmishes with "Savages" of the Powhatan tribe, which left them uncertain whether "great smokes of fire" they saw in the nearby woodlands were because of food planting, or were the Powhatans giving a sign to their compatriots to unite in attacking the settlers. After this, though, they made contact with some other Indians "which directed us to their Town, where we were entertained by them very kindly". Their hosts

> would not suffer us to eat unless we sat down, which we did on a Mat right against them. After we were well satisfied they gave us of their Tobacco, which they took in a pipe made artificially of earth as ours are, but far bigger, with the bowl fashioned together with a piece of fine copper.

The settlers had arrived in May, too late in the season to plant crops, and many of the men were unused to physical labour, at least of the kind necessary to carve out a new colony. Their mission was based on an assumption that they would be able to trade trinkets for food with the Indians. The captain departed for England the following month and, by August, Percy was recording a litany of deaths from "the bloudie flux" (dysentery), fever (probably malaria), woundings by the "Savages" and other causes. More than half the men died within a year. Only support from the Indians, who brought them bread, corn, fish, and meat "in great plenty", helped them survive.

Women and children were permitted to join the nascent colony in 1609, but although the population grew to 500 that year, the bulk of them fell victim to the "starving time" the following winter.[50] Governor Thomas Dale, arriving in 1611, was dismayed to find colonists had given up agriculture, spending their days instead "bowling in the streetes".[51] Desperate measures were called for – tobacco appeared to be the only cultivar that could survive the journey back to Europe and attract a high enough price to be economical.

Coates writes "with the exception of tobacco, the plantation staples of the south-eastern states – rice, cotton, and sugar cane – are all naturalized exotics".[52]

Strictly speaking the overwhelming amount of tobacco grown in the USA and Canada today is equally exotic. North America was the 2,000-year home of *N. rustica*, a variety high in alkaloids with a bitter taste unpopular with European consumers. It was for this reason that in 1613 the Jamestown settler John Rolfe (famous for marrying Pocahontas, chief Powhatan's daughter) obtained some *N. tabacum* seeds from Trinidad. How these seeds came into his possession is uncertain. Trinidad and its resources were jealously guarded by the Spanish, but there was a lot of contraband traffic. [53] Rolfe personally shipped the first crop he grew to London – in the company of Pocahontas – in 1616.

Fair stood the wind for further shipments after this voyage, since this source of tobacco was not dependent on the goodwill and tariffs of the Spanish colonies. Tobacco was to go on to become the mainstay of the early colonial economy. In 1616, 1,250 pounds of tobacco in total were exported; in 1628 this had increased to £370,000.[54] The arrival of the colony's new governor in 1617 revealed the extent to which tobacco had taken hold. He reported finding in Jamestown "but five or six houses, the Church downe, the Palisadoes broken, the Bridge in pieces, the Well of fresh water spoiled" but, in a sign of success, "the market-place, and streets, and all other spare places planted with Tobacco".[55] "The discovery that tobacco could be successfully grown and profitably sold was the most momentous single fact in the first century of settlement on the Chesapeake Bay", writes one historian; "tobacco had guaranteed that the Jamestown experiment would not fail".[56] According to another, tobacco not only made the settlements possible, but "none of those founded South of the Potomac before 1640 could have survived without it". [57]

Conditions for these early settlers were pretty dreadful, and death rates were high. The ideas the Virginia Company had for organizing and running the colony were more akin to operating a military barracks than a frontier community. Lack of women was one of the chief complaints of the early (male) settlers and, in 1619, 90 "maids" (as they were known) were shipped to Virginia from Bristol, with a hundred more the following year.[58] Maids reaching Bermuda (another dominion which owed its successful colonial settlement to the production of tobacco) were sold for £100 of tobacco each.[59] In Virginia, the rate set by the Virginia Company in London was £120, although fluctuations in the market value of tobacco meant that the company insisted that if a maid died on the transatlantic crossing "there must be proportional addition [of tobacco by weight] upon the rest".[60] White women were not the only people regarded as chattels during this period. The same year as the first consignment of maids arrived from Bristol, John Rolfe reported purchasing "20. and odd Negroes" from a Dutch man-of-war ship.[61] But the price of tobacco in England was high in the first decades of the 17th century, and this encouraged new measures to expand production. One of these was to bring over more labourers. Tobacco had become a mover of people as much as people had become movers of tobacco, its success leading to at least 5,000 English people migrating to the Chesapeake region between 1617 and 1623.[62]

Conditions remained perilous, however. In early 1622, 347 white settlers were massacred by the Powhatan Indians, largely in reaction to the great expansion of settler lands for larger and larger acreages of tobacco.[63]

John Donne extended his interest in all things "tobaccaean" through a keen interest in the work of the Virginia Company, applying unsuccessfully to become its secretary in 1609.[64] He preached a placatory sermon for the Company at St Paul's Cathedral following the Powhatan massacre, in which he professed himself "an adventurer; if not to Virginia, yet for Virginia; for every man that prints, adventures".[65] He inveigled himself onto the Council of the company later that year.[66] His second-born son George followed his father's interests by becoming Charles I's "muster-master general and marshal of Virginia" and travelled to the colony in 1637. He was shocked at the settlers' mercenary attitudes and lack of compassion; sick and hungry servants were regularly dumped on the shores of Chesapeake Bay. In Breen's words: "The colonists and the merchants who transported these servants to the New World were so consumed with making money that they had overlooked the fact that these immigrants were royal subjects and human beings, not simply a cheap economic resource".[67]

Between 1634 and 1640, exports from Virginia to England doubled from £500,000 to more than £1 million annually. By the late 1670s, Chesapeake planters were exporting more than £20 million a year.[68] Prices collapsed proportionately.[69] Additional labour was needed to assure the continued well-being of what might be called the emergent 'plantocracy', but options were rather limited. The indigenous native Americans had been all but decimated by the combined effects of being forced off their lands by the colonists and their lack of immunity to the diseases the Europeans had brought. As mentioned in Chapter 2, Columbus had brought a lot more than just people across the Atlantic with him. Indigenous Americans had had no previous exposure to diseases common in the 'Old World' such as smallpox, chickenpox, measles and influenza, to which they lacked immunity.[70] Furthermore, the small numbers in the original bands that had come from Beringia into the continental American landmass some 15,000 years earlier (Chapter 1) meant they lacked the genetic diversity which might have given them a wider array of biological defences against the illnesses the Europeans introduced. The consequences of the west-east passage for native Americans were devastating.

In the Chesapeake region, tobacco planters replaced Indian villages with farmsteads dispersed across the landscape, but primarily along the rivers and waterways so that they could be near trade routes and able to profit from the best soils. At the end of the 17th century, a newly appointed minister in Calvert County, Maryland, was concerned that, with two or three families on each square mile of taxed land, "we are pretty closely seated, yet we cannot see our next neighbours house for trees. In a few years we may expect it otherwise", the reverend went on, "for the tobacco trade destroyes abundance of timber both for making hogsheads and building of tobacco houses;

besides cleareing of ground yearly for planting".[71] Labour was required to effect these substantial changes to the landscape. The Spanish and Portuguese in the 16th century had shipped hundreds of thousands of slaves from Africa to their plantations and mines in Mexico and South America. However, English colonists lacked access to this trade and, without a reliable indigenous workforce, they initially sourced the labour tobacco demanded through a system of indenturing, organized through the Virginia Company. However, the stable, hierarchical model of society on the Chesapeake it upheld was based on a utopian model of English rural life that proved unworkable.

The indentured labour system that was established saw workers arriving from different parts of the British Isles for periods of between four and seven years. After the servant had repaid the cost of his passage, he was in principle free to become a planter himself. Between 1630 and 1680 some 75,000 British emigrants came to the Chesapeake region, most of them poor unskilled youths. Many died in the first few years of their service, but those that succeeded frequently rented or purchased their own land to set up as small planters themselves. Conflict between the established planters and the newly freed servants was almost inevitable.[72] Freed servants and tenants were amongst the most vigorous supporters of Nathaniel Bacon's violent rebellion of 1676 against the then governor's authority and supposedly 'soft' policy against the Indians. "The social mobility of ex-servants, along with their short life span, led to a feverish search for profits that left little time for the imposition of social control upon servants, poor people, and women similar to that practiced by gentlemen and patriarchal husbands in England".[73] This indentured labour pool, the mainstay of the early development of commercial cultivation in the Chesapeake and elsewhere, dwindled during the latter decades of the 17th century.[74] Yet, although indentured migration rates from England started to fall, only then, with a decline in the desperate rates of mortality, did population levels start to rise – from an estimated 13,000 settlers in Virginia in 1625 to 63,000 by 1700.[75]

The demise of the home-grown

The increasing strength of Virginia as a colony founded on tobacco, supported by a company modelled on the EIC, had its consequences back in the United Kingdom. One of the strengths of a species like *N. tabacum* is its ability to grow in a diverse range of environments.[76] In 1615, an instructional book *An Advice how to plant Tobacco in England...with the Danger of the Spanish Tobacco* was published in London by someone with the initials 'C.T.' Whoever they were, C.T. clearly had first-hand knowledge of growing and curing tobacco in the West Indies:

> The naturall colour of Tobacco is a deepe yellow or a light tawnie: and when the Indians themselves sold it us for Knives, Hatchets, Beads, Belles, and like merchandise, it had no other complexion, as all the

Tobacco this day hath...where we buy it from the naturall people; and all these sorts are cleane, and so is that of St. Domingo, where the Spaniards have not yet learned the Art of Sophistication.

Note the use of the word "naturall" to describe the Indians. By "learned" in this context, C.T. means 'taught', and "Sophistication", as we saw in *The Alchemist* (Chapter 2), is the addition of supplements to 'sophisticate' tobacco. C.T. clearly thought little of Spanish efforts to enhance the product in this way:

[their] Tobacco is noynted and slubbered over with a kind of iuyce, or syrope made of Saltwater, of the dregges or filth of Sugar, called Malasses, of blacke honey, Guiana pepper, and leeze of Wine...This they doe to give it colour and glosse, to make it the more merchantable.

By the time the first large-scale cultivation of tobacco in England had been established in the Vale of Tewkesbury in Gloucestershire (first recorded in 1619), the influence of the Virginia Company and the extraordinary about-turn of James I meant tobacco had become vitally important to the success of both the nation's colonial interests and its tax revenues. Attempting to control imports by sea was easier, for revenue purposes, than trying to control what was grown and transported on land. Interestingly, many of the people who got into the business of tobacco cultivation in England – or at least, who tried to do so – also had connections with Virginian tobacco. One of the families involved, the Tracys, had links with the Virginia Company through a younger scion, William. He had actively recruited men for the Virginia plantation, and sailed to Virginia himself with his wife and two children in 1620 where he became a member of the Council of Estate.

Another Gloucestershire venture was started by a partnership of two Londoners, John Stratford and Henry Somerscales. Somerscales appears to have done the planting and curing, while Stratford, a London merchant exploiting his county connections, transported the crop to the capital for sale. Stratford offered landowning gentlemen and yeomanry four-year, bonded, high-rent leases for the privilege of growing such a profitable crop. However the success of the enterprise was stymied when, as a result of successful petitioning by the Virginia Company, the government's Privy Council imposed a ban on English tobacco cultivation. Stratford tried to change the terms of his leasing agreements. One of his leases, John Ligon, had been reluctantly persuaded by a tenant, Ralph Wood, to allow ten acres of his land near Cheltenham to be used for tobacco. Ligon's reluctance was due to the land being good pasture, near to the farmhouse and with little other grazing nearby. A substantial orchard also needed felling to make way for the new crop. However, the rent offered – £80 per year, compared to £13 paid him by Wood – was persuasive. After a successful 1619 harvest, however, the prohibition on further cultivation meant Stratford was only able to plant barley on the land, after which he abandoned the project. This left Ligon with a weed-infested plot which his tenant was only willing to carry on renting for £6.10s. per annum.

England was unique in the way mercantile interests influenced government: "in no other European country did merchants and planters manage to secure a total prohibition on domestic cultivation for the sake of colonial trade".[77] But there was also an air of wild speculation about the merchant-landlord-cultivator triumvirates reminiscent of the 'tulipmania' that overtook Holland at about the same time.[78] The usual profit from an early 17th century farm in a reasonable farming area has been estimated at around 10s. an acre. The profit on an acre of tobacco was potentially between £26.9s. and £100, depending on the quality of the crop. Stratford was bankrupted by the government's actions.

The Privy Council's edict was only intermittently enforced, however. Tobacco cultivation spread to Worcestershire, Wiltshire, Jersey, Guernsey and Monmouthshire. The English Civil War from 1642 to 1651 made governance arrangements problematic, and thus gave growers a decade of relative peace from prosecution and, we may assume, profitable harvests. However, in 1652, Oliver Cromwell's Council of State passed a new Act which again banned tobacco cultivation. Following growers' protests, a new law was passed in 1653 which allowed them to continue growing the crop as long as they paid excise duty on it. This displeased the Virginia merchants who pressed for the original Act to be reinstated and enforced, arguing that tobacco growing was harmful to local agriculture. By this stage, tobacco had spread to 14 English and Welsh counties and there was little enthusiasm for carrying out the terms of the Act. Many of the Justices of the Peace (JPs) who would be expected to carry out the government's laws were themselves landlords involved in tobacco growing.

One disconsolate soldier, expected to take responsibility for destroying tobacco around Cheltenham in 1658, wrote that he was stationed without a superior to turn to for advice, a cornet "who would not act", and JPs around who "refuse to give warrant for the peace and. . .[are] rather a hindrance than always helpful". Many of the horsemen from the county, he complained, were "dealers and planters" themselves, and so had to be hand-picked in consequence". In order to spread the risks of tobacco growing in these precarious circumstances, sharecropping arrangements were common, with tenants allowing labourers to do the intensive work of planting and crop husbandry to bring the crop to fruition, in exchange for half the tobacco produced. It was thus the poorest men and women, scraping a living by growing tobacco, who frequently ended up intimidated and their crops destroyed by the measures. Not until William of Orange assumed presidency of the Privy Council in 1688 was the campaign against tobacco growing quietly dropped. "William III came from a country [Holland] where tobacco supported many small peasants, and where, far from being an illegal crop, it was the basis of a modest but flourishing industry".[79]

Conclusion

This chapter has demonstrated some of the resistances, rocks, and eddies impeding tobacco's flow across the emergent supply chains that, with relative peace between European nations, were starting to span the globe at the beginning of the 17th century. The published arguments against tobacco were by turn medical, moralistic or (frankly) racist. James I incorporates all three in his famous *Counterblaste*. The strength of resistance to tobacco amongst rulers around the world indicates something which was a perceived threat to their 'divine right' or spiritual power. However, the compromises demanded in order to realize tobacco's potential as a revenue source meant such qualms had to be put to one side. Tobacco, through its success in supporting the early settlers in and around Jamestown, Virginia, became intrinsic to the development of an English 'common-wealth', even when this meant the suppression of cultivation in England itself. There was more to tobacco's success than its contribution to tax and business revenues, however. Its 'enchantment' of the world also took place at physiological, cognitive and relational levels. These will be the subject of the next chapter.

Notes

1 Goodman (1993: 13).
2 Charlton (2005: 103).
3 Philaretes (1602).
4 Laufer (1924: 22).
5 Others followed James' lead in disparaging the plant – too many to elucidate here. In 1606, for example, Warner wrote disparagingly of "An Indian weede, That feum'd away more wealth than would a many thousands feed".
6 Laufer (1924: 26).
7 Ibid. (65, 26, 29-30).
8 Davison et al. (1992).
9 Ibid. (682).
10 Hughes (2003: 133).
11 Bednarz (2004). Reid (2014: 2) argues that "these days, few bona fide early modernists would lend much credence to the idea that this clandestine, Elizabethan coterie once existed, nor would they regard this belief as much more than a curiosity in the history of twentieth-century scholarship – an academic flash in the pan that, in retrospect, may have been separated by only the narrowest of margins from the realm of crackpot theory".
12 Parsons (1592: 18).
13 Deacon (1616: 81-2; 174-6).
14 Knapp (1988: 58n. 53).
15 Flynn (1995: 197n. 15).
16 Hoby (1613: 39).
17 Dobson and Wells (2001: 480-1).
18 Harley (1993: 35).
19 The weed is only "black"' in the 1st Folio Edition. Thereafter no colour is given.
20 Kezar (2003: 31) claims Othello is "all about tobacco", although this statement is qualified by his weasel words, "I sponsor the reading that, however, untenable,

must be right. Doing so, I promote a reading that, however tenable, must be wrong". He does, however, point out how the question "what is the matter?" appears over twenty times in the play, and suggests this might be interpreted as oblique references to tobacco as 'thing' as much as to the desire and jealousy that is the protagonist's downfall.

21 As Oscar Wilde claimed at his trial in 1894.
22 Quoted in Hill (1975: 206). Note the strong sense of both binary distinction and conjoinment in this statement.
23 Hill (1975: 198). The Ranters' greeting "fellow creature" could be applied not only to mankind but the whole of creation.
24 Hill (1975: 201). Fox was displeased when a large company of Ranters came to see him in prison in 1655. "A good deal of drink and tobacco was consumed...and some familiar ranter tenets were vented" (ibid., 213)
25 These quotes are taken from Hill (1975: 15 and 14).
26 Hill (1975: 199). The additional quote is from Maurice, H. (1695) *An Impartial Account of Mr John Mason of Water Stratford*: 52.
27 Hill (1975: 200).
28 Ibid. (201-2).
29 Marston ([1599]/2005: 79-80).
30 Ibid. (113).
31 Ibid. (151).
32 Anon. (1675: 1).
33 Harley (1993: 45-6).
34 He expanded membership of the Privy Council from 12 to 35, for example (Travers 2003: 18).
35 Asch (2014: 46).
36 Proctor (1997: 437).
37 Robins (2006).
38 See Gokhale (1974).
39 Matthee (2004: 58).
40 Matthee (2005: 127-8).
41 Grehan (2006: 1362).
42 The preacher's name was Mehmed Efendi Kadizade.
43 Grehan (2006: 1363).
44 Similar anxieties existed in England – see Cowan (2005).
45 The Company of Merchant Adventurers to New Lands (a shortened version of a much longer full name) was the first colonial joint stock company, established in London in 1551. It sought a north-east passage to China beyond the North Cape of Scandinavia, in order to avoid Portuguese and Spanish maritime activities in southern waters. Unfortunately the leader of the company's first expedition in 1553 had no previous maritime or navigational experience. Russian fishermen discovered his vessel, full of frozen corpses, at the mouth of the Varzina River near present-day Murmansk the following spring. Another company ship reached a harbour near present-day Arkhangelsk from where the captain made the 1000 km journey to Moscow. The then Czar, Ivan IV, was looking for an alternative route to the Black Sea and was willing to give trading privileges to the English. However the Dutch were also in search of new lands and trading routes. Willem Barents discovered Spitsbergen (now called Svalbard) in 1596 and claimed the waters south of the islands on behalf of New Holland. Traders found themselves in constant conflict with the Dutch and were never able to make a success of the enterprise.
46 Romaniello (2007: 915).

47 Cited in Romaniello (2007: 920).
48 Hakluyt (1599-1600) cited in Clucas (2009: 18).
49 It has come to be known as "The Lost Colony" – see Miller (2000).
50 Goodman (1993: 134).
51 Reported in Morgan (1975: 73).
52 Coates (2007: 81).
53 Goodman (1993: 135-6).
54 Ibid. (135).
55 Quoted in Knapp (1992: 12).
56 Robert (1949: 15).
57 Davies (1974: 147).
58 Ransome (1991).
59 Davies (1974: 144).
60 Linton (1998: 127). This was somewhat ironic considering the monarch after whom the Jamestown settlement was named.
61 Elliott (2007a: 556).
62 McCusker and Menard (1985: 118-9).
63 In his sermon for the Virginia Company preached at St Paul's Cathedral in November 1622, Donne counselled against retribution towards the Indians, arguing it was as important to ask how many of them had been converted to Christianity as what "Trees, or druggs, or Dyes" a Ship coming into harbour might have brought (quoted in Johnson 1947: 135). Doubtless he would also have had a personal interest in the tobacco on board. Johnson gives more detail on this sermon, and Donne's connections to the Virginia Company.
64 Had his application been successful, he would probably have sailed with Sir Thomas Gates that year and suffered a shipwreck in the Bermudas (which became the basis for Shakespeare's *The Tempest*) – another lucky deliverance for Donne (Hadfield 2006: 49).
65 Quoted in Armstrong (2007: Ch. 1).
66 Johnson (1947).
67 Breen (1973: 452).
68 Kulikoff (1986: 32).
69 Goodman (1993: 153).
70 Crosby (2003).
71 Quoted in Kulikoff (1986: 30).
72 Kulikoff (1986: 35).
73 Ibid. (37).
74 Various explanations have been discussed. One was the severe depression in the tobacco economy between the 1680s and 1715, when prices dipped below 1d. per £1. The only way planters could make a profit was by increasing output per hand, which is something it was easier to make slaves do than reluctant, indentured servants.
75 Goodman (1993: 169).
76 Today some may be surprised to learn that tobacco is successfully grown in Poland and Southern Ontario, Canada, for example – areas with seasons very different to those of tropical Amazonia!
77 Thirsk (1974).
78 On tulipmania see, for example, Dash (2000) and Goldgar (2007).
79 Thirsk (1974: 281).

Chapter 4

Tobacco and Enlightenment

Introduction: explaining the 'Enlightenment'

This chapter argues that the arrival of tobacco on European shores and the emergence of the philosophical and cultural epoch known as the 'Enlightenment' may be more than just coincidental. Enlightenment is a word first recorded in the English language in 1621, about the same period that tobacco was making substantial inroads into European life. Its first use, however, had a very ecclesiastical meaning, suggesting that the Spirit [of God] was necessary to 'enlighten' God's Word [the Bible], otherwise it "is as good Seede sowne on untilled ground". Yet the term subsequently came to designate something much less ecclesiastical, a philosophy "which typically emphasized freedom of thought and action without reference to religious and other traditional authority".[1] It was matched by comparable names in different countries – *Lumièrie* (France), *Ilustración* (Spain), *Illuminismo* (Italy), *Aufklärung* (Germany). These synonymous words point to its pan-European quality as well as the potential for there to be national differences and competing schools of thought within it. Yet Enlightenment is a term which, although it still retains respect and caché in some Eastern religions, in the west "is a phrase that now appears mostly in contexts of condemnation or contempt".[2] It is also, for some, a contentious term when applied to world history.

Philosophers and historians spend much time debating the existence, size, shape and extent of an epoch called the Enlightenment, as well as its sources and precursors.[3] Academics have tended to focus on elements salient to their own disciplinary interests when seeking to explain what was happening and why during the period. Thus philosophers argue for intellectual factors (the 'great-book, great-man' view of history) while literary scholars argue for the development of print media (perhaps as a proxy for 'knowledge'?). Historians and sociologists argue for political, economic and social changes being the crux of the matter, while anthropologists look to cultural changes (in some ways, an amalgam of all the above arguments) in their explanations. In this chapter I suggest that the biotic, specifically the arrival and circulation of tobacco, offers a further explanatory dimension and is an element overlooked in previous analyses.

In proposing this, I am not suggesting that other explanations are wrong or misguided. It is easy to criticize any of the explanatory arguments for the Enlightenment (including my own) when they are made in isolation. We can justifiably criticize the 'great-book, great-man' view of the Enlightenment, the 'greats' in this case being primarily white literati or *philosophes*, moulded by historians into a mythological 'intellectual history' divorced from the social, political and economic circumstances of their day.[4] Another much derided intellectual approach charts the development of Enlightenment thought in terms of a history of ideas, one idea (rather than men or their books) affecting the development of others in a similarly decontextualized bubble. In attempting to swing the pendulum back towards greater inclusion of socio-economic and political contexts in any explanation of the origins and development of Enlightenment thought, the rediscovery of pre-Christian antiquity and the tensions that developed between Catholic and Protestant forms of Christianity (which found expression through Martin Luther in 1517 but which had abated somewhat by the latter half of the 17th century) have been identified as key drivers.[5] Other factors seen as causative include the socio-cultural changes engendered by the cessation of many of the military operations that had been draining of manpower and Treasury coffers through-out 16th and early 17th century Europe, and the increased opportunities for trade which followed. The rise of the natural sciences was also significant, based on careful observation and mathematical reasoning rather than rever-ence for old tomes and classical traditions, and an increasing sense that the everyday world and the lives and activities of ordinary people were as important as those of priests and princes.[6] Other historians lay claim to what they call an 'anthropology' of the Enlightenment, arguing for the importance of the development of 'cultural perspective' in its formation.[7]

Use of the word 'perspective' is interesting given the 'cosmological perspectivism' we encountered in Amerindian thought in Chapter 1 – the ability to see things from another person, creature or thing's point of view – and the possible links between perspectivism such as this and the shamanic use of tobacco. The Renaissance is commonly seen as the age of oceanic discovery and the development of artistic perspective. For Larry Wolff, the Enlightenment was when the implications of all this voyaging – what he calls a 'cultural perspective' derived from a growing sense of global diversity, the need to re-interpret the nature of human societies, and of cultural difference – became manifest. For Wolff, 'cultural perspective' is epitomized in Jonathan Swift's *Gulliver's Travels* with its comparison of the Houyhnhnm horses (their behaviour "so orderly and rational, so acute and judicious, that I at last concluded, they must needs be magicians, who had thus metamorphosed themselves upon some design") and the savage Yahoos. Gulliver considered his own family, friends, countrymen and race were "Yahoos in shape and disposition, [but] perhaps a little more civilized". So smelly were the Yahoos, indeed, that Gulliver could only tolerate them by keeping his "nose well stopped with rue, or sometimes with tobacco". In these ways, "the experience of travel in the Age of Enlightenment would increasingly become the stimulus to question cultural presumptions, and to place the traveler's own native customs and satisfactions – whether narrowly English or more broadly European – in the critical context of multiple and various cultures".[8] Wolff sees such a perspectival shift as fundamental to an increased sense of self-consciousness generated by the growing awareness of an 'us' and 'them' (transmogrified into the heightened sense, perhaps, of 'self' and 'other'). Might tobacco, in addition to stopping up the nose as in Gulliver's example, have contributed more to the development of this sense of individualism and the binary oppositions that flow from it?

For Tim Ingold, books (particularly the translation of the scriptures into English and other languages) were a crucial factor. He compares the European Medieval concept of the book of the universe or nature with what happened in the post-reformation era with the translation of the scriptures. Those hearing the *voces paginarum* (voices of the pages) in Medieval times are said to have felt nature was speaking to them directly as monks read aloud. Post-reformation, scripture shifted from something figurative or allegorical to "an authoritative record of historical truth", with a much more rigorous defence accorded the meanings of individual words. Nature, in this scheme, became a closed book, one "whose secrets could be prised out ['de-scribed'] only through rigorous investigation".[9] Through this change, Ingold argues, facts became separated from values, and nature from human society. Information took pride of place over wisdom, and suddenly dragons, previously living beings like any other, became a figment of the imagination rather than something that might potentially be experienced 'in real life'.

Francis Bacon, in the 1620s, was one of the new breed of philosopher-scientists whose arguments exemplify the trend towards the bifurcation of 'facts' and 'values', 'reality' and 'fantasy'. Bacon criticized 'traditional' modes of knowledge because of their tendency to continually mix up "the reality of the world with its configurations in the minds of men".[10] The 'cracks and deformities' of the mind, he argued, prevented it reflecting 'the genuine ray of things'. The only option, in Bacon's view, was to 'dissect the nature of this very world itself' by seeking out the facts about everything. For 20th century ecofeminist and science historian Carolyn Merchant, this process of closing the book on Nature also turned it from a feminine entity commanding respect into a feminine object ripe for violation and exploitation. This new outlook "sanctioned the domination [by men] of both nature and women". Merchant sees this shift in perspective as both reflected in and driven by the change from organic to mechanistic metaphors in 17th century science,[11] particularly criticizing Bacon for his language of sexual aggression, torture and inquisition, while for Ingold, "Bacon's injunction, which modern science has taken to its heart, has had fateful consequences for human life and habitation, cutting the imagination adrift from its earthly mooring and leaving it to float like a mirage above the road we tread in our material life. With our hopes and dreams suffused in the ether of illusion, life itself appears diminished".[12]

Jonathan Israel is the historian par excellence who has shifted the pendulum back towards the middle ground, seeing socio-political and economic context and Enlightenment ideas themselves in a two-way relationship that drives change.[13] In this he is following early Marx, who "before arriving at his more dogmatic formulations of dialectical materialism", admitted "it is by no means obvious why a thoroughgoing materialist and naturalist account of the world should be unable to accommodate a balanced interaction, or two-way traffic, between physical reality and human consciousness".[14] Israel argues for the need to disaggregate the Enlightenment, presenting it not as a single entity (as in "there were many *philosophes* in the eighteenth century, but there was only one Enlightenment", as one major work has claimed)[15] but recognizing it as comprising at least two major and in many respects antagonistic strands of thought – one moderate, one radical.[16]

For Israel, moderate and radical strands of Enlightenment philosophy both sought an "amelioration of the state of mankind",[17] and accepted that "all Enlightenment, by definition, is closely linked to revolution".[18] However the radical wing sought to establish reason alone as the supreme value in human life, while more moderate – some would say conservative – Enlightenment philosophers sought to reconcile reason with faith and tradition.[19] Radical thinkers differed over the contentious issue of whether a critique of religion was required as well as law and politics in order to establish the supremacy of reason. Outram talks darkly about the potential for "contradiction between unrestricted inquiry and the need to assure stability in state and society".[20] In some circles the somewhat paradoxical notion of 'Enlightened absolutism', in which rulers govern according to Enlightened ideas, held sway.

I am not seeking to reconcile these competing arguments and different viewpoints about where the Enlightenment originates, and whether there was one Enlightenment or many. Rather, I am arguing for the inclusion of what is in many ways a much more mundane but in my view significant 'game changer' in the intellectual and socio-political changes taking place in European society during this time, namely the ingress of tobacco. For along with the factors outlined above, it seems to me remarkable that no-one, to the best of my knowledge, has commented on the arrival and increasingly prodigious quantities of tobacco consumed across Europe from the start of the 16th century onwards. This presence, I argue, could have been just as mutually constitutive of the intellectual and socio-cultural foment of the period as the exposure to people 'from other lands', the printing press, religious reform or urban life. Tobacco, I will argue, has had profound influences worldwide, not only on health, well-being and the economy, but also on sociality and cognition. I shall end by suggesting a conspiratorial element in human-tobacco relations, one that the Enlightenment itself helped to engender, and one which I suggest needs overturning or reformulating in order to establish what might be called a 'post-Enlightenment' view of tobacco.

Enlightened aristocracy?

Let us move now to the situation in Europe in the 17th century where, I shall argue, the increasing consumption of narcotic and intoxicant tobacco must have had at least some influence on human experience and intellectual thought. Unlike James I, some members of the European aristocracy, both male and female, developed more positive attitudes to the use of tobacco, with addiction probably a powerful motivating force. Two examples of changing attitudes, both of them linked to different aspects of Enlightenment philosophies, are demonstrated in the courts of Catherine, Duchess of Savoy and of Peter the Great of Russia.

In 1650, a ballet was performed at the court of Catherine, the Duchess of Savoy in Turin, on the occasion of the marriage of Adelaide, sister of the Duke Carlo Emanuele II, to Prince Ferdinand of Bavaria. The subject of the ballet, *Il Tabacco*, was somewhat unusual for its composer, Filippo d'Agliè, since he more usually dealt in Greek mythology or pastorals. Rather than tobacco being regarded as an object of fun (as it was in Tomkis' play *Lingua* in Chapter 2), in d'Agliè's ballet a group of townspeople dressed in native costumes danced and sang their thanks to God for having given humanity such a wondrous plant. In the second act, another troupe performed, dressed in costumes from all over the world. In a pageant that a spectator today might find strangely reminiscent of Disney's *It's a Small World After All*, representatives of all the world's cultures gathered together and set off for a 'School for Smoking' where, in marked contrast to James I's views on 'beastly Indians', they asked the Indians to instruct them in tobacco's virtues.[21]

The trials and tribulations faced by the English Muscovy Company in its efforts to sell tobacco legally in Russia (Chapter 3) only ended with the accession of Tsar Peter the Great (1672–1725) as sole ruler in 1696.[22] Peter the Great saw himself as a true child of the Enlightenment, a tireless reformer who attempted to establish social and political systems that were western, scientific and secular. In contrast with the trials and tribulations the English Muscovy Company had faced in its efforts to sell tobacco legally in Russia over the preceding century and a half, the year after his accession Peter signed an agreement with William III of England permitting the importation and sale of tobacco, in lieu of payment for a naval yacht.[23]

Peter was a true aficionado. Snuff was coming into vogue in aristocratic circles (see Chapter 5) and so the tsar had his waistcoat pockets made sufficiently big to hold the quantities of snuff he considered worthy of a great man, and began a collection of snuff boxes.[24] A Hapsburg Secretary to Muscovy in 1698-99 reported an extraordinary ritual inversion of which Christopher Marlowe or the radical Ranters (Chapter 3) would have been proud, involving an Orthodox ceremony being turned into a celebration of Bacchus rather than the Christian God. As well as wine, beer and spirits, revellers "carried great dishes of dried tobacco leaves, with which, when ignited, they went to the remotest corners of the palace, exhaling those most delectable odors and most pleasant incense to Bacchus from their smutty jaws". Two tobacco pipes set crosswise "served the scenic bishop to confirm the rites of consecration".[25]

However, Peter was out of step with wider public opinion. The 'Old Believers' were a sect who had rejected a reform of Orthodox Church rituals in the 1660s, associating them with "Greek" (Orthodox) innovations. They denounced Peter's broader reform efforts as the work of an anti-Christ using tobacco as one of his weapons against the faithful. In one legend they propagated, tobacco was an ancient evil associated with Jezebel's daughter. When she rejected an opportunity to repent, God cast her down into the earth

> with the Devil in her belly and the cesspool of filth in her bosom. And then it rained over her grave, and on the very same spot the dirt spewed a weed. The Greeks, in compliance with the Devil's plan, will adopt this weed and plant it in their gardens, and call it "tobacco".[26]

For these and other reasons, only 5,500 of the agreed 8,000 hogsheads (large barrels) were imported during the first two years of the contract between Muscovy and William III. Twenty years later, availability of tobacco in the Russian provinces continued to be a problem for those in need of it. An Ottoman envoy, Nişli Mehmed Ağa, on a visit to Russia in 1722, described meeting Cossacks on the way to Moscow who begged him for tobacco. He used the occasion to comment on how in the Sultan's lands, unlike Russia, everything was available and how if his party had not shipped their provisions in advance, they would have had nothing left to be desired.[27]

Soaring up

Despite the handicaps to onward trade with Muscovy, as we saw in Chapter 3, exports of tobacco to England from Virginia were skyrocketing. Much of this increase was due to onward exportation to other European countries, for which England acted as an entrepôt. Domestic demand was also rising. At the turn of the century, the average price of Spanish American tobacco sold in London was about £1.10s. per pound weight (and labourers' wages were about 8d. per day). However, as production and supply of cheaper Virginia tobacco grew (along with some local cultivation during the disruption of the English Civil War – Chapter 3), consumption in its turn began to go up around 1640. By 1700 it is estimated that 26 million pounds of tobacco were being imported into England every year. About 60 per cent of this was still re-exported to other parts of Europe, including Russia by this time (above).

However, the 10.4 million pounds remaining still meant a generous one-and-a-half pounds weight of tobacco per inhabitant per year – enough for 25 per cent of the adult population to enjoy a pipe and a half each day.[28] The Dutch were consuming tobacco in similar proportions.[29]

Modes of consumption were likely to have been very different to the accustomed ways tobacco is used recreationally in most parts of the world today. One contemporary, but typical, description of tobacco as a product whose "divine breath…doth distill eloquence and oracle upon the tongue",[30] may seem strange to 21st century sensibilities. Simon Schama writes of the Dutch artist Adriaen Brouwer who, in the 1620s and 1630s,

> took great care to record the expressions of deep inhalation or drowsy puffing peculiar to the serious pipe smoker. Some of their figures appear so stunned and insensate with smoke that it has been argued – speculatively – that their tobacco might have been spiked with some sort of opiate or narcotic.[31]

However, I don't think that speculation needs to dwell on adulterants as the source of people's dazed faces. The amount of tobacco being consumed was enough to generate the same kind of narcotic intoxication as that experienced by shamanic practitioners in lowland South America with the heavy ingestion of *N. tabacum* to this day. An amusing and somewhat moralistic account of 'Sam Scot's Smoking Club' in mid-18th century London describes its members – a linen draper turned dancing-master, a city musician, an engraver and a Scottish writer – as a group that "had acquired such an expeditious Way of consuming a Pipe of Tobacco, that when they were met together, they would make no more of smoking a Pound in an hour".[32] Accepting the probability of some humorous hyperbole, this is tobacco consumption of shamanic proportions. The account goes on to explain how, due to the prodigious amounts of smoke they produced ("like a Yarmouth herring-house"), the group was frequently forced to alter the venue of their meetings, shifting between victuallers, alehouses, and coffee shops because of the complaints about the effects of their smoking by other customers.

Figures 4.1 and 4.2 were both etched and engraved in the same year (1794). Figure 4.1 could well be a portrayal of Sam Scot's club. Figure 4.2 makes the point about how quiet the environment is. Cowan quotes a Russian historian who visited England in 1790:

> I have dropped into a number of coffeehouses only to find twenty or thirty men sitting around in deep silence, reading newspapers, and drinking port. You are lucky if, in the course of ten minutes, you hear three words. And what are they? "Your health, gentlemen!"

Figure 4.2 implies that many of the customers the visitor encountered may well have been stupefied by tobacco!

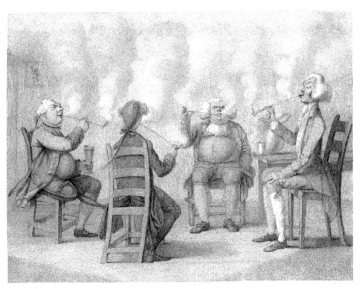

A SMOKING CLUB.

Fig. 4.1 'A smoking club'

Source: Courtesy of the Wellcome Collection

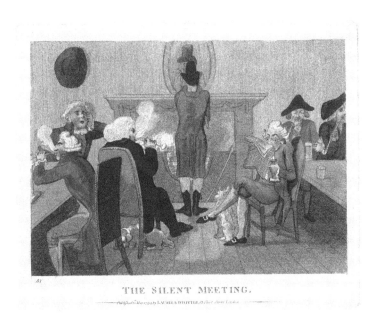

THE SILENT MEETING.

Fig. 4.2 'The silent meeting'

Source: Courtesy of The Lewis Walpole Library, Yale University

Tobacco and imagination

Taverns and alehouses had long been places of conviviality across Europe, and the addition of tobacco to these venues, as reflected in the play *Wine, Beere, Ale and Tobacco* (Chapter 2), helped sustain their bacchanalian traditions. Withington, writing in relation to early modern English society (just prior to the Enlightenment) detects a connection between the use of intoxicants (such as beer, wine and tobacco), the development of the notion of good fellowship and company, and the growth of 'societies' or clubs for English gentlemen within which the main activity was consuming these intoxicants.[33] In such gatherings men of discretion, good judgement, and wit benefitted from the ways in which alcohol and tobacco might stimulate the 'fancy'. Withington argues, with reference to the philosopher Thomas Hobbes, that the exercise of "wit" was dialectical – involving the "constant negotiation between fancy and the passions on the one hand and judgement and discretion on the other, with individuals perpetually poised between their thoughts, feelings and imaginings and their understanding of the civil proprieties of any given society".[34] Ingold's "imagination cut adrift" rings very true in such accounts, except that, rather than opposed, "fancy and the passions" are seen as balanced with "judgement and discretion" in the production of "wit".

The creative imagination, argues John Engell, was the most important and powerful notion to develop in the 18th century. "The pre-1600 world was more interested in man's relationship to external nature and to God than it was in internal processes of thought and feeling that sustain a comprehensive and aesthetic view of the world", he writes.[35] According to him, only in the 17th century did a tradition of empirical psychology become established which started to ask questions and find out about the formation of passions, thoughts, perceptions and mental knowledge. Some would challenge such dichotomizing of people's cognitive and intellectual capacities by era in this way (not all would agree with Ingold that there was a 16th and early 17th century rupture between the real world and our imagination of it, for example). One anthropologist goes so far as to claim "the specifically human capacity for imagination" is a human cognitive universal.[36] However, might there have been shift in the qualities of the imagination around this time? If so, what were the qualities of this shift? And was it more than coincidence that it correlated with the arrival of tobacco in large quantities through ports across Europe? What were the consequences of this? Does the tobacco ideology of Amerindian societies explored in Chapter 1 – tobacco constitutes persons, tobacco changes perspectives and tobacco generates dualisms – resonate with Euro-American activities and behaviours associated with tobacco?

Tobacco and curiosity

Tobacco was not only consumed in taverns, however. As the 17th and 18th centuries progressed, coffee houses developed across Europe to rival the tavern as meeting places.[37] The first in Britain opened in Oxford in 1650, and others followed soon after, becoming known as the 'Penny Universities' from their penny admission charge. Coffee houses offered a place for gentlemen to congregate, to read, as well as learn from and to debate with each other. They were associated with the 'virtuosi', a social category to rival the 'gallants' and 'guls' but composed of men at the margins of the social elite who "shared a distinct sensibility, a set of attitudes, habits, and intellectual preferences that, unlike the gallants, they labelled 'curiosity' rather than 'dandyism'".[38]

According to Cowan, "no other country took to coffee drinking with quite the same intensity that Britain did in the seventeenth century. London's coffeehouses had no rival anywhere else in the world, save perhaps Istanbul. In 1700, Amsterdam could boast of only thirty-two coffeehouses, while London had at least several hundred".[39] Paris was not far behind – its first coffee shop (Café Procope) opened in 1686 and by the 1720s there were 400 of them. "Along with its drinks, the coffeehouses offered a place to smoke tobacco...Judging by the presence of pipes in nearly every representation of the early coffeehouses, smoking was a natural complement to drinking coffee".[40] The coffeehouses, more than the taverns and alehouses, were seen as places of learning and discourse about affairs of the day. They were also "the incubators of capitalism and modern politics", places where "commercial transactions took place and news was collected and distributed".[41] They were centres for debate, doubt and difference, fuelled also by the explosion of newspapers and magazines around the turn of the 18th century. As such, it is tempting to see them as Habermas' "public sphere" writ large, a domain marked – ideally – by a disregard of status and a will to inclusivity, where people could come together to discuss problems of the day and take collective political action to ameliorate them. Such spaces, Habermas argues, were crucial for the rational, critical and open discussion of ideas as the Enlightenment developed.[42] Thus coffee houses were "establishments that threatened the social and political order by potentially gathering together men of various social estates to share a common table, and what was worse, perhaps even common discourse over matters of state".[43] In the Middle East, where they had been in existence much longer, Matthee argues "coffee houses...played a similar 'modernizing' role in the sense that they contributed to the creation of a cultural public sphere separate from the mosque".[44]

Whether in Britain or the Middle East, coffee houses were not necessarily inclusive in their clientele, however, or disregarding of status. Women tended to be absent (except in serving roles), as were members of the 'lower orders'; indeed, for many Enlightenment thinkers the word 'public' was often used as a contrast to 'people'.[45] However, while predominantly bourgeois in their manifestations, coffee houses and taverns alike did offer greater opportunities for social interaction to take place, in some cases between people whose paths might otherwise not have crossed.[46] Tobacco was well ensconced in such locations. According to Macaulay's *History of England*, the coffee houses of the period "reeked with tobacco like a guard room; and strangers sometimes expressed their surprise that so many people should leave their own firesides to sit in the midst of eternal fog and stench".[47] This description is corroborated by John Gay's account of Will's coffee house in 1715 as choked in "clouds of Tobacco".[48]

Tobacco and sociability

Tobacco was also an important defining element in the new philosophical traditions that sought to facilitate the flourishing of individuals and societies. It is interesting that the word 'modern' – in relationship to a remote past rather than simply a present existence, only came into use in English and other north European languages towards the end of the 16th century and the beginning of the 17th, just at the time tobacco was taking hold.[49] Withington includes "modern" with "society", "company" and "commonwealth" in a list of "powerful ideas" that became popular in Britain in the 1570s and were incorporated into vernacular thought after that.[50] It was also a time when pleasure became an acceptable aim in life rather than a vice. Tobacco was central in the emergence of both notions of sociability and pleasure.

Porter talks of British pragmatism embodying "a *philosophy* of expediency, a dedication to the art, science and duty of living well in the here and now".[51] He goes on, "to be enlightened, a gentleman had to be sociable, or in Johnson's coinage 'clubbable'".[52] Israel is somewhat dismissive of writers who make too much of "new eighteenth century social spaces and practices, such as the salons, in generating Enlightenment ideas",[53] but not all the elements of the public sphere were necessarily as high-brow and exclusive as Israel contends. This was particularly the case in Scotland, from whence came the Scottish writer in Sam Scot's Smoking Club (above). In Scotland, arguably, the institutions of urban life were more egalitarian in their ethos than comparable institutions elsewhere in Europe. According to the Professor of Moral Philosophy at Glasgow University in the early 18th century, "ethical feelings and moral judgements could be cultivated through communication", while "men and women are not only naturally benevolent but also sociable beings who love nothing better than to convey their discoveries to one another and to create harmony through shared judgements and ideals".[54] His successors took a similar tack. David Hume commented on the extensive network of clubs and societies that were "every where formed". These were many and varied, made up of university professors, philosophers, scientists, church ministers, lawyers, writers, artists and merchants. According to Hume: "Both sexes meet in an easy and sociable manner; and the tempers of men, as well as their behaviour, refine apace...Thus *industry, knowledge*, and *humanity*, are linked together, by an indissoluble chain".[55]

In these groups, "polite and free conversation – the give and take of social exchange – produces a kind of knowledge in which feeling and logic constantly check one another".[56] Tobacco, I propose, was in no small measure integral to the development of the easy and sociable manners and the refinement of temperament of which Hume speaks, the balancing of Hobbes' "thoughts, feelings and imaginings" of the individual and the proprieties of the group on the other. Let us go on to look at the formation of the sense of the individual as a person with 'thoughts, feelings and imaginings' in more detail.

Tobacco and individuality

'Tobacco constitutes persons' applies to bodies in lowland South America (Chapter 1). Its reception may have done something similar with regard to minds in western Europe. The subjective and objective consciousness of a sense of 'self' has come to be known as individualism and, as with the imagination, there are major disagreements about what it is and when it developed. To suggest that individual consciousness developed during the 16th and 17th centuries is as contentious as Ingold's suggestion that the imagination was cut loose from the earthly moorings of material life during much the same time. For some scholars, "development of the individual" was a defining feature of the Renaissance,[57] the humanist trend away from Man cowering in God's shadow towards Man as a unique, all powerful entity.[58] From roots in classical and biblical times, as well as medieval mysticism, Steven Lukes considers the Renaissance, Reformation and Enlightenment periods the crucible for the development of the much wider range of political, religious, ethical and economic strands of individualism, as represented by post-1500 writers such as Hobbes, Luther and Calvin.[59] Riesman and colleagues see two periods in the development of modern individualism – its 15th and 16th century emergence from older 'tradition-directed' social forms, and an 'inner directed' stage of intense individualism which occurred between the 16th and 19th centuries.[60] Alan Macfarlane, meanwhile, puts the "origins of English individualism" way back to at least the 13th century.[61]

Clearly many different factors were in play in the development of individualistic thought processes and the question of where and when they operated is a difficult one to answer. All I propose here is further to my argument that the sudden and unexpected arrival of tobacco on the global scene during the 16th century was a pluripotential factor that has generally (and to my mind unjustifiably) been ignored. Its presence corresponds particularly closely with the advent and development of Riesman's 'inner directed' individualism, as well as with what John Martin distinguishes as the "performative or prudential" sense of selfhood in Renaissance Europe (Table 4.1).

Martin sees the three different types of selfhood he distinguishes – "communal" or "civic", "performative" or "prudential", and the "porous" or "open", as elements which individuals would have combined to different degrees during the era. They are "a far cry...from the autonomous and self-

Table 4.1 Martin's three basic types of selfhood in Renaissance Europe

Type	When?	Characteristics	Comments
Communal or civic	Throughout period	Group or collective identity, often based on family or lineage	Often based on family or lineage
Performative or prudential	Appeared quite suddenly in early 16th century	Individual as expressive, self-reflective subject	Increasingly conscious of need to assume different roles based on context
Porous or open	Late medieval and early modern	Body as porous, open to strong 'spiritual' forces from outside	Often through witchcraft or possession

Martin 2002: 210.

contained individualist…often assumed to have been a defining characteristic of the self in this era".[62] For him, then, "the idea that the Renaissance was the period in which individualism first emerged from its previously dormant state and became a defining aspect of the modern western world is dubious at best".[63] Martin points out the significant regional variations between and within countries in the production of what he calls 16th and 17th century "ego documents" in support of his claim. Such documents were particularly common in early modern England (as epitomized by the prolific diarist John Pepys) and the maritime provinces of the Dutch Republic (Friesland, Zeeland, Holland) – variations he describes as "baffling".[64] Yet, as we saw above, these were precisely the two areas of Europe where tobacco use was particularly heavy at this time!

One of the most fundamental aspects to the generation of individuality, it seems to me, is the development of a reflective sense of 'self' and 'non-self', something which the narcotic effect of tobacco is likely to encourage. The "individual as expressive, self-reflective subject" in Martin's formulation of the performative type of selfhood, and the shades of cosmological perspectivism in a self "increasingly conscious of need to assume different roles based on context" both seem highly likely to have been encouraged by the nicotian influence of tobacco. However, other dualisms apart from 'self' and 'non-self' appear to have become prominent in European thought at a time directly corresponding to tobacco's arrival. Withington highlights the "perennial tensions" (dualisms all) that came into play as the word "modern" sidled in with "society", "company" and "commonwealth", all of them at much the same time as tobacco became a significant feature of the European intoxicant landscape. They include tensions "between received wisdom and personal experience; between reform and resistance; between public service and private profit; between the common good and its political organization; between idealism and power; between the social and the natural worlds".[65]

In his view, "early moderns highlighted these polarities but never resolved them. Neither, I suspect, will we".[66] Latour argues that such distinctions – like the binary oppositions between "nature" and "culture", "religion" and "science", and "subject" and "object" – are creative fictions generated by the word "modern" (and its correlate, modernity) rather than mundane fact. He argues that the differentiation of the "moderns" as special and distinctive compared to people of other times or places is a fantasy of the moderns' own making.[67] Nothing really changed as a result of the Enlightenment, he says. He goes on to make the challenging observation that, as quickly as one tries to become "modern" by splitting the world into binaries such as "nature" and "culture", hybridity comes to reassert itself more strongly with nature coming to assume some of the attributes of culture, and culture developing attributes of nature. We shall see more evidence of this tendency in Chapter 5.

The greater sense of individual selfhood which tobacco helped to engender was mirrored by "a host of new disciplines of the flesh" such as dieting, deportment, exercise, greater hygiene levels and the avoidance of "self-pollution". [68] New beliefs about Man and his fate were also adjustments to socio-cultural change. England was fast urbanizing; "its expanding middle classes were possessed of some learning in their heads and money in their pockets, and its propertied élite was newly basking in civilized refinement".[69] The more peaceful conditions and greater levels of prosperity led to changes in beliefs and preoccupations concerning human temporalities. For some, the question of fundamental importance changed from the theological one of whether they would be saved (and go to heaven) to the more immediate concern of how they should be happy in the present world. All were not necessarily equal in the gardens of pleasure, however. "Élite drives for the reformation of popular culture equated the flesh and the plebs, and hence made the bodily connote all that was vulgar, disorderly, contagious and threatening".[70]

Tobacco and attention

The Metropolitan Museum of Art, New York, has a collection of Dutch brass tobacco boxes including one featuring the Scottish financier and speculator John Law (Fig. 4.3). Law was a forward-thinking economist, one of the first to develop the notion of establishing banks that could issue paper money. Unfortunately this led to the development of a series of rash speculative bubbles culminating in setting up a private bank that was permitted to issue paper money to fund French colonization of the Mississippi Valley.[71] The underside of the tobacco box is a satirical commentary on what became known as the "Wind Trade". "I walk with windmills" (i.e. "I am crazy", like Don Quixote) states an inscription next to Law's hat. A cat disappears into the heavens attached to balloons. "Wind is the beginning, wind is the end" reads the inscription at the bottom; a rebus (a mixture of words and symbols making up a hidden message) on the top and bottom of the box translates as "Take time and get to know the world". This can be interpreted two ways – either as a caution, since Law did not apparently take time to understand the workings of the speculative venture that ruined thousands (himself included), or as a meditative reflection on how to approach the contents of the tobacco box. I prefer the latter interpretation.

One of tobacco's main cognitive effects is to enhance attentiveness through acting as a stimulus barrier, screening extraneous and distracting stimuli from the tobacco user's awareness. Interestingly enough, the 18th century was marked by the development of a new poetic genre, one which has been labelled "the poetry of attention". It is marked by "a commitment in much of the period's poetry to teaching readers how to attend closely".[72] "This preoccupation is related to a more widely recognized impulse in eighteenth-century poetry to describe details and to proliferate objects...to focus on the minute, the miscellaneous, the detailed, the domestic".[73] This description could apply as much to the still-life paintings so popular in the Dutch Republic at the time (and equally, perhaps, reflecting a new attention to detail brought about by tobacco).

Do we also, perhaps, start to see evidence of cosmological perspectivism arising at this time too? According to Koehler, "less has been said about this poetry [the poetry of attention]'s renderings of corollary states of awareness. The fascination with ordinary, literal surroundings requires a particular state of mind: methodical, experimental attentiveness. How does the world look from a cat's vantage? What response does the ringing of a bell evoke from hungry sparrows?...In these poems the ordinary is defamiliarized; it is particularized according to the perception of one attentive viewer".[74] A cat's vantage point? The perspective of one attentive viewer? There are smoky whiffs here of the cosmological perspectivism characteristic of lowland South American life and thought. Does the presence of tobacco – a relative new-comer to the cognitive realm outside of the Americas in the 17th and 18th centuries – offer an explanation for the changes in literature and the arts in Europe at this time which, like the plant itself, have remained largely 'hidden in plain sight'?

For another example of what I mean, we can return to the English poet John Donne. We saw in previous chapters how his early poems display a studied aversion to tobacco and how, despite having been accused by an opponent of being a "Tobaccaean writer", he had various reasons for keeping quiet about his 'tobacco habit'. However, one can argue that his later writings display traces of the Amazonian perspectivism or 'other points of view' recognizable in the shamanic cosmologies and ideologies associated with tobacco's origins. These transfer adroitly into the fluid, heterogeneous per-spectivism of some of Donne's later work, through which he constantly

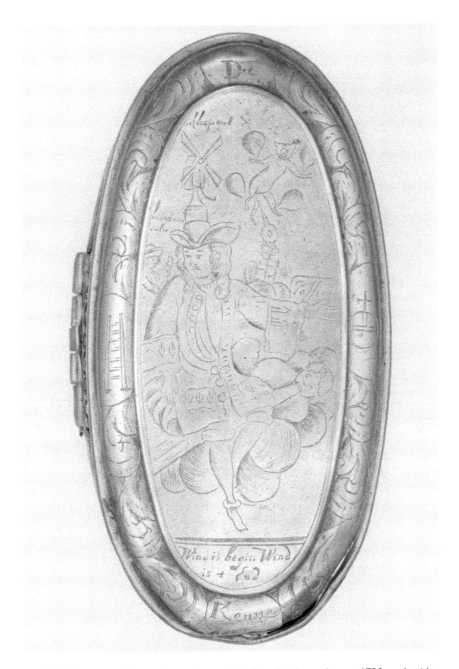

Fig. 4.3 'Take time and get to know the world' – Dutch tobacco box, c. 1720, underside
Source: The Metropolitan Museum of Art, New York

challenges his readers to perceive reality anew. We can also see evidence of a keen sense of the new individualism and the 'self-reflective subject' in various of his works. Could tobacco have had an influence in his penning of the following lines in his 'First Anniversary', for example?

> And new philosophy calls all in doubt
> . . .all coherence gone;
> All just supply, and all relation:
> Prince, subject, father, sone, are things forgot
> For every man alone thinks he hath got
> To be a phoenix, and that then can be
> None of that kind, of which he is, but he.[75]

More perspectival in their approach are the well-known lines of his 17th Meditation:

> No man is an iland, intire of it selfe; every man is a peece of the Continent, a part of the maine; if a clod bee washed away by the Sea, Europe is the lesse, as well as if a Promontorie were, as well as if a Mannor of thy friends or of thine owne were; any mans death diminishes me, because I am involved in Mankinde; And therefore never send to know for whom the bell tolls; It tolls for thee.

"No man is an island, entire of itself". The shift in viewpoint occasioned by the use of the word 'itself' rather than the expected 'himself' is remarkable. Then comes a 'microcosm'/'macrocosm' moment when we are told: "If a clod be washed away by the sea, Europe is the less, as well as if a promontory were, as well as if a manor of thy friend's [perspective shifting again] or of thine own were". Finally, "[a]ny man's death diminishes me, because I am involved in mankind, and therefore never send to know for whom the bell tolls; it tolls for thee". In the final sentence we move from another (dead) man to the speaker ("I") who is involved in all mankind; we then shift quickly to a vocative "never send", the bell, and back to the reader for whom it tolls (as well as the person who has died, to whom the speaker is linked).[76]

According to Brook,

> if Donne in 1623 was excited to discover that no person was an island, it was because, for the first time in human history, it was possible to realise that almost no one was. No longer was the world a series of locations so isolated from each other that something could happen in one and have absolutely no effect on what was going on in any other. The idea of a common humanity was emerging, and with it the possibility of a shared history.[77]

The notion of common humanity reflects the sociality which tobacco engenders – perhaps a growing sense of concern for others. However, the piece can also be read from the point of view of its style as well as its content. Knowing what we do about the shifting perspectives occasioned by tobacco, what I have suggested is a heightened awareness of, and attentiveness to, 'individual' and 'world'. Tobacco had a role in shaping the relationship between the two. Is it more than idle speculation to think that the style of the Meditation owes much to the arrival of tobacco on European shores and the new sense of spatial, temporal and psychic perspectivism it precipitated amongst users like Donne?

Literary sources help us appreciate tobacco's potential role in changing perspectives and helping users to see things, as in Amazonia, from the other's point of view. Tobacco also plays a part in aiding concentration and attention in the everyday here and now, as reflected in the poetry of attention and the development of still-life paintings in the 17th century Netherlands and the UK. From the metaphysical poetry of the 'tobaccaean' John Donne to the 20th century perspectivalism of T.S. Eliot, English poetry has smacked of nicotian influences, just as tobacco and its paraphernalia has been the subject (and sometimes the speaking object) of its prose. Not all writers have been as benignly disposed towards the outcome of these tobaccaean influences, however. Samuel Johnson found metaphysical poetry annoying for the way in which "the most heterogeneous ideas are yoked by violence together; nature and art are ransacked for illustrations, comparisons, and allusions; their learning instructs, and their subtlety surprises; but the reader commonly thinks his improvement dearly bought". Dryden was similarly critical of Donne's cerebralism (cognitive preoccupations heightened by the effects of tobacco, perhaps?). He criticized Donne for how he managed to "affect the metaphysics", focusing particularly on Donne's satires and on his amorous verses intended for the "fair sex" where, according to Dryden, "nature only should reign". Furthermore, "he perplexes the minds of the fair sex with nice speculations of philosophy, when he should engage their hearts, and entertain them with the softnesses of love".

It was only in the 1920s that Donne's reputation, and that of the other Metaphysical poets, came to be reinstated. T.S. Eliot appreciated Donne's capacity for "a direct sensuous apprehension of thought, or a recreation of thought into feeling". The Metaphysicals could "devour any kind of experience", in the process affecting a "unification of sensibility". The English novelist and poet A.S. Byatt expresses Donne's capacity to "feel thoughts" somewhat differently. "It's being aware of, and delighting in, the electrical and chemical impulses that connect and reconnect the neurones of our brains",[78] she says. What could have been causing such stimulating neuronal activity, one wonders? T.S. Eliot himself was an inveterate tobacco user (he died of emphysema in 1965) and was clearly aware of its narcotic effects: "Let us take the air, in a tobacco trance", he writes in 'Portrait of a Lady' (1920).

His famous ability to shift voice and hence perspective in the course of a poem is well demonstrated in 'Burnt Norton' – first from a narrator who speaks to the audience directly, then through the urgings of a bird to follow echoes that inhabit the garden "into our first world", to roses that had, "the look of flowers that are looked at/There they were as our guests, accepted and accepting", "leaves…full of children", and on to the London Underground where technology dominates. All these shifts speak to me of his tobacco use and addiction. While Eliot's shape-shifting multiperspectivalism is more developed than we find in Donne, such are the affinities between the two poets that one commentator has suggested that "Eliot wants not so much to understand Donne as to *be* him…Eliot would ultimately convert to Catholicism (the parallels or inverse parallels indeed tempt one to believe in reincarnation)".[79]

Tobacco and Enlightenment

Social anthropology has a tendency to see ideas as constructed within a specific cultural setting which may be contested even within that setting and whose cross-cultural validity is dubious. While this chapter isn't saying that tobacco was the sole means whereby the Enlightenment came into being, my argument is that tobacco, hidden in plain sight yet again, has been ignored as an agent in helping to explain why the Enlightenment occurred as and when it did. Neither am I saying that the Enlightenment is somehow exclusive as an historical epoch, or that similar cognitive trends to those associated with the ingress of tobacco were absent in eras which, in European terms, were before the fateful day in 1492 when Columbus had first contact with tobacco (Chapter 2). Greenblatt, rather like Ingold (above), suggests the Renaissance began early in the 15th century with "something that surged up against the constraints that centuries had constructed around curiosity, desire, individuality, sustained attention to the material world, the claims of the body".[80] He attributes the change to the effects of the discovery of a book by the Latin writer Lucretius, *On the Nature of Things*. The Renaissance? A book? Whether amplifying trends that had already been set in motion earlier, or causing a transformation of life and thought afresh, tobacco seems at least an equally plausible explanation for the "curiosity, desire, individuality, attention and claims of the body" that Greenblatt attributes to Lucretius' book.

In this chapter I have raised the possibility that the 16th century transit and insinuation of tobacco – from West to East and from spirit to mind – had hitherto unacknowledged consequences that were cognitive, psychological and philosophical as well as physiological, social and economic. The understanding of the world they presage was as likely a by-product, or at the very least supported by, the increasingly prodigious use of tobacco as an intoxicant of choice (and, subtly, addiction) during the period in question. Serious exceptions must be made to avoid the danger of being accused of a material determinism in my portrayal of the agency of tobacco. In scientific terms, tobacco may have influenced, but did not cause, the changes highlighted. There are no definitive records for exactly which scholars imbibed tobacco and who did not. René Descartes went into voluntary exile from France in 1628, appalled by the increasing religious intolerance being shown there and mindful that the Italian philosopher Lucilio Vanini (1585-1619) had been burnt at the stake for proposing that the cherished miracles of the Catholic Church could be explained by natural forces. Descartes' theory of Cartesian body-mind dualism, produced by sitting in an oven in order to seek confirmation of his existence, led him to decide he could only be sure of that which he knew empirically, personally, individually. In this, despite some half-hearted protestations to the contrary, he was another philosopher implying doubt about the existence of God and the immortality of the soul – in his case, requiring him to take urgent exile from the salons of Paris to the marshlands of the Dutch Republic. Here he was surrounded by what (apart from Britain) was perhaps the greatest concentration of tobacco-persons anywhere in what, from the perspective of tobacco, was the 'new' world at that time.

To the best of our knowledge, however, Descartes was not a tobacco user. His 'I think therefore I am' statement suggests a concern not to addle his thinking persona with untoward substances. Furthermore, given his anxiety (in the first of his 'Meditations on First Philosophy', subtitled 'Concerning those things that can be called into doubt') that all perception and cognition might be in error (due to such diverse things as madness, dreams, and bad eyesight), it is little wonder that he forsook anything that might have affected his brain. The Dutch Republic and Britain were the countries that experienced the earliest unfolding of Enlightenment thought, and likewise are where widespread tobacco use first occurred and where it was most prodigiously consumed. Descartes would thus have been no stranger to fellow *philosophes* who were willing and able partakers of tobacco and its associated cognitive influences. After Descartes, Kant (with his 'think for yourself' philosophy) thought for himself and was fervently against tobacco, as were Goethe, Heine and Schopenhauer after him. Perhaps by the time he had his oven thoughts, so pervasive had the influence of tobacco become that Descartes' philosophy did not need to derive from nicotian dreams. The mind was separate from the body; the imagination could be liberated from its material moorings, and reality.

Despite its mixed reception, "whenever tobacco showed up, a culture that did not smoke became a culture that did...Not all the original meanings of Native smoking made the jump to other cultures, of course. But many did, including the notion that tobacco opened a door to the spiritual realm".[81] From an object of fun in Tomkis' *Lingua* in London in 1607, by 1650 tobacco had become the subject of a reverential ballet in Turin. Transculturation (Chapter 2) is much evident in such shifts. I have argued in this chapter that cultural change of this sort involves not simply socio-economic and political change but cognitive changes as well. The Enlightenment, I have proposed, should be considered an outcome of the transculturation of tobacco as much as the indigenous development of print media, the amelioration of religious tensions and the development of trade and transport. In comparing aspects of Enlightenment thought with the cosmologies of Amerindian societies characterized by a 'tobacco culture' we can see traces of the cognitive universe offered by the ingestion of tobacco to an intoxicating degree.

The discovery of a 'New World' (in addition to the passage of tobacco out of its millennia-old crucible) engendered a sense of cultural perspective. The argument this chapter supports, however, is that the changes wrought by a sense of cultural perspective were not simply the result of the discovery of a human 'Other'. After all, in the European context, human 'Others' were nothing new (as witnessed, for example, in the European encounters of the Crusades or the travels of Marco Polo) and, as we shall see in the next chapter, Europeans were only too willing to accord those they encountered in the 'New World' the status of 'less than human'. Rather, it was the ingress of a botanical 'Other' into western life that led to a sense of perspective, both cultural and cosmological, and this, I argue, was a crucial component in the development of Enlightenment thought. The intoxicating effects of tobacco, taken in the amounts that were common in the 17th and 18th centuries, undoubtedly facilitated the development of the reflective capacities that such realizations of difference required. However, an interest in the interpretation and comparison of human societies, religions and ways of life – all hallmarks of the Enlightenment era – could as easily lead to a denigration of the objects of comparison, their inclusion in the domain of 'nature' rather than 'culture'. The consequences, as we shall see in the next chapter, were frequently terrible for the people concerned. Some disputed the idea that the inhabitants of the New World shared a common humanity, for example, and many more were happy to categorize the different groups (or 'races') found there – and elsewhere in the world – according to an evolutionary hierarchy. The conclusions people came to as a result of a growing awareness of global diversity and cultural difference, then, were by no means favourable to a multicultural approach. Nor is this supposed hallmark of western intellectual thought a ubiquitously shared perspective today.

There were other ways, in addition to its potential contribution to the Enlightenment, in which tobacco's agency served to link the experiences of tobacco users around the world. Mintz regards "tobacco, sugar, and tea as the first objects within capitalism that conveyed with their use the complex idea that one could become different by consuming differently...it is closely connected to England's fundamental transformation from a hierarchical, status-based medieval society to a social-democratic, capitalist, and industrial society".[82]

> The spread of smoking was a major cultural watershed that was both profoundly liberating and unsettling. It helped to accelerate cultural transformations that earlier generations could hardly have foreseen. In its strictly physical aspects, it brought about a revolution in the use of the

body, which in the act of inhaling smoke now performed an operation that medieval populations across the planet would have found startling and perplexing. More troubling were its hedonistic overtones. In the long term, smoking would help to redefine patterns of social interaction, promoting more relaxed attitudes about pleasure and opening up new avenues for leisure and escapism.[83]

This is written about the Middle East, but the description of tobacco's effects could be applied to life pretty much anywhere in the world. In all places, tobacco "helped to frame a distinctively early modern culture in which the pursuit of pleasure was thereafter more public, routine, and unfettered".[84] According to Sahlins, with the Enlightenment,

> although it could never quite shake its aura of wickedness, self-pleasing came out of the shadow of its sinful ancestry to assume a moral position nearly 180 degrees removed. The individual's singular attention to his own good turned out to be the basis of society rather than its nemesis – as well as the necessary condition of the greatest wealth of nations.[85]

The particular characteristics of the act of smoking provided a distinctive environment for human interaction and exchange: the reflective pauses it demands in conversation to enable smoke inhalation and expiry; the shared substances – breath and smoke – visibly mingling (some would say conspiring) in an Enlightenment fug.

Conclusion

There are interesting similarities and differences to be observed between embodied cognition in the indigenous Americas (with its extensive, if ill-defined 'tobacco ideology') and the places to which tobacco transited and transculturated from the 16th century onwards, hence affording indigenization opportunities of a different kind. I have suggested tobacco is a common factor in the multinatural perspectivism of some (but not all) Amerindian thought, as it became in the multicultural perspectivism of some (but not all) western thought. There are also parallels that can be discerned with tobacco constituting persons and fabricating conviviality, as well as the binaries, so fundamental to much Enlightenment thought, that arise out of a heightened sense of 'self' and 'other', 'subject' and 'object'. While there are multiple reasons why the Enlightenment occurred when it did, and it would be foolish to attribute everything to tobacco, this chapter has argued it would be equally foolish to deny the possibility that tobacco might have had a hand in the significant intellectual changes that took place during this era. Indeed, it is tempting to suggest that, as much as tobacco affecting the intellect, the intellectual changes themselves had a role in perpetuating and expanding the place of tobacco.

I would like to finish with an extract from a poem by the 17th Century Chinese poet, Wang Lu.[86] To my mind it perfectly captures the qualities of tobacco which have been highlighted in this chapter, including the poet's willing subservience to it and the easy transculturation evinced by the line "long I have known your name". It is arguably one of the finest eulogies to the herb ever penned:

> Thin mists and light clouds waft imperceptibly
> The friends who have gathered here pass the pipe around
> I know that there is no constancy in what is possible and what is not,
> Yet I do not believe that fire and ash are only fragments of time.
> As dawn sits astride the aboriginal hills, it disperses the miasmic vapours,
> As night frames the window where banana leaves rustle, it aids my
>   thoughts.
> *Danbagu*: long I have known your name;
> Burning and dying out: you alone are my master.

The remaining chapters in Part I will go on to look at what has happened as a result of the Enlightenment; the increasing pleasure and commitment given by people around the globe to this 'master', and the consequences as Enlightenment science came to question the effects of the plant to which so many had given their hearts and minds for so long.

Notes

1 Oxford English Dictionary (2018).
2 Fleischacher (2013: 1).
3 Israel (2006: v) bemoans the fact that "there still remains great uncertainty, doubt, and lack of clarity about what exactly the Enlightenment was and what intellectually and socially it actually involved".
4 Israel (2006: 15-26).
5 Gay (1966).
6 Fleischacher (2013: 3) calls it "a great, hitherto unnoticed value in the details of quotidian human life".
7 Wolff (2007: 3).
8 Wolff (2007: 7).
9 Ingold (2013: 742).
10 Ingold (2013: 734).
11 Merchant (1990: xxi). She argues that "the female earth was central to the organic cosmology that was undermined by the Scientific Revolution and the rise of a market-oriented culture. . .for sixteenth-century Europeans the root metaphor binding together the self, society and the cosmos was that of an organism. . .organismic theory emphasized interdependence among the parts of the human body, subordination of individual to communal purposes in family, community, and state, and vital life permeating the cosmos to the lowliest stone" (Merchant 1990: xx, 1).
12 Ingold (2013: 735).
13 Israel (2006: 15-26).
14 Israel (2006: 21).
15 Gay (1966: 3) criticized by Israel (2006: 25).

16 Israel (2006: 10).
17 Bage (1792, vol. 3: 125) quoted in Israel (2010: 1).
18 Israel (2011: 7).
19 Israel (2010: 10).
20 Outram (1995: 3).
21 As described in Brook (2008: 150-1). For more information on this fascinating ballet, which presents it as a somewhat less plebeian affair, see Grammeniati (2011).
22 Romaniello and Starks (2009).
23 Ryan (1983).
24 Kiernan (1991: 173).
25 Romaniello and Starks (2009: 1).
26 Romaniello (2007: 936).
27 Klein (2010: 93).
28 Davies (1974: 146).
29 Goodman (1993: 60).
30 Anon. (1630). See Chapter 2 for the literary ethnographic context of this statement.
31 Schama (1987: 212).
32 Ward (1745: 276).
33 Withington (2011: 651).
34 Ibid.
35 Engell (1981: 11).
36 Bloch (2012: 107).
37 Cowan (2005).
38 Cowan (2005: 11).
39 Cowan (2005: 30).
40 Cowan (2005: 82); he points out that "while coffeehouses offered many drinks in addition to coffee, it seems that coffee was not sold in other drinking establishments".
41 Matthee (2014: 113).
42 Habermas (1989).
43 Cowan (2005: 42).
44 Matthee (2014: 113).
45 The French philosopher Condorcet is a particularly noteworthy champion of an exclusively bourgeois 'public'.
46 The situation regarding taverns was interestingly different in the Middle East, where, since it was formally outlawed, "alcohol could never become the subject of a public discourse, just as the tavern, operating in the shadows, could never become part of a quasi-public sphere" (Matthee 2014: 104).
47 Macaulay (1849: 288).
48 John Gay, letter to Congreve, quoted in Nokes (1995: 191).
49 Oxford English Dictionary (2018) "modern, adj. and n." [accessed 19th February 2018].
50 Withington (2010).
51 Porter (2000: 15), his italics.
52 Porter (2000: 22).
53 Israel (2011: 2n. 4).
54 Dwyer (1993: 1).
55 Hume quoted in Porter (2000: 246).
56 Dwyer (1993: 4).
57 Burckhardt (1958, vol. I: 143). Burckhardt points out that late Medieval Italy in particular was full of people writing letters, diaries, memoirs, journals and the like.

58 Opie (1987) talks of the "man-intoxicated" spirit of the Renaissance.
59 Lukes (1973).
60 Riesman et al. (1950).
61 Macfarlane (1978).
62 Martin (2002: 211).
63 Ibid. (209).
64 Ibid.
65 Withington (2010: 239).
66 Ibid.
67 In other words, *We Have Never Been Modern* (Latour 1993). The translation of this title is somewhat misleading given the way it attributes a concrete nature to modernity, since the adjective 'modern' is actually a plural noun in the original French which is hard to translate directly into English – 'modern people' or 'moderns'.
68 Porter (2003: 25).
69 Porter (2003: 22).
70 Porter (2003: 26).
71 Kisluk-Grosheide (1988: 206).
72 Koehler (2012: 2)
73 Ibid.
74 Ibid.
75 Donne (1896). *The First Anniversary* was written in 1611 and the extract comes from vol. II: 205-18
76 Perhaps Donne's sense of compassion and interrelatedness was inherited by his second son, George (see Chapter 3).
77 Brook (2008: 221).
78 Byatt (2006: 248).
79 Sugg (2007: 21).
80 Greenblatt (2011: 9-10).
81 Brook (2008: 126).
82 Mintz (1985: 185).
83 Grehan (2006: 1353).
84 Grehan (2006: 1377).
85 Sahlins (2008: 84).
86 Quoted in Brook (2004: 88). Steve Connor (2011: 160) focuses on the pipe in this poem and the reflections it prompts on the material and the immaterial, the constant and ephemeral.

Chapter 5

Enslavement of all sorts

Introduction: dissolving the boundaries of nature and culture

In the previous chapter I argued for the hitherto unacknowledged contribution of tobacco to the intellectual and social developments known – somewhat contentiously – as the Enlightenment. I suggested the arrival of tobacco on European shores may have contributed to a heightened sense of perspectivalism and binaries similar to ideas characteristic amongst people in lowland South America, the region where tobacco's entanglement with people has been longest (Chapter 1). However, whereas the multinaturalism characteristic of lowland South America incorporates a large number of 'other' non-humans into the realm of 'culture', the Enlightenment in Europe seemed, at least at first, to generate an increasing sense of a multicultural universe in which cultured humans were set apart from all other animals. Man became master of his own destiny in Enlightenment thought; his stewardship or control of an impassive Nature offering a triumphalist sense of human dominance over the non-human. In contrast to the situation in indigenous South America, in 18th century Europe "the syncretic master opposition between nature and culture"[1] became the site for the emplacement of increasingly large numbers of 'other' humans into the realm of 'nature'. In this chapter, we will see how the consequences of this dehumanization of people into goods and chattels – the fundamental premise of the slave trade – played out in the tobacco plantations of North America, and in the process further strengthened the importance of this product in the emergent capitalist economy.

We can also see converse evidence of the 'humanization' of nature. There is a fascinating but relatively under-researched English literary genre that erupted in the 18th century, the non-human 'object'- or 'it'-narrative. It is hard not to see elements of the cosmological perspectivism characteristic of lowland South America (Chapter 1), the fluidity of form and purpose between the human and the non-human, in this genre. This chapter will explore the implications of things speaking in 18th century literature, and the curious fact that tobacco steadfastly stayed out of this talking game. In fact, tobacco was withdrawing from the talking, visible world in other ways too; shifting its shape with changing patterns of commodity use and increasing its power and influence as it did so. The 18th century was one in which snuff, involving the nostril insufflation of tobacco dust rather than oral inhalation and exhalation of tobacco smoke, became a mark of discretion, distinction and refinement in European society. The state and elite producers in the USA were also dependent on tobacco, but their reliance on the commodity risked being undermined by poor control of its quality. Efforts to ensure the continued large revenue stream (on which both had come to depend) were reflected in the building of King's Pipes at entry points for tobacco around Britain so that surplus and damaged tobacco could be destroyed and the buoyancy of the market maintained. In these ways tobacco grew from individual intoxicant and social lubricant to a mainstay of trade and the plantation economy.

The complex relationship between Man and Nature, the human and non-human, in these and other developments is reflected in the philosophical dissolution of 'nature' and 'culture' in Locke's *Essay Concerning Human Understanding*, published in 1690. Using arguments reminiscent of Lucretius, the rediscovery of whose work in the Middle Ages Greenblatt contends introduced some of "the key principles of a modern understanding of the world",[2] Locke argues we cannot determine whether thought occurs in our souls, or in "some systems of matter fitly disposed", such as our brains. Nor is it possible to make such a determination "by the contemplation of our own ideas, without revelation".[3] This was a controversial proposition at the time – not so much for what it suggested about the functions of the brain *per se*, but for what the implications of these might be for the concept of the soul and the divine.[4]

The 'sentient matter' question, as it came to be known, revolved around whether sentience derived from a soul (as the immaterialists believed), or whether man was nothing more than matter whose thought occurs in and through the brain (as the so-called 'free thinkers', or materialists, argued). The immaterialists, attempting "to maintain the ontological privilege of humanism",[5] could only accept matter as passive. A 1692 sermon by Richard Bentley, part of a lecture series endowed by the chemist Robert Boyle with the intention of reconciling science with the rational belief in God against the "vulgarly received notion of nature'" espoused by the materialists, was titled "Matter and Motion cannot Think: or, a confutation of atheism from the faculties of the soul". "Sensation and Perception are not inherent in matter as such", Bentley argued, "for if it were so; what monstrous absurdities would follow? Every Stock and Stone would be a percipient and rational creature".[6]

Could tobacco have played a part in creating the potential for Bentley's "monstrous absurdities"? Pushing Locke's reasoning further, is the brain the only form of apparently senseless matter capable of some degree of sense, perception and thought, or might we be able to find other "systems of matter fitly disposed" to do so, particularly in hybrid entanglements? Rather than treating "senseless matter" as belonging to an exclusively non-human realm, Locke was arguing for the investigation of material things having attributes traditionally viewed as part of the exclusive realm of the human. This was the cue (if one were needed) for the development of the peculiar literary form, the 'object'-narrative.

Things start speaking as never before

Whatever the origins and implications of the 'sentient matter' question, it is extraordinary to observe how, in 18th century English literature, things started speaking as never before. Holbraad (Introduction) alerted us to "the possibility – and in so many instances the fact – that the things we call 'things' might not ethnographically speaking be things as all",[7] something he frames through the philosophical, and superficially avant-garde, question "can the thing speak?"[8] Well, in 18th century literature things were positively gabbling. 'Object'- or 'it'-narratives were satirical pieces of prose, the protagonists and narrators of which were "not humans, but, rather, mundane material objects such as banknotes, corkscrews, shoes, and coins that circulate through human society, commenting upon and damning it as they go".[9] These were not children's stories, at least not initially – their targeted audience was unreservedly adult. They were immensely popular: one of the first, Charles Johnstone's *Chrysal: Or the Adventures of a Guinea*, went into a third edition within three years of its original publication in 1760.[10] Locke's views, rather than Bentley's, seem to be the imaginative touchstone for these remarkable stories. A total of 284 published object-narrative prose works are recorded between 1700 and 1900.[11] With them come terms and ideas which seem consonant with contemporary notions of material agency (Introduction). Indeed the term "material agency" was first used in William Jones' 1762 essay *First Principles of Natural Philosophy* in a manner remarkably similar to how it is used by science and technology studies scholars today.[12]

A diverse range of things speak in object narratives, and they go to many places – mobile objects are an advantage. A banknote circulates "within the space of five pages from a milliner, to a bishop's wife, to the bishop, to a bookseller, to a printer, to a pastry cook, and to a seller of dead dogs".[13] The alternative is objects, often places, such as a Covent Garden pub or the Bank of England, that are static while their human characters pass by. The rupee in *Adventures of a Rupee* spends most of its time in a pawnbroker's, the novel presenting a series of portraits of visitors to the shop, whose stories are told to the rupee by the spirits of gold.

Various explanations have been posited for the eruption of these stories and their success with the reading public. Lynch, for example, suggests they were an attempt to soften (through humanizing) the new market system "which made English men and women uneasy".[14] Flint argues, less convincingly in my opinion, that speaking objects reflect authors' anxieties over the public exposure of their books.[15] However, as well as reflecting the impact of markets or books, object narratives can also be seen as creative explorations of the philosophical issues arising out of the Enlightenment's increasing interest in the material world – a trend established, paradoxically, by an increasingly strong dissociation of the human from the non-human from the 17th century onwards, a trend in which, I have argued, tobacco played a strong fomenting role.

Paradoxical, however, is the curious lack in this material babbling of any extant narratives by tobacco or its paraphernalia. Despite the acculturation of things ('nature') through narrative, tobacco, although apparently eminently appropriate for such a task, appears to have remained steadfastly silent in making its own voice heard, at least in prose. Perhaps the reason is a practical one. Unlike a coin of the realm (for example) tobacco is an inherently unreliable speaking object, since it is less likely to be passed on from person to person than to go up in smoke (in the hands of a smoker) or (as became increasingly popular during the 18th century) up the nostril, as snuff. But a pipe, a tobacco box, pouch, or snuff box would appear ideal objects to offer their perspicacious observations in the manner so evidently enjoyed by readers of other 'it-narratives'. It is of course much harder to explain why something doesn't happen than why it does – consider, for example, Sherlock Holmes' nicotine-fuelled ruminations about the dog that did not bark in the night a century later (Chapter 6). Perhaps, given its close association with metaphysical things in the previous century, tobacco and its objects were regarded as too problematic to be the basis of an object narrative. Or perhaps, simply, no-one thought to create a story along these lines.

Tobacco's silence is doubly surprising considering it had already been a speaking character in the plays we saw in Chapter 2, composed well before the start of the period defined by its 'object narratives'. A reprint of *Lingua* in the book *A Select Collection of Old Plays* in 1780 triggered a modicum of interest in the play amongst the literati. A gentleman styling himself 'William Whif' wrote to the editor of *Gentleman's Magazine* remarking on the appearance of tobacco in the play: "were a modern poet to introduce Mr. Tobacco (smoaking personified) as one of his characters upon the stage (and, Heaven knows, we have strange characters enough now and then)...the Managers would be at a loss to know how to dress the worthy gentleman". He goes on "Can any of your correspondents make sense of Tobacco's language, or suggest why he uses it? The editor [of the reprint] takes no notice of it".[16] Whif's query epitomizes the changing perspectives of the 18th compared to the 17th century. The 17th century was still the era of spectacle and phantasmagoria; I don't think anyone would have seriously entertained the idea that tobacco really was speaking a potentially intelligible or translatable language at that time, and would have been happy to accept unquestioned Phantastes' opinion that this was an Antipodean language, or Memoria's opinion that it was the language of Arcadia whose people existed "before the Moone".[17] William Whif reflects the changes occasioned by the development of Enlightenment science and the accompanying belief that things (in this case the language of a speaking plant, anthropomorphized as the "King of Tobacco") needed to be decoded or 'de-scribed' rather than taken – as Tomkis surely intended us to do – as just a bit of nonsense. No correspondents to *Gentleman's Magazine* attempted to answer Whif's query – or if they did, the editor did not publish their responses.

If not tobacco, a tobacco-related object spoke at least once in 18th century English literature. A tobacco pipe converses with a perfumed wig in a "poetic fable" published by Christopher Smart in 1752. The wig, described as of the "flaunting French" sort that was so popular in genteel society at that time, is critical of the tobacco pipe's "barb'rous English! horrid Dutch!" polluting breath. The pipe retorts:

> Know, puppy, I'm an English pipe,
> Deem'd worthy of each Briton's gripe [grip],
> Who, with my cloud-compelling aid
> Help our plantations and our trade[18]

Compare this to the discourse of the "great Emperor tobacco" in *Lingua*. No longer a King that had "conquered all Europe, in making them pay tribute for their smoake", as Tobacco was seen 150 years earlier, the tobacco pipe (a human artefact rather than an exotic plant) was "deem'd" [by people] worthy of each Briton's grip. And, rather than being the source of exploitative tribute or taxes, as was the case in *Lingua*, the pipe – through its "cloud-compelling aid", is the help-mate of "our plantations and our trade". Tobacco had shifted from an exotic, monarchical presence to an everyday product, the consumption of which was fundamental to supporting the national interest.

Trade had become the *sine qua non* of British colonialism in the 18th century. Unlike dominion, trade was seen as an unequivocally benign, morally upright activity. According to the essayist and politico Joseph Addison, writing in 1716,

> it is our Business to extend to the utmost our Trade and Navigation. By this means, we reap the Advantages of Conquest, without Violence or Injustice; we not only strengthen ourselves, but gain the Wealth of our Neighbours in an honest Way; and, without any Act of Hostility, lay the several Nations, of the World under a kind of Contribution.[19]

Tobacco was the second-most important trading commodity in the world after sugar. At the beginning of the 18th century, over 30 million pounds' weight of tobacco was being imported into the British Isles annually from the Chesapeake Bay colonies (Maryland and Virginia) alone.[20] It served a domestic market that encompassed all regions and social classes. Indeed, the universalistic quality of tobacco is one of the most common themes in poetry about tobacco from this century.

Less genteel than tea, more genteel than gin (a drink associated primarily with the urban poor), as the supposedly more cultured gentry moved to snuff, smoking was conversely imagined as an activity that united the nation. The 'Convert to Tobacco', in *A Collection of Merry Poems* (1736), describes tobacco offering contentment to the Welsh farmer trudging barefoot through the snow ("With thee he warms his dripping Nose,/And scrubs, and puffs, and on he goes"), as well as to the "Justice grave", who partners tobacco with ale to hold court at his table after dinner "Whilst sober whiff fills each Hiatus". Tobacco is described as "Assistant Chief" to a "Country vicar"; "If text obscure perplex his Brain, He scratches, thinks, but all in vain; Till lighted Pipe's prevailing Ray,/Like *Phoebus*, drives the Fog away".[21] Such egalitarianism, and cognitive insights, reflect the increasing extent, diversity and normality of tobacco use, amongst all sections of society. In fact, whereas in the 17th century tobacco had been "contending for superiority" over "wine, beere and ale" (Chapter 2), an 18th century poem was titled 'The Triumph of Tobacco over Sack and Ale'. It, like the 'Convert' poem, emphasized the social unity tobacco engendered:

> Tobacco engages
> Both Sexes, all Ages,
> The Poor as well as the Wealthy,
> From the Court to the Cottage,
> From Childhood to Dotage,
> Both those that are sick and the healthy.[22]

Inspired by tobacco

Tobacco was thus firmly ensconced across social classes and geographical areas. Literary circles in early 18th century London were steeped in tobacco, and virtually every prominent male author of the period – such as Addison, Pope, Prior, Steele, and Swift – was at least an occasional user of the drug. But tobacco use in 18th century Britain also extended far beyond the metropolitan elite. For one Scottish Secessionist minister, Ralph Erskine (1686–1752), smoking was a spiritual experience which brought the mind closer to God. His 'Smoking Spiritualised' derives from a much earlier poem that compared tobacco's effects on the body and the Holy Spirit's action on the soul. For Erskine, tobacco had a "medicinal effect" which paralleled the greater healing power of "Jesse's Flower"; the fire inside the pipe evokes the hell-fires waiting for the sinner's soul while tobacco smoke, suggestive of the vanity "Of worldly stuff/Gone with a puff", manifests the soul's future ascent to heaven.

In vain th'unlighted Pipe you blow,
Your pains in outward Means are so,
Till heavenly fire,
Your heart inspire.
Thus think and smoke Tobacco.
The Smoke, like burning Incense, tow'rs.
So should a praying heart of yours
With ardent cries
Surmount the skies.
Thus think and smoke Tobacco.[23]

Another enthusiastic endorsement of tobacco came from the Oxfordshire poet John Philips, for whom the weed was a recurrent theme both in his life and poetic career. Samuel Johnson, writing about him in *Lives of the Poets*, remarks on his "addiction to tobacco" and how he takes any opportunity to celebrate "the fragrant fume". In company he was said to be "silent and barren, and employed only upon the pleasures of his pipe".[24] One of his last poems, 'An Ode to Henry St. John, Esq' (1707)[25] is a thank-you to this gentleman for a gift of pipe tobacco and alcohol. The poem perpetuates the familiar refrain of tobacco offering solace and metaphysical inspiration.

O Thou from India's fruitful Soil,
Who dost that sov'raign Herb prepare;
In whose rich Fumes I lose the Toil
Of Life, and ev'ry anxious Care:
While from the fragrant lighted Bole,
I suck new Life into my Soul.

However, Philips' "Muse from Smoke" is inferior to a classical Muse: even as it elevates the mind, it weakens the body. In preparing to sing his gift-givers' praises, he experiences a fit of breathlessness:

But, O! as greatly I aspire
To tell my Love, to speak thy Praise,
Boasting no more its sprightly Fire,
My bosom heaves, my Voice decays;
With Pain I touch the mournful String,
And pant and languish as I sing.

Philips died in 1709, age 33, his death attributed to a "lingering consumption, attended with an asthma".[26]

William Cowper's poem 'To the Rev. William Bull' praises tobacco for its divine inspiration in cases of writer's block – those times when "what we would, so weak is man, Lies oft remote from what we can". The sun was once seen as the inspiration "setting genius free", but this had become disregarded. A substitute for the sun was needed "t'accelerate a creeping pen". For the poet, "this oval box well fill'd/With best tobacco, finely mill'd" was the means "To disengage the encumber'd senses".[27]

A more satirical approach to the 'inspiration' – spiritual or otherwise – offered by tobacco is contained in six satirical poems by the barrister, politician and poet Isaac Hawkins Browne (1706–60).[28] United by the topic of tobacco, each one parodies the style of a different contemporary poet, including Addison, Pope and Swift. Public enthusiasm for this scurrilous anthology is reflected in the fact it featured in two pirated miscellanies published in the same year. The authors whose styles are represented may claim more refined sources of poetic inspiration, but the reality for Browne is that the "light from smoke" upon which they rely is tobacco. Like Philips (above) tobacco is a disreputable cousin to the classical Muses. While offering a sublime heightening of perception and thoughts, the inspiration she offers is debased by fleshly cravings, foul-smelling fumes, and addiction. At the same time tobacco offers not only distraction, but also potentially distance from both the cares of the world and the opposite sex. Thus Swift is moved to retreat to an Irish village as yet unmolested by government troops, where he can live and "Doze o'er a Pipe, whose Vapour bland/In sweet Oblivion lulls the Land", while Philips' erstwhile paean to womanly beauty becomes an erotic ode to his tobacco pipe, a "Little Tube of mighty Pow'r,/...Object of my warm desire" leading to "the sweetest bliss of blisses/breathing from thy balmy kisses". Another poem describes "Tobacco, Fountain pure of limpid Truth" and implores it to remain "*my great Inspirer*, Thou/*My Muse*; Oh fan me with thy Zephyrs Boon,/While I, in clouded Tabernacle shrin'd,/Burst forth all Oracle and mystic Song". Another alludes to the need to taste tobacco unblemished by the corrupting effects of the heavy fiscal penalties for its use: "come to thy Poet, come with healing Wings,/And let me taste Thee *unexcis'ed* by Kings".[29]

Musicians also used tobacco in their compositions and, presumably, creative musings. Handel and J.S. Bach both liked their pipes. Bach invited visitors to soothe themselves with a pipe of tobacco after one of his dazzling harpsichord displays.[30] Mozart was a keen snuff user, having found being in a room with thick tobacco smoke difficult in his early years, although latterly he enjoyed a solitary pipe. In one of his last letters to his wife, he described playing two games of billiards, after which "I told Joseph to get Primus to fetch me some black coffee, with which I smoked a splendid pipe of tobacco; and then I orchestrated almost the whole of Stadler's Rondo" – the Clarinet concerto he was writing for Anton Stadler.[31]

Triumph of tobacco, sex and gender

The literary discourse had moved on from the 17th century 'Women's complaint against tobacco' (Chapter 3). Whereas that piece ended with the women of "gossips' hall" convincing their menfolk to eschew the weed or face the carnal consequences, the 'Convert to Tobacco' poem describes a man getting the better of *Buxoma*, a banker's widow, on this score. The widow, who had vowed "Never to wed with filthy Smoaker", tested her many suitors by offering them pipes and tobacco at the end of their meal. She was thus able to summarily reject the amorous overtures of those who partook of her offer. After she had packed off up to 20 lovers (some indication of the popularity of smoking at this time), a "Swain of *Irish* race" made his appearance, who had bribed her maid into betraying her mistress' vow. Thus, when asked, the Irishman claimed "He wou'd not smoke, to save his Life". But on their wedding day, after the guests had withdrawn, the groom roared for a pipe. The shocked woman lay awaiting "the happy Consequence" of matrimony, but all kisses and "th' ensuing Bliss" were preceded by pipe smoking, her husband being one "so stout/To take a fifth 'ere he gave out". The poem ends with her awed admonition "What! Yet again? The Devil's in thee,/*Nat*, Fetch the Pound of *Sly's Virginia*,/All the new Pipes, and a fresh Light,/Your Master says he'll smoak all Night".[32] Sex and smoking come together here in a trope around pleasure which was to continue into the 20th century.

The bondage of Britons to sensual pleasures was not without its critics, however. For historian Roy Porter, a

> materialistic worldliness was to spread in the bubbling commercial atmosphere of the eighteenth century and the birth of 'the consumer society'. With the growth of prosperity and creature comforts, the moneyed became absorbed in the here-and-now, in matters tangible, buyable, disposable; in items of fashion and taste, manufactures, commodities, privacy, domesticity and a new sexualisation of existence.[33]

There was a growing backlash against such materialism, at least when applied to the body.

> The 'body' remained hardly less puzzling than the soul and, if more concrete, far more objectionable. . .Meanwhile, élite drives for the reformation of popular culture equated the flesh and the plebs, and hence made the bodily connote all that was vulgar, disorderly, contagious and threatening.[34]

Snuff offered itself as a product that enabled greater opportunities for distinction between people to occur.

Snuff: refinement, distinction, and resistance

Perhaps it was the increasingly common use of pipes across the social class gradient, the glimmerings of health concerns about smoking, or the earthy tenor of everyday art as it became enmeshed with tobacco, that led to the need for an alternative to smoking. For despite the eulogies to smoking in the above examples, this was the era in which a new form of tobacco consumption was rising to social prominence. Perhaps the attraction of it came from a desire amongst the elite for a product which involved less of a shared fug and more of an individual experience. The French king, Louis XIV (1638-1715), was the first monarch to establish the distribution and sale of tobacco as a state monopoly. Although he was another despotic monarch who despised tobacco, he still made sure there was plenty available for the French military. His disapproval of pipe smoke may have been partly responsible for the growing preference for snuff, which gained in ubiquity.[35] A Parisian text published in 1700 records how:

> One takes snuff at court as well as in the city; princes, lofty lords, and the people all take snuff. It ranks among the favourite occupations of the noblest ladies, and the middle-class women who imitate them in every-thing follow them in this activity as well. It is the passion of prelates, abbés, and even monks. Despite papal prohibition, priests in Spain take snuff during the Mass. The snuffbox lies open before them on the altar.[36]

Snuff gave the French aristocracy ample opportunities to show their cultivation and refinement. Offering and taking snuff correctly became one of many ways of demonstrating one's command of ritual etiquette and of assessing that of others. A French instruction manual from the mid-18th century turned snuff-taking into a ritual of 14 discrete actions:

1   Pick up the snuffbox with the fingers of the left hand.
2   Place it into the correct position in the hand.
3   Tap the snuffbox with your finger.
4   Open the snuffbox.
5   Offer the snuffbox to the others in your company.
6   Take back the snuffbox.
7   Keep the snuffbox open all the while.
8   Make a pile of the tobacco in the snuffbox by tapping on the side of it with a finger.
9   Carefully take up the tobacco in the right hand.
10 Hold the tobacco for a moment between the fingers before bringing it up to the nose.
11 Bring the tobacco up to the nose.
12 Take in the snuff evenly with both nostrils, without making a grimace.
13 Sneeze, cough, expectorate.
14 Close the snuffbox.

An anonymous 1706 satire 'On the great Mode of Snuff taking' argues that the fashionable powder had reduced all London to the level of the "Man of Mode":

> The Gentleman bedaubs his Snout
> With Thee, i'th' inside and without;
> The Footman too with's Plague and Pox,
> At ev'ry Oath must ope his Box,
> And's mangy Thumb and Finger thrust
> To pinch from thence a Shoal of Dust;
> Then smears his Nose and Stale-beer Beard,
> So justles in 'mongst Modish Herd.[37]

While it is not the object (snuff) speaking, the voice in this poem is interesting – it speaks *to* snuff ("The Gentleman bedaubs his Snout/With Thee, I'th'inside and without") rather than describing snuff in the third person ('With It'). While snuff can be addressed almost as an equal, the implication appears to be that people are in charge, not the other way round. The foppish modes of taking snuff were severely criticized in a 1722 essay, not because of the overblown mannerisms snuff-taking entailed as much as its growing popularity amongst the lower classes and women. This, it was claimed, had created a "Sham-Gentry", ready to "sin as ingeniously as the expertest Fop that ever appear'd in the Side-Boxes and Pit of a Play-House".[38]

The snuffbox became an important decorative element in Rococo apparel. Count Heinrich Brühl, director of the Meissen porcelain works in German, is recorded as having had over 600 snuffboxes, many of them covered in precious stones, each designed to match a different suit of clothing.[39] The refinement that snuff-taking came to represent is reflected in how rare it is, despite its relative popularity, to see examples of pipe smoking in official portraits of gentlemen in the 17th and 18th centuries; in contrast, there is a painting by Gainsborough in the North Carolina Museum of Art showing the aristocratic Ralph Bell carrying his snuff box. The Meissen figure of a monkey taking snuff is another interesting commentary on the snuff craze – the monkey as a sentient being aping (literally) the behaviours of human society (Fig. 5.1).[40]

Alexander Pope contrasted the elaborately decorated snuff box and the self-conscious rituals for the extraction of its contents, with the wit of its owners. His mock-heroic poem *The Rape of the Lock* (1712) ends with the depiction of a lunar terrain where "Heroes' Wits are kept in pondrous Vases,/And Beaus' in Snuff-boxes and Tweezer-Cases" (V.115-16). Perhaps the most telling portrayal of the 'tobacco-human' hybrid from this era, however, is James Arbuckle's conclusion to his 1717 homage to snuff. He presents us with an image of his body buried and decaying in the fields where tobacco, "the blest Plant in native Beauty grows". In his vision, his corpse becomes absorbed into the growing plant. Thus his body "as it moulders, shall it kindly feed,/And with its Substance cloath the embryo Seed./The earthly parts shall to the Stem adhere,/The rest exhale in aromatick Air".

The poem 'Hail Indian Plant', published in *The London Medley* in 1731, praises tobacco as "the Old Man's Solace, and the Student's Aid" and suggests

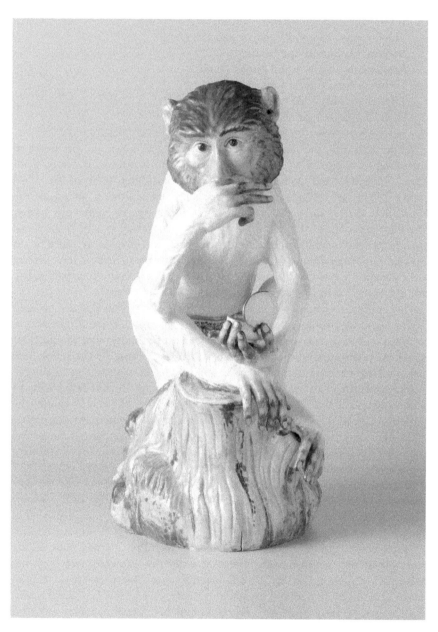

Fig. 5.1 Monkey with snuff box, attributed to Kändler, c. 1731
Source: Rijksmuseum, Amsterdam

that, when pulverized into "smart Rappee" (a form of coarse snuff), tobacco can invigorate even "Sir Fopling's Brain, if Brain there be" since, on taking it, "He shines in Dedications, Poems, Plays".[41] Yet such ready access to the brain came at a recognized, if unproven, price – a loss of the faculty of smell. For one Scarborough "Country Parson", the snuff box was the "Box of Pandora" since "Politeness, which Men in this Age so admire,/Hath taught us in Snuff against Health to conspire".[42] However, loss of the sense of smell might, if anything, have been an appealing adjunct to snuff's stimulating effects on the brain. Given the hygiene standards of the time, one commentator remarks, "for members of courtly society...loss of the sense of smell was no catastrophe; on the contrary, it may have come as a relief".[43]

Resistance

There was medical resistance to the over-use of snuff, such as John Hill's 1761 booklet *Cautions Against the Immoderate Use of Snuff*, an account, its author claimed, "founded on the known qualities of the tobacco plant, and the effects it must produce when this way taken into the body". This was the continuing narrative trope about the health consequences of tobacco, here shifted to snuff.[44] Hill was concerned that the nose offered a direct path to the brain, its nostrils "covered, in a manner, with branches of nerves: and these so thinly guarded from the air, that the brain itself may be said to lie almost naked there". This gave the nose the unwarranted reputation as a sensitive organ and the organ of reason.

Arbuckle comments on the likeness between the tobacco leaf and the brain:

> What curious Lines compos'd of many a thread
> From the great Stem in vagrant branches Spread
> The secret Conduits where the fragrant Soul
> Transfus'd, perspires and vegetates the whole;
> Which in their Texture, and their Use contain
> An apt Resemblance of the Humane Brain.[45]

He goes on to praise snuff for its arousing and calming abilities and, like the smoking poems discussed earlier, welcomes its stimulation of the creative muse. The poet:

> To calm his Thoughts at length a Pinch he takes
> The Force of Thought the dark Amusement breaks
> The Soul recruits, then with new Vigour flows;
> Now Images that long had molding been
> With mighty pain, Jump ready molded in;
> [...]

What Tuneful Odes to thee, O Snuff belong,
To whom he owes the Musick of his Song![46]

More general concerns were also being raised, however, about the addictive qualities of tobacco, as they had been all along. A physician writing in 1750 commented "the greatest Inconvenience arising from habitual Smoking is, that the Herb is of such an infatuating Nature, that those accustomed to it cannot leave it off without the greatest Mortification, and a kind of Violence or Force done to their Inclination".[47] Such assertions were tempered by arguments that health issues were less important than the fact one was smoking for one's country, as Smart's talking pipe averred. In addition to trade, tobacco consumption was contributing substantial amounts to English tax revenues as well.[48] However, much of the profit occasioned by tobacco was dependent on the alienation of labour that was slavery.

Virginia – enslaved to production

The agency and powers of expression occasioned by the hybridity of tobacco and its users in Europe – the non-human/human assemblage – came at the price exacted by the dehumanization that was colonial slavery. Tobacco is a plant greedy of labour. As Goodman puts it, "[u]nlike other staples of the period, tobacco was unique in that a sustained labour input was required constantly, different kinds of skills were called for at different times of the year, and each stage had to be accomplished with the utmost care".[49] The distinctive characteristics of tobacco meant "its cultivation required continuous personal attention: at every stage the planter made crucial judgments about the crop's development. His attention throughout the year was focused not upon whole fields or even specific plants but upon individual leaves",[50] what Hahn calls a sequence of distinct stages or "task complexes".[51]

Slavery would probably never have taken off the way it did had it not been for the intensive labour requirements and exacting tasks demanded by the Virginian tobacco crop in the late 17th and 18th centuries. Chesapeake planters turned increasingly to the nascent trade in African slaves for this purpose.[52] This had the indirect effect of bringing the different groups of white settlers together in opposition to the black slaves, whom they held to be inferior, partly because they had become enslaved in the first place.[53] The Royal African Company was set up in London in 1672 (following on from a company established by royal statute in 1660) with a monopoly on what was euphemistically called the "Guinea" or "African" trade. This trade was opened up to all-comers in 1698 when any trader exporting from Africa undertook to pay a 10 per cent levy to the company. A triangular system was established, with raw materials (sugar, cotton, tobacco) being brought from the colonies for processing in the Mother Land, and manufactured goods (including cloth and tobacco) being taken from the English ports south to West Africa where they were traded for slaves.

The notorious "Middle Passage" then ensued, in which slaves were transported, in rows with no more than two feet in between them, shackled and naked, in the lower holds of ships. These people, many of them destined for American tobacco plantations, were sometimes given tobacco and pipes to 'placate' them during voyage.[54] Diseases such as dysentery were rife; while mortality rates varied depending on port of origin and year of passage, anything up to 25 per cent of those transported died during the voyage.[55] Most of the first generation slaves in the Virginian colonies had come from markets in the Caribbean; direct transport from Africa came later, from 1680 onwards. Although slavery of indigenous peoples also occurred in the North American colonies, its scale was less. Unlike indentured labour, slave status for Africans was almost invariably permanent and hereditary: children born into slavery became slaves themselves.

Between 1670 and 1730, the proportion of the Virginia population who were enslaved increased from five to 26 per cent.[56] By 1700, the majority of unfree labourers were black. "Slavery, from being an insignificant factor in the economic life of the colony, had become the very foundation upon which it was established".[57] Slaves were "the strength and sinews of the Western World" wrote one scholar a century later.[58] Another comments how slavery formed the backbone of capitalism.[59] An observer in the early 18th century remarked on just how insignificant the numbers of white servants had become "compared with the vast shoals of Negroes".[60] The word "shoals" is significant – the increasing numbers led to a greater sense of dehumanization – from people to fish. With the increasing numbers came a number of Codes and Acts designed to suppress any attempts at rebellion. Slaves on the tobacco plantations were divided into small work groups or 'gangs', as befitted the intensive labour required. Pacesetters were selected from amongst the hardest-working slaves while supervisors utilized sufficiently brutal methods of labour control to ensure reluctant compliance. Slaves had little incentive to work at anything other than the slowest pace possible, since there was only ever more work to do. Their reluctance was easily and conveniently interpreted by the planters and supervisors as fecklessness, shiftiness and irresponsibility – so furthering a view of slaves amongst the tobacco masters that conveniently promoted their 'less-than-human' status.[61]

The trade perpetuated

As the demand for slaves increased, rising prices for tobacco made the trade an increasingly lucrative and attractive proposition on all sides. This had repercussions for all three corners of the trading triangle. In Africa, as the scale of slavery increased, a number of large and powerful kingdoms developed, such as the Yoruba kingdom of Oyo on the Guinea coast, the Asante (Ashanti) kingdom on the Gold Coast, Dahomey (now Benin), and the Chokwe chiefdoms in what are now Angola and the Democratic Republic of the Congo.[62] Europeans rarely entered the interior of Africa, due to fear of disease and the danger of counter-attack from resistant Africans. They left the task to the formidable armies and increasingly sophisticated firearm technologies of the African states which, through territorial warfare and raiding by predatory local strongmen and their militias, generated the human captives required for the burgeoning trade. Sometimes leaders were able to rig their judicial systems to enable individuals and families from amongst their own people to be sold to European traders in exchange for trade goods. Tobacco was a popular commodity in this trade.

The slave trade reached its zenith in the late 18th century, when most slaves were captured by raiding expeditions into the interior of West Africa. It is estimated that over the centuries, 12 to 20 million people were shipped as slaves from Africa by European traders. Britain was second only to Portugal in the number of slaves shipped, accounting for roughly a quarter of the total. It may seem strange that England, a country that had long lost any economic and imaginative attachment to slavery, should so quickly embrace the practices and profits of the African slave trade. There were thriving commercial links between English merchants and traders and their counterparts in Portugal, Spain and Italy, where slavery was much more strongly in evidence. Merchants in Lisbon, for example, saw the importation of Africans as early as the fifteenth century, and were well versed in the opportunities it offered.[63] Robert Thorne, a former mayor of Bristol, England, ran a soap factory in Seville, Spain with his brother. Seville was the centre of a trade in "blacks, Muslims and Canary Islanders", and Thorne was listed as one of the major slave traders in that city.[64]

The precedents for slavery set by other European countries were used as an excuse for England (and, after the Act of Union in 1707, Britain) to avoid losing not only its favourable position as an imperial power, but also its ability to impart the 'true' form of Protestant Christianity on heathen tobacco producers. Trade, religion and an increasingly derogatory regard for other races thus became three frequently invoked ideological justifications for the slave trade, along with some other racially motivated theories such as the argument that African labourers were better suited to labour in more tropical climes than whites, an erroneous claim that hardly fitted the situation in Virginia. By these means the baser economic need by tobacco growers for slaves was buttressed on political and moral grounds. The profits to be made from investing in the slave trade were likewise attractive in Britain too, where, although there was resistance to such investments in some quarters, the prevailing arguments – such as 'everyone's doing it'; 'if I don't, someone else will profit'; or 'they are less than human anyway' – held sway.

There was also a convenient masquerading of tobacco's production methods in the advertisements that became increasingly prominent during the 18th century. Trade cards, receipts (known as billheads) and tobacco wrappers were engraved or etched with advertisements for the shop from which they hailed and the product that was sold there. Of the 400 18th century tobacco advertisements in the collections of the British Museum analysed by Catherine Molineux, about half included black people.[65] They were presented in a myriad of ways – as feathered royals, working in bucolic pastoral landscapes, or in situations of trade or camaraderie with white people. In the Bradley Russel Street advertisement (Fig. 5.2), for example, the white merchants join the black man at a cloth-covered table to inspect and enjoy the "sweet scented" produce. The implied sovereignty of the regal black producer over the tobacco plantations in the background and the implication that the three are trading partners belies the brutal realities of slavery. The closest one gets to some kind of acknowledgement is in another image, for Archer's Best Virginia, where a white overseer leans languidly against a hogshead barrel smoking his long-stemmed pipe, a dog jumping at his coat tails, while in the distance semi-naked black men and children work industriously preparing the leaves and sealing and rolling the hogsheads down to a ship waiting off shore.[66] The exoticism of heathen tobacco, far from the threat it presented in the 17th century, had become part of its allure; its trade cards permitting consumers an imaginary scenario that softened the harsh reality of the slavery system.

Beyond the pale: reverberations in West Africa and elsewhere

The international slave trade, purloining labour from West Africa for a life-time's toil on the American tobacco fields, had lasting effects upon the cultural

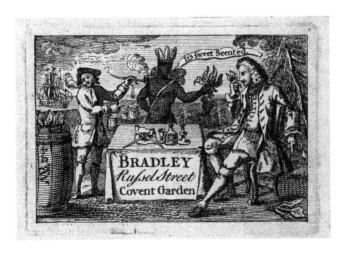

Fig. 5.2 Tobacco-paper for Bradley, tobacco and snuff seller, Russel Street, Covent Garden, London

Source: Heal Collection, 117.15, British Museum (CC BY-NC-SA 4.0)

landscape of Europe and West Africa as well as North America. The participation of cities like Bristol, Liverpool and London in 'the African trade' led to a remarkable rise in housebuilding, refinement and gentility.[67] There was some shame in the connections of many wealthy port city families to the slave trade; linkages could be well-known, but not openly discussed. There were an estimated 20,000 black people living in the British Isles in the latter half of the 1780s, their status vis-à-vis slavery ambiguous in some cases.[68] English poet William Cowper claimed

> We have no slaves at home – Then why abroad?
> [. . .]
> Slaves cannot breathe in England; if their lungs
> Receive our air, that moment they are free.
> They touch our country, and their shackles fall.
> That's noble, and bespeaks a nation proud
> And jealous of the blessing. Spread it then,
> And let it circulate through every vein.[69]

Cowper's claims that the very air of England made slaves free are purely rhetorical: there were certainly examples of slaves in English society. But rather than their status ever becoming the subject of serious scrutiny they have always been, as they remain today, largely hidden in plain sight like the tobacco with which they were imbricated.

The effects of the slave trade have reverberated across West Africa in various ways to this day. A late 19th century tobacco pipe in the Metropolitan Museum of Art in New York comes from the Chokwe savannah area in what is now the Democratic Republic of Congo and is in the form of a beaded rifle.[70] Chokwe chiefs were increasingly involved in trade with Europeans seeking rubber, wax and ivory as well as slaves. Exchanging slaves for firearms ensured more successful raids on neighbouring peoples and a steady flow of captives for European traders. The museum suggests the pipe was used with expensive imported tobacco exchanged for slaves, although there is no reason to assume locally grown tobacco was unavailable in the area by this time.

Those areas in West Africa hardest hit by endemic warfare and slave raids experienced general population decline which still has its demographic trace. It is believed that the shortage of men in particular changed the structure of many societies, thrusting women into roles previously occupied by their husbands and brothers. Additionally, some scholars have argued that the violence and banditry lives on in collective memory through a variety of metaphysical fears and beliefs concerning witchcraft. In many parts of West and Central Africa, witches are believed to kidnap solitary individuals to enslave or consume them.[71] Finally, the increased exchange with Europeans and the fabulous wealth it brought enabled many states to cultivate sophisticated artistic traditions employing expensive and luxurious materials. From the fine silver- and goldwork of Dahomey and the Asante court, to the virtuoso woodcarving of the Chokwe chiefdoms, these treasures are a vivid testimony to this turbulent period in African history.

There is another contemporary resonance, however, more directly aligned to the subject of this book. Tobacco use rates amongst former West African slave-trading countries like Ghana and Togo are well below the average for low- and middle-income countries (LMICs) and are hard to explain. A common pattern seen by those working in global tobacco control is that, as legislation increases and smoking rates decline in industrial and post-industrial societies, so the industry redoubles its efforts to market its products in the LMICs.[72] Countries in the World Health Organization's Eastern Mediterranean Region, for example, now have growth rates for cigarette use that are amongst the highest in the world, with cigarette consumption having increased by more than one third since 2000. In West Africa, by contrast, rates appear to be holding steady at a relatively low level. Is it too far-fetched to wonder whether memories of the slave trade and its reasons may be acting as some kind of inoculant against tobacco for some contemporary West African peoples, making them less susceptible to the glamorous appeal of a product that is able to seduce populations of similar economic status in other parts of the resource-poor world?

Indebted to tobacco

If the collective memory of enslavement has left West African societies resistant to the easy hybridization of people and plant, in North America, such hybridized senses of personhood were ebullient. For tobacco planters, tobacco became "an extension of self. . .the highest praise one could bestow on an eighteenth-century planter was to call him 'crop master', a public recognition of agricultural acumen".[73] The demands (or excuse) of tobacco cultivation meant there was little Sunday church-going. When Richard Lee, a well-known defender of American liberties in the period leading up to Independence, wrote an essay "The State of the Constitution in Virginea", the main topic of his tract was the agricultural practices by which Virginians cultivated tobacco. He felt it important that people who did not understand the culture should find out "how much labour is required on a Virginean estate & how poor the produce". Breen argues "the staple [as people called it] provided a medium within which the planter negotiated a public reputation, a sense of self-worth as an agricultural producer".[74] One 1799 visitor was struck by "how much the subject of this staple [tobacco] was interwoven in the spirit of the time; and how nearly the history of the tobacco plant is allied to the chronology of an extensive and flourishing country".[75]

White planters became an increasingly differentiated group. Some were able to capitalize on their assets while others, primarily those freed from the restraints of indenture, struggled to gain a foothold as small farmers in the region (Chapter 3). Wealthier tobacco planters purchased slaves, but small planters could not afford to do so. Colonists who owned slaves produced more tobacco, with the profits from which they were able to buy additional Africans. The process continued until "some planters...literally possessed hundreds of unfree workers".[76] Financial arrangements were also important. The wealthier planters sold their tobacco by a system known as consignment. They would send their own produce, and sometimes harvests they had bought off their poorer neighbours, to merchants in Britain who would sell the consignment on at the best prices they could obtain. The merchant would also buy and send by return various manufactured goods the planter had ordered. Through the provision of luxury goods, enjoyed in opulent plantation homes, the planters aspired to live like English gentlemen.[77] Increasingly grand Georgian mansions built along Virginia's river banks in the 1720s and 1730s symbolized both tobacco's success and the increasing wealth inequalities between its producers. It was wealth, however, based on the "symbolic annihilation" of the labours of the enslaved Africans whose productivity, like the tobacco they were producing, remained largely "hidden in plain sight".[78] The same could be said of the houses many traders were building on the other side of the Atlantic.

Amongst the wealthy, access to consumer goods continued to proliferate. One commentator reported how, by 1766, in planters' homes "nothing are so common as Turkey or Wilton Carpetts, the whole Furniture of the Roomes Elegant & Every Appearance of Opulence".[79] Yet both slavery and consumerism, according to Breen, "created staggering financial risks". Particularly for small planters, the death or sickness of a slave could result in bankruptcy.[80] When the bottom dropped out of the tobacco market in Europe again in the 1760s, the planters' position became increasingly perilous. Enslavement worked in many different directions: "we all know that we are slaves to the power of the merchants" wrote a planter in the *Virginia Gazette* in 1771.[81] Tobacco was at the heart of some quite heartless power relationships generated by and through its systems of production and consumption. All the while the boom and bust economy typical of capitalist world systems led to an increase in profits amongst the largest planters who could weather such storms, and diminishing wealth amongst the smallholders who could not.

Scottish merchants became particularly prominent figures in the North American tobacco landscape after the Act of Union in 1707. Glasgow merchants in particular competed with each other to service planters with credit in order to ensure their future access to the tobacco crop.[82] The Scots tended to provide credit to smaller planters, purchasing directly from them, their stocks passing with increasing regularity straight to France, which had a state monopoly system that accepted lower quality tobacco in exchange for the ability to buy in bulk. Such a system of increasing indebtedness didn't matter too much in a growing market; planters could simply buy more slaves to increase the productivity of their lands. However, an economic depression developed in the

1720s and, as it got worse, wealthier planters became increasingly keen to differentiate themselves from the others by ensuring the effective monitoring of all exported tobacco. A warehouse-based Inspection Act, introduced in 1730, was intended to limit exported tobacco to stuff that was "good, sound, well-conditioned, and merchantable, and free from trash, sand, and dirt". The notes given to planters whose tobacco passed these stringent inspections could be used as legal tender to pay taxes and debts, while unsuitable tobacco was burnt.[83] The net effect of the Act was to increase dissent and dissatisfaction amongst those unable to meet the exacting standards, leading to a series of 'tobacco riots' where warehouses across Virginia were razed to the ground.

There were other sorts of resistance to the productive power of tobacco. A US writer wrote of tobacco in 1773 that "our staple commodity, seems completely adapted for restraining the Progress of Population, and of natural Wealth; as it is a mere Luxury, affords no Aliment, extremely impoverishes the Soil, and requires considerable Extent for it[s] Cultivation".[84] A sense was developing that tobacco was a plant of colonialism. Resentment amongst the plantocracy about their indebted status contributed to the forging of emergent ideas of freedom and independence that helped fuel the American Revolution. In 1791, a report to President George Washington stated "people are generally exchanging tobacco for wheat; I flatter myself the face of our Country will soon assume an appearance that will not only do honor to our climate but ourselves".[85]

King's Pipes, state of tobacco and tobacco state

Efforts by the North American planters to maintain production standards and hence their wealth were mirrored at national level in Britain. We saw in Chapter 3 how quickly a nation could become fiscally dependent on tobacco, regardless of its leaders' views about tobacco use. Once it arrived on British shores, tobacco became enmeshed with the growing physical, state and economic structures created to deal with the burgeoning transatlantic colonial trade. English customs duties on tobacco increased from 2 to 5 pence in 1685. The need to maximize the revenue from tobacco accruing to the public purse was paramount. Acts could be passed by Parliament, but much of the day-to-day organization of the trade and interpretation of the Acts took place through the office of the Commissioners for Trade and Plantations in London. They adjudicated disputes and requests from merchants concerning practical issues in the tobacco trade, such as standardizing the size of barrels used.[86]

There was a problem with maintaining the quality of tobacco reaching Britain and what the Commissioners should do with damaged or spoiled tobacco, or tobacco which was seized as contraband. Transportation was not reliable, and a significant proportion of the tobacco that arrived in Britain from the colonies had started to rot. One option that was tried was to sell damaged tobacco at public auction, but poor quality tobacco brought down prices overall and the Virginia planters, whose profits were already reduced due to the War of Spanish Succession (1701-14), felt their livelihoods threatened. Furthermore, with no provision made to destroy damaged tobacco, a commonly executed fraud involved declaring tobacco unfit for human consumption intentionally in order to avoid paying customs' duties. Destroying inferior tobacco, in order to keep the quality and costs of what was legally sold high, was as advantageous to the state as it was to the Virginia planters. A British law enacted in 1714 thus required all damaged and seized consignments of smuggled tobacco to be burnt, to prevent either from re-entering the market without duty.[87]

In London, a 'Tobacco Burning Ground' was set up at Rotherhithe on ground leased from the Duke of Bedford. An inspector appointed in 1717 was expected to "give constant attendance there, and take care that the watchmen do their duty".[88] Whitehaven built a pipe, which came to be known as 'The King's Pipe', on an isolated hill to the north of the town.[89] Falmouth in Cornwall also constructed a pipe, its position facing seaward, intended to signal to the maritime community the controlling power of the state over trade.[90] Such was the strength of this association in people's minds that "if smoke was seen billowing from the pipe, it was commonly said that 'The king is having a smoke today'".[91] The contrast with the political symbolism of the 17th century and King James' *Counterblaste* could not have been more stark – although it was James I himself who had started the process of extracting revenue for the state from tobacco (Chapter 3).

Liverpool did not fare as well as London, Whitehaven and Falmouth, however. In 1715, one Mr Moorecroft, landlord of the Custom House on the dockside, was presented at the "poomoot" court (predecessor of the magistrate's court) for having recently erected a tobacco pipe "to the manifest prejudice of the Town".[92] In what might be interpreted as a kind of spectral revenge for the source of their wealth, it continued to cause great distress to the inhabitants of some of Liverpool's most affluent streets and squares for 70 years. In 1784, for example, when a large import of damaged tobacco was being burnt, petitioners to the Customs Board complained that

> the volumes of dense smoak which issue from this chimney cloud the streets to the annoyance of all passengers and fill the rooms of every house in the line of its direction to a degree perfectly offensive and intolerable.[93]

Their chief concerns were that, should the nuisance remain:

> Our Lands and Houses must sink in value, within the reach of the Smoak the Furniture of our Houses is spoiled, Life is rendered comfortless to all, many are afflicted with Sore Eyes and only the young and Healthy at some times can breathe.[94]

Three years later, though, little appears to have been done. The junior mayor of Liverpool and 35 other gentlemen wrote to the Customs Office in London requesting again that "a proper building for that purpose to be erected in a more convenient situation". While in their view, "everything has been done by him [the Controller], which human invention can devise", wind direction and strength make the tobacco pipe a "Nuisance beyond human prevention". They complained how "for above three weeks past this smoke has particularly tormented several of us, and filled the houses, day and night within the direction of it, from the Garrets to the Cellars, with Clouds of dank Smoke in every respect intolerably offensive". They bemoaned the competition between revenues and their personal comfort, and prayed "you will not only order the Building to be erected elsewhere, but forbid the burning of any more Tobacco within the Custom House Yard". Yet clearly at some point the hand of the customs' office was forced, because the remains of a King's Pipe today is at Stanley Dock, some two miles north of the old Customs' House. It was apparently rebuilt there sometime in the early decades of the 19th century.

Conclusion

This chapter has charted the increasing shape-shifting of tobacco in the 18th century, reflected in the refinement and gentility associated with the use of snuff. We can see tobacco's power reflected in many of the writings, artefacts and architectural legacies of the time. The subjugation of Nature and its bounty – supported by a humanist Enlightenment philosophy that put a certain type of aristocratic white male very much in the driving seat of history – proceeded hand-in-hand with the dominion over certain types of people, who became commodities just like tobacco appeared to be. Plantation agriculture in the USA is remarkable for the subjugation of successive types of people – 'Indians', women, indentured servants and slaves – a sequence following on from tobacco's transformation from a colonial plant to a globally traded commodity. Dependencies of a different sort were evident in various English sea ports where the need to maintain state control over the quality of tobacco was reflected in the building of numerous 'King's Pipes' which 'smoked' in order to dispose of spoiled tobacco or tobacco on which excise duty had not been paid. In the course of these developments, unlike the 'things' that became favoured with speech in 18th century English literature as if participating in a multinatural universe, tobacco, mysteriously, went silent. Perhaps it did not need a voice – its power and position, quite literally, went without saying. Perhaps it was a source of embarrassment to its literary adherents who were delighted to let other things speak, scurrilously and in a jocular fashion. Yet tobacco had further to go in establishing world domination. The next chapter looks at what happened in literature and life in the 19th century, when snuff became superseded by the power of the cigar.

Notes

1 Viveiros de Castro (2012b: 46n1).
2 Greenblatt paraphrases Lucretius as follows: "there is no master plan, no divine
   architect, no intelligent design…There is no reason to think that the earth or its
   inhabitants occupy a central place, no reason to set humans apart from all other
   animals, no hope of bribing or appeasing the gods, no place for religious
   fanaticism, no call for ascetic self-denial, no justification for dreams of limitless
   power or perfect security, no rationale for wars of conquest or self-aggrandize-
   ment, no possibility of triumphing over nature, no escape from the constant
   making and unmaking and remaking of forms" (2011: 5).
3 Locke (1690, Section 4.3.6).
4 Nowka (2006: 26).
5 Nowka (2006: 59).
6 Bentley (1692: 13).
7 Holbraad (2011: 12).
8 In this he is taking his cue from Spivak (1988)'s "Can the subaltern speak?"
9 Nowka (2006: 7).
10 Douglas (2007: 147).
11 Bellamy (2007).
12 Nowka (2006). An example is provided by Pickering: "scientists maneuver in a
    field of material agency, constructing machines that … variously capture, seduce,
    download, recruit, enroll, or materialize that agency" (Pickering, 1995).
13 Bellamy (2007: 118).
14 Lynch (1998: 96).
15 Flint (2007).
16 Whif (1788).
17 There are shades in Memoria's remarks of a South American Tupi myth on the
    origins of the night, which was preceded by a time when in was daylight all the
    time and "everything had the power of speech", including, we assume, tobacco
    (Lévi-Strauss, 1973: 417).
18 Smart (1752: 211-13) The poem is titled 'The Bag-Wig and the Tobacco-Pipe: A
    Fable'.
19 Addison (1716: 243).
20 Price (1964: 497).
21 Anon. (1736).
22 Anon. (1725: 154).
23 Erskine (1870).
24 Johnson (1779: 10).
25 Philips (1736: 9-23) 'An Ode to Henry St. John, Esq.'. The poem was originally
    written in Latin, in partial imitation of Horace, but was translated into English
    and published with a prefatory letter by Thomas Newcomb.
26 Griffin (2004).
27 Cowper (1995).
28 Browne (1736).
29 Italics original. For more on the poetics of 18th century tobacco, see Williams
    (2011).
30 Bach wrote a poem about smoking which has a melancholy tone to it, meditating
    on the parallels between him and his clay pipe, both of which will one day return
    to the earth. The tobacco it contains will likewise turn to ash, and his body to
    dust. He sees the fruitful meditation his pipe-smoking engenders as akin to
    worshipping god.
31 Quoted in Karhausen (2011: 253).

32 Anon. (1736: 111-14).
33 Porter (2003: 24).
34 Ibid. (26).
35 Reid (2005: 170).
36 "Le Bon usage du Tabac en Poudre" (1700) quoted in Schivelbusch (1992: 131).
37 "'On the great Mode of Snuff taking", *The Poetical Courant*, no. 6 (2 March 1706: n.p.).
38 "The Foppish Mode of Taking Snuff", in *Whipping Tom: or, a Rod for a Proud Lady*, 4th ed. (London, 1722: 8–10).
39 Schivelbusch (1992).
40 Or human society becoming more like apes, a point made by Norton (2008: 191-2).
41 'Hail Indian Plant', in *The London Medley* (London, 1731: 8–9).
42 Anon. (1732: 38).
43 Schivelbusch (1980: 146).
44 Withey (2014).
45 Arbuckle (1719: 28).
46 Ibid. (6).
47 Short (1750: 250).
48 Soto (2009) points out that England/Britain was at war for about half the 18th century. Customs duties on tobacco fluctuated, while excise duties (on domestically manufactured tobacco products) rose substantially during this period. See also Price (2007).
49 Goodman (1993: 170).
50 Breen (1985: 57).
51 Hahn (2011: 20).
52 According to Walsh (2001: 144), 90 per cent of Chesapeake slaves were shipped from Africa, either directly or via the Caribbean.
53 Think of James I's derogatory remarks about the "slavish Indians" (Chapter 3), their enslavement to the Spaniards being regarded by him as further evidence of their "beastly" natures.
54 Fox (2015: 80).
55 See Klein et al. (2001) for further detail on variations in mortality statistics.
56 Kulikoff (1986).
57 Wertenbacker (1922: 131).
58 Sainsbury (1880), cited (as Saintsbury) in Dresser (2001: 7).
59 Williams (1964).
60 Jones (1724), quoted (as James) in Dresser (2001: 41 fn 32).
61 Morgan (1998: 191).
62 Other jurisdictions based on slavery that are often listed include the Kong Empire, the Imamates of Futas Jallon and Toro, the Kingdoms of Koya, Khasso and Kaabu, and the Fante and Aro Confederacies.
63 Guasco (2014).
64 Dresser (2001: 9).
65 Molineux (2007: 330 fn 5).
66 Molineux (2007: 333).
67 See, for example, Dresser (2001) on Bristol.
68 Creighton (2008: 21, 11).
69 Rhodes (2003: 84).
70 A picture and account of the 'Pipe:Rifle' can be seen at https://www.metmuseum.org/art/collection/search/310440
71 Shaw, R. (2002).
72 Gilmore et al. (2015).
73 Breen (1985: 61).

74 Breen (1985: 58).
75 Tatham (1800: 184).
76 Breen (1985: 35).
77 English snobbery remained, however. One visitor in 1736 expressed shock at how "every considerable Man Keeps an Equipage [team of horses], tho' they have no Concern about the different Colours of their Coach Horses, driving frequently black, white, and chestnut, in the same Harness" (quoted in Breen 1985: 37).
78 Dresser (2001); Baptist (2014: xix); Yuhl (2013).
79 John Wayles quoted in Breen (1985: 131).
80 Thomas Jefferson was amongst those planters opposed to slavery for this reason (Breen 1985: 132).
81 Breen (1985: 196).
82 Devine (1975: 60).
83 Kulikoff (1986: 110).
84 Breen (1985: 200).
85 Stuart quoted in Breen (1985: 205).
86 For example, tobacco was carried in large barrels called hogsheads, but Maryland hogsheads were 48 inches long and 32 inches in diameter across their lids, significantly larger than the Virginia ones, a challenge for the Commissioners for Trade and Plantations to resolve.
87 The law also called for a public spectacle to be made of the destruction of the smugglers' assets. From 1746, when smuggling became a capital offence, the public spectacle became the execution of smugglers themselves.
88 Willis (2009: 63).
89 Rideout (n.d.).
90 Willis (2009).
91 Ibid. (60).
92 Rideout (n.d.).
93 Ibid.
94 Ibid. This is also quoted by Willis (2009: 58).

Chapter 6

Vogue: tobacco worlds in 19th century Europe

Introduction: the age of diversification

Tobacco became increasingly diversified and commercialized during the 19th century, a process that culminated in it becoming incorporated (literally) by the formation of companies that were to become increasingly global tobacco corporations. I argue for the importance of material factors in the spread of tobacco; qualities deriving from the material agency of the plant itself in hybrid relations with its human associates and the expanse of non-human worlds this generated. The material subjects discussed in the first half of this chapter are cigars, chewing, and pipe tobacco. They index an era of diversification in their own right, but other major changes were afoot in the realm of tobacco paraphernalia and the development of brands that had profound implications for the commercialization of tobacco in the 19th century. I shall encapsulate all these under the heading 'Material worlds'.

However, there are worlds other than those of material tobacco to consider. The section on tobacco hybrids looks at the continuing theme of tobacco in people's inner lives and creativity. As in previous chapters, an ethnographic approach explores the existing and emergent worlds that tobacco's non-human/human relationships created in and outside Europe at this time. It is an approach that incorporates arts and literature as well as semiotic and structural analyses in coming to an understanding of tobacco as agent, so vibrant indeed that it speaks in the ephemeral forms of smoke and cigar. 'Tobacco and the colonial encounter' offers another example of the role of tobacco in transgressing boundaries between 'human' and 'non-human', 'subject' and 'object' in the objectification and commodification of the person. In Chapter 5 this was slavery; in this Chapter it is the use of tobacco as a 'drug food' amongst so-called 'native populations' in the colonial domain. The importance of tobacco in missionary life is particularly interesting in this regard; another underexplored way in which tobacco shaped and reinforced human power relations. Meanwhile, 'Objecting to tobacco' looks at the discordant mix that was the anti-tobacco movement during the 19th century.

The impact of the Bonsack machine in reducing the price and increasing the volume of cigarettes in an exponential way is the subject of the second half of this chapter. One of the worlds thus created is that of the tobacco corporation. Our stories shift back across the Atlantic from W.D. and H.O. Wills in the UK to 'Buck Duke' and the American Tobacco Corporation, formed in Durham, North Carolina, in 1890, and the tobacco corporation 'par excellence' with global implications.

Material worlds of the 19th century

If the 18th century was the century for snuff, "the 19th was the era of the cigar".[1] In the United States, meanwhile, chewing tobacco held sway. A diversity of technologies and techniques preceded the development of the cigarette as a machine-made commodity, discussed in the second half of this chapter. Meanwhile, the development of branding gave tobacco fresh opportunities to become embodied in named physical products that required no necessary connection to the physical reality of their contents. Tobacco spearheaded this transformation in the methods of retailing.

The age of the cigar

Cigars were the first method of tobacco consumption that Europeans encountered in their New World forays.[2] After tobacco's initial crossing of the Atlantic from Mexico to Spain, cigars were manufactured in Cadiz and latterly Seville. Yet the spread of tobacco in this form elsewhere in Europe was relatively slow. According to Ortiz, "it was. . .after the conquest of Havana by the English in 1762, that Havana cigars set out to conquer the world".[3] A cigar factory was established in Hamburg by H.H. Schlottmann in 1788 and cigars became especially popular in Germany. Soldiers returning to other parts of Europe from the Peninsular War in Spain[4] brought cigars with them that they had encountered there, while "the Duke of Wellington's triumphal return from Waterloo [in 1815] was a triumph also for the cigar".[5] Originally nicknamed 'the Spanish vice', their use in Britain increased exponentially in the first half of the 19th century, rekindling some old debates about the moral and physical effects of both snuff and smoking.[6] The labouring classes went on with their clay pipe smoking (and snuff when they could get it) pretty much as they always had, men and women alike; only in more genteel circles was there stronger differentiation of tobacco use by gender, with women almost invariably discouraged from smoking compared to men.

Chewing tobacco

The situation in the United States was somewhat different. Yankee soldiers had participated in the battle for Havana and brought cigars home with them, too. But chewing tobacco was a far more important form of tobacco consumption in the US. Charles Dickens, visiting Washington in 1842, disparagingly called it "the head quarters of tobacco-tinctured saliva".[7] Gately cautions that "some of his prejudice resulted from falling out of his bunk on a canal boat into a pool of tobacco spit",[8] but Dickens found "the prevalence of those two odious practices of chewing and expectorating...soon became most offensive and sickening".[9] He went on,

> In all the public places of America, this filthy custom is recognised. In the courts of law, the judge has his spittoon, the crier his, the witness his, and the prisoner his; while the jurymen and spectators are provided for, as so many men who in the course of nature must desire to spit incessantly. In the hospitals, the students of medicine are requested by notices upon the wall, to eject their tobacco juice into the boxes provided for that purpose, and not to discolour the stairs. In public buildings, visitors are implored, through the same agency, to squirt the essence of their quids, or "plugs", as I have heard them called by gentlemen learned in this kind of sweetmeat, into the national spittoons, and not about the bases of the marble columns...The thing itself is an exaggeration of nastiness, which cannot be outdone.[10]

Diversified paraphernalia

Tobacco paraphernalia – things and technologies associated with both pro-duction and consumption of tobacco, continued to diversify during the 19th century. The friction match, invented by a chemist in the northern English town of Stockton-on-Tees in 1824,[11] was exploited commercially in London from 1832 onwards by a firm that became known as Bryant and May. Matches made it easier for tobacco to be kept alight in smokers' pipes and to light up other forms of smoked tobacco products. Better tobacco processing machinery was needed to keep up with the advances in market-ing and transportation that took place from the 1850s onwards. A new kind of cutting machine was introduced in 1853, and a packaging machine followed soon after. Briar pipes, originally made from highly resilient gorse root, were introduced from the late 1850s and started to replace the traditional clay; vulcanite mouthpieces were added in 1878. Human tastes for tobacco were also shifting from the stronger shags and roll tobaccos to the milder Virginias that had always been more popular in London. Tobacco smoking was becoming more acceptable, particularly amongst the middle and upper classes; as it did so, demand for smoking apparel – jackets and caps – increased. On the railways, smoking carriages were introduced for gentlemen in 1868.[12]

Cigarettes

Cigarettes, complementing pipes, snuff and cigars, probably first came into England in the late 1840s, with a few manufacturers taking up their production, by hand, in small quantities.[13] Cigarettes gained some popularity amongst British soldiers who had seen Turkish soldiers using them during the Crimean War (1854-56). A number of cigarette makers from eastern and south-eastern Europe migrated to Britain after this time.[14] However, cigarettes had only novelty appeal at first, as the most commonly used dark air- and fire-cured tobaccos tended to be too strong for them. Not even the arrival of cigarettes made from best quality Turkish tobaccos and with fine textured paper managed to capture the market, despite their exotic, aromatic flavour. Flue curing, involving heat without smoke, permitted the production of a different kind of leaf, popularly known as Virginia Bright, which was milder, more acidic and with relatively less nicotine. This came into Britain in the late 1860s, and was taken up by the Bristol-based firm W.D. and H.O. Wills and other manufacturers. Virginia bright was perfect for the cigarette, as it permitted the option of inhaling.

Tobacco brands and their implications

Changes were also afoot in the marketing and distribution of tobacco. On New Year's Day, 1847, Wills pioneered giving brand names to some of its products. Two of the firm's cut tobaccos were initially introduced and marketed in branded form – Best Bird's Eye and Bishop Blaze.[15] Some snuff products had previously been branded, but with the aim of making them more exclusive rather than for mass consumption. The idea of branding products to make them objects of mass consumption was a novelty. While some ancillary materialities went hand-in-hand with branding, such as the development of packaging to preserve the quality of tobacco,[16] the basic intent of companies like Wills was to appeal directly to consumers and escape the 'middleman' role of the shopkeeper. Tobacconists had been amongst the earliest examples of specialization in retailing, one that was "based on tobacconists' expertise in blending tobaccos and snuffs to meet local tastes, and bore no relation to selling standardized products to a mass market",[17] and required "forging personal relationships with one's customers".[18] The introduction of branding for tobacco products, however, meant "the guarantee of quality now came from the product, not the assurance of the retailer".[19] In a manner reminiscent of Ingold's description of the imagination becoming cut adrift from its earthly mooring (Chapter 4), tobacco was free to adopt a myriad of forms, the meaning of which "no longer had to be communicated by word of mouth but was, instead, embodied within the physical product itself".[20] Initially, brands matched different consumer groups in British society, but in due course, as they were promoted in new ways, they structured the consumption patterns of society itself.[21] Tobacco's reach and diversity increased exponentially through such means.

Wills' innovative marketing strategies included exclusive deals with 'sole dealers', direct advertising through show cards and ordinary packet labels, and advertising in local newspapers. As trade expanded, the necessity to protect their brands with a 'house' trade mark (a star) became apparent. Branding, and the associated relationship evoked with the customer, became more popular amongst many branches of commerce in the 1870s. As disputes arose between firms concerning particular brand names or designs, the Trade Marks Act was passed in 1875, giving firms the exclusive right to registered trademarks by law. The first manufactured cigarettes in the UK, with the brand name 'Bristol', were made by hand in W.D. and H.O. Wills' London factory in 1871.[22]

Early brands drew strongly on literary associations such as 'Three Castles'[23] ("There's no sweeter tobacco comes from Virginia, and no better brand than the Three Castles" from Thackeray's *The Virginians*) and 'Westward Ho!' ("When all things were made, none was made better than Tobacco, to be a lone man's Companion, a bachelor's friend, a hungry man's Food, a sad man's Cordial, a wakeful man's Sleep, and a chilly man's Fire. There is no herb like it under the Canopy of Heaven", Charles Kingsley). This blending of literary and marketing techniques was taken to a new level by the Cope's company in Liverpool. Cope brothers began manufacturing cigars in 1848; by 1876 their factory employed around 2,000 workers, 1,500 of them women, and produced around 36 million cigars annually. The printing and lithographic office began producing *Cope's Tobacco Plant*, a monthly journal with the motto "Tobacco; all about Tobacco, and nothing but Tobacco", in 1870. It contained a miscellany of literature about tobacco, including some commissioned works. One of the contributors, James Thomson, described it as "one of the most daring and original publications of the day, a periodical which actually loves literature, though it has to make this subordinate to the Herb Divine".[24]

Tobacco thus became both the subject and object of print media. For Thomson, his

> love of literature was almost equalled by his love of smoking, so the task of writing for the Tobacco Plant was a thoroughly congenial one. Thomson himself declared that "I have not had to violate my conscience by writing what I don't believe, for I *do* believe in Tobacco".[25]

There were plenty of advertisements for Cope's products in this publication. The articles it contained came from a range of sources and were extensively recycled in a variety of different formats. One of the *Cope's Smoke Room Booklets*, published between 1890 and 1894, attempted to reproduce a guide to John Ruskin's *Fors Clavigera*. It had to be withdrawn when Ruskin (a non-smoker) sued for copyright infringement.

Tobacco hybrids in the 19th century

With some notable exceptions,[26] tobacco assumed powerful bonds in male political, scientific, literary and artistic circles across 19th century Europe. Napoleon was never without his snuff box on the battlefield. Bismarck argued that a man should not think of dying before having imbibed at least 5,000 bottles of champagne and 20 times that number of cigars.[27] General Gordon of Khartoum ended his days chain-smoking "fat cigarettes, rolled by a *cavasse* standing behind his chair with one ready to slip between his fingers when he silently held up a hand for it".[28] As Sudan fell to the Mahdi and the rebel hosts closed in on Khartoum, Gordon continued his habit. "The day before his death he sat all day in his palace, and then on till midnight, smoking".[29] Charles Darwin learned to take snuff while a student at Edinburgh University, and to smoke while working with gauchos in South America. He carried on smoking only when resting, but used snuff for its stimulating qualities during working hours – indeed, he wrote in a letter after giving up for a month that he felt "most lethargic, stupid and melancholy".[30] Sometimes he kept his snuff jar outside his study. This, he felt, served to curb any over-indulgence, since he had to stand up and go out to get a pinch.

Marx and Engels were both enthusiastic smokers and tobacco arguably played a big part in the formulation of Marx's ideas. "*Capital* will not even pay for the cigars I smoked writing it",[31] he reported to his son-in-law. Perhaps the influence of tobacco can be found in his strong belief in the apparently magical power of things. Just as 'primitive' people were said to attribute mystical powers to objects such as stones, wood carvings or weapons, so were economists motivated by a belief that spirits lurk in physical currency and move markets by magic – mysterious forces beyond human control. The elaborate symbol systems they used, such as money, debt, property rights, and prices meant they could conveniently ignore the labour that produced commodities, and hence the nature of the profit through which a small class of property owners acquired political and economic dominance through selling them. "A commodity appears, at first sight, a very trivial thing, and easily understood. Its analysis shows that it is, in reality, a very strange thing, abounding in metaphysical subtleties and theological niceties", he wrote.[32]

Marx's particular contribution was 'commodity fetishism'; how commodities were "like gods" with mystical, spectral, magical powers that lie outwith concrete experience – things created by people, but an alien force which rules people's lives. Thus, a table, once it has passed out of the carpenter's hand and become a commodity, "changes into a thing which transcends sensuousness. It not only stands with its feet on the ground, but, in relation to all other commodities, it stands on its head, and evolves out of its wooden brain grotesque ideas, far more wonderful than if it were to begin dancing of its own free will".[33] There is an element of 'tongue-in-cheek' humour in Marx's account (his description owed much to the 'table turning' séances that were all the rage amongst some sections of Victorian society),[34] but Marx would accept, as Willburn puts it, that just as "subjects might become objectified, commodities might become subjectified".[35] The parallels with the 'it-narratives' of the 18th century are obvious.

Marx should be considered in conjunction with his colleague and collaborator, Friedrich Engels. Engels edited all but the first volume of *Capital*, which entailed considerable eyestrain. However, he attributed his ocular problems to excessive fertilizer use in the tobacco fields from which his cigars originated, and switched to other brands. Two years later, having been able to smoke only a gram of tobacco every other day, Engels decided to take a summer break by the seaside (Eastbourne on the south coast of England was a favoured haunt). He wanted to regain his health sufficiently that he might once again smoke a cigar, something he had not done for two months.[36]

Other European countries shared the vogue for tobacco. Coleridge wrote in 1799 to his wife from Ratzeburg in Germany that "a common amusement at the German Universities is for a number of young men to smoke out a candle! That is, to fill a room with tobacco smoke till the candle goes out",[37] while in France the motto of a Parisian journal devoted to smoking was "*qui fume prie*", ("smoking is praying").[38] The French writer Baudelaire wrote a poem in the voice of his pipe: "I am an author's pipe; from contemplating my Abyssinian or Kaffir appearance one sees that my master is a mighty smoker. When he is sorrowful I smoke like a chimney where food is prepared for the labourer's return. I wrap up and cradle his soul in the wafting blue smoke which rises from my lit mouth, and spin a powerful balm which charms his heart and heals his spirit from its exertions".[39]

Tobacco speaks as smoke and cigar

The 'Pre-Raphaelite Brotherhood' (PRB) were a group of British artists and literati deeply committed to the experiential life,[40] although concerns about mechanization and industrialization, the effects of its "vomiting smokestacks" on Nature, led some of them to develop a more ambivalent relationship to tobacco and its smoke than many other artists and writers of the time. The 'it-narrative' tradition (Chapter 5) found continued expression in their number. John Tupper, a respected poet and artist, wrote a poem for their mouthpiece journal *The Germ* in the voice of tobacco smoke which reflects Victorian preoccupations not only with smoke/death but with the supernatural/the afterlife. "I am king of the *Cadaverals*,/I'm *Spectral* President. . .- Look at me and you shall see/The ghastliest of the ghastly".[41] Other members of the PRB continued a tradition of attending to detail and 'truth to Nature' deriving from Dutch still-life paintings and the 18th century English 'poetry of attention' (Chapter 4). All these, I suggest, are tobacco-inspired.

The PRB was criticized by Robert Buchanan, himself no stranger to tobacco, as made up of "Fleshly Poets", "young gentlemen with animal faculties morbidly developed by too much tobacco and too little exercise".[42] One of the leaders of the group, D.G. Rossetti, was delighted to visit Alfred, Lord Tennyson and find his hero was not "more partial to tobacco than I already was, and have since then increasingly continued".[43] It is perhaps not a complete coincidence that Rossetti, with his love of nicotine, has been described by one critic as "better able than any poet since Keats to identify himself with the physical reality of the object he chose to portray. His insistence that art demanded 'an inner standing-point' must surely have implied a willingness to suspend judgment, to grasp his subject dramatically on its own terms".[44]

Tobacco speaks again in *Chambers' Journal*, as a cigar who explains to its readers the distinguishing characteristics of tobaccos around the world. The American branch of the family is "supposed to be the best", while Brazilian tobacco "is a very short scrappy-looking leaf...covered with the sands of the plains". Havana "is unquestionably our ancestral seat; the heads of our family there reside, respected and esteemed, and emitting a most agreeable odour". Turkish tobacco is brightly coloured, sweet-tasting but weak, while Latakian is "aristocratic, enervated, [and] listless". Holland is "respectable", Java "volcanic", and German "a poor relation whom we are loath to own, with a most prolific growth – which poor relations always have". There is also some knowing commentary on how "boxes, brands, and labels are all imitated, or made up by the junior clerks out of the Spanish dictionary", and how "there is quite a Borgia system of poisoning administered to the British public, under pretence of the pipe of peace".[45]

Like travel guides, which were becoming equally popular in this period, this kind of didactic narrative aims at preventing a male reader becoming the victim of "some adulterated fraud cast upon him by a market which had identified him as an easy, ill-informed dupe".[46] The narrative ends back at the "very private, self-indulgent form of consumption" which the public face of the male role is intended to sublimate. Knowledge and satisfaction meld in the final sentences with the author "joining the reader and lighting one up themselves".[47] For the talking cigar, however, the narrator joins the reader only to be consumed by him: "Alas, alas I am in the hands of a purchaser; it is well that my story is told; for my existence will be but for a few minutes longer, and then my ashes will be scattered on the winds!"[48] As well as turning the reader into a knowledgeable, competent male, these accounts transform tobacco from object and passive commodity into humanized subject, animated and empowered by its hybrid relationship with those who consume or otherwise become entangled with it. The reader, meanwhile, is stilled, rooted to his armchair from whence he can be "an 'ardent votary', a worshipper, disciple and true friend of 'the divine lady nicotine'".[49]

Tobacco and creativity

The mobilization of tobacco for creative purposes continues a common theme amongst writers and musicians into the 19th century. The disengagement of the senses and stimulus to the imagination provided by the Nicotian muse was praised by the American poet James Russell Lowell:

> The unspoken thought thou canst divine;
> Thou fill'st the pauses of the speech
> With whispers that to dreamland reach,
> And frozen fancy-springs unchain
> In Arctic outskirts of the brain.[50]

Nineteenth-century composers who used tobacco to help thaw the "Arctic outskirts" of their brains included Schubert (pipe), Schumann (cigar) and Wagner (snuff). Carlyle, Dickens, Thackeray, Tennyson and Kingsley all "extolled the virtues and delights of smoking".[51] Only Thomas Hardy of the Victorian 'greats' was an abstainer, and smoking is rarely to be found in his novels.[52]

J.M. Barrie is perhaps the iconic English Victorian male writer on tobacco. In 33 essays in the *St James' Gazette*, he paid homage to smoking and addressed some of the arduous problems involved in giving up. These were compiled into a collection, *My Lady Nicotine*, published in 1890. The materiality of smoking and its paraphernalia is heralded by chapters with headings like 'My Pipes', 'My Tobacco Pouch', 'My Smoking Table' (as well as 'The Grandest Scene in History', mentioned in Chapter 3). There is even a chapter written in the voice of a rose used as a buttonhole during an unsuccessful courtship, the wire surround of which eventually – and symbolically – becomes used as a pipe cleaner. The choice of an ideal blended pipe tobacco (in his case, 'The Arcadia Mix') was also a serious business, not to be divulged lightly since to do so "would be as rash as proposing a man with whom I am unacquainted for my club. You may not be worthy to smoke the Arcadia mix".[53] The responsibility of introducing one to the mixture was also great, since:

> This mixture has an extraordinary effect upon character, and probably you want to remain as you are. Before I discovered Arcadia, and communicated it to the other five…we had all distinct individualities, but now, except in appearance – and the Arcadia even tells on that – we are as like as holly-leaves. We have the same habits, the same ways of looking at things, the same satisfaction in each other…when we are together we are only to be distinguished by our pipes.[54]

This is camaraderie, common perspectives and identity forged by, with and through a particular tobacco mixture. Barrie continues about his smoking companions that "any one of us in the company of persons who smoke other tobaccos would be considered highly original".[55]

Tobacco features in 49 of the 60 cases of Sherlock Holmes.[56] "Tobacco simultaneously frees Holmes's mind to soar and encages him in the armchair, where nicotine in the blood will supply the answers he seeks", writes one critic, describing Holmes as "part genius, part nicotine junkie".[57] "What are you going to do, then?" asks Dr. Watson when *The Red-headed League* case appears intractable. "To smoke", answers Holmes "...it is quite a three pipe problem". Meanwhile in *The Man with the Twisted Lip*, Holmes "sits cross-legged all night on an Eastern divan, smoking an entire ounce of strong shag tobacco".[58] Watson's description of Holmes as a "self-poisoner by cocaine and tobacco" is tempered as their adventures develop and tobacco becomes the mediator for the solution of great mysteries. Holmes' "ratiocinations" are based on astute, empirical observations; he is in many ways the apogee of the empirical, attentive, Enlightenment scientist for whom, rather like Bacon (Chapter 4), nature is the source of 'data' to solve 'cases'.

It is not only literary detective work that reveals tobacco's mediatory role in creativity, however. The Edwardian composer Edward Elgar was relaxing at his piano with a cigar after a tiring day travelling around giving violin lessons in October 1898.

> In a little while, soothed and feeling rested, I began to play, and suddenly my wife interrupted by saying "Edward, that's a good tune". I awoke from the dream: "Eh! tune, what tune!" And she said "Play it again, I like that tune". I played and strummed, and played, and then she exclaimed: "That's the tune".

The result was the Enigma Variations.[59]

Tobacco and the colonial encounter

Tobacco was more than a matter of consumption and gentlemanly finesse in the imperial heartlands, however. It is perhaps a measure of how much tobacco was equated with modernity that European explorers, missionaries and colonialists were often surprised to find that tobacco had reached their destinations before them, in ignorance of the strong direct trade there had been between Bahia in Brazil and southern Africa since the 17th century, for example.[60] David Livingstone, exploring in what is now Zimbabwe in 1860, wrote "large quantities of tobacco are raised on the lower banks of the Zambezi during the winter months, and the people are perhaps the most inveterate smokers in the world". He goes on to describe what the people he encountered think "is an improved method for smoking. They take a whiff, puff out the grosser smoke; then, by a sudden inhalation contrive to catch and swallow, as they say, the real essence, the very spirit of tobacco, which in the ordinary way is lost". Livingstone goes on to describe how

> Batoka tobacco is famed in the country for its strength, and it certainly is both very strong and very cheap: a few strings of beads will purchase enough to last any reasonable man for six months. It caused headache in the only smoker of our party, from its strength; but this quality makes the natives come great distances to buy it".[61]

It is perhaps significant to note, given the claimed ubiquity of tobacco in the Victorian novel,[62] that only one man in Livingstone's party was actually a smoker.

In central New Guinea, an explorer observed the Motu people's behaviour regarding tobacco. The Motu word for tobacco was *kuku* and people

> would pawn their very clothes for it if they wore any...I never knew a people so fearfully fond of this weed. *Kuku* is their god, whom alone they worship and adore. The word *kuku* escapes their lips more than any other in the course of the day, and is ever in their thoughts. Its praises are sung in their *hehonis*, or night-chants, and your health is smoked with it in the day time...It is the cause of joy, the cause of sorrow, the cause of friendship, the cause of enmity, the cause of content, and the cause of discontent.[63]

Tobacco as 'drug food'

Both Batoka tobacco and *kuku* (above) have acculturated well. Yet while it may be ethnographically captivating to encounter the "very spirit of tobacco" in vignettes such as these, they are not necessarily the most important or historically informed stories about tobacco in the colonial world. The slave economy continued to develop on the eastern seaboard of the US and elsewhere into the 19th century. Production methods – one of the contexts the tobacco world engendered – were part of Chapter 5. Here, the focus is on what tobacco did in terms of generating a "psychoactive revolution" and its role as a "drug food"[64] in stabilizing the colonized-colonizer relationship more generally and the nascent forms of European capitalism this permitted.[65] A 'drug food' was a substance which could be used to encourage and, subsequently, through the chemical dependency it fostered, compel native populations to undertake new forms of labour when the population in question neither needed nor embraced the established status symbols of the colonial order. Tobacco was ideal for such a task, since it stimulated cortical alertness without hallucinations, while engendering a high degree of dependency. Tobacco was frequently sold to establish economic relations and dependencies with native peoples (irrespective of whether they had a tobacco culture or economy already).

Tobacco shapes missionary work

Tobacco was popular in missionary work. "They are beginning to learn the use of tobacco" wrote one Anglican missionary of the inhabitants of a village in what is now eastern Papua New Guinea in 1890. Tobacco most probably first came into the north and south coasts of New Guinea in the early 1600s, via ancient trade routes dating back at least 5,000 years.[66] However, the European colonists and missionaries who began arriving in large numbers towards the end of the nineteenth century were largely ignorant of this extensive trading history. This, and the myths that were related by some of the New Guineans concerning indigenous tobacco and ancient culture heroes, led to the erroneous assumption that the tobacco being cultivated and used was native to the region.[67] In fact, the introduction of 'twist' or 'trade' tobacco "provided the Europeans with a means by which to manipulate indigenous populations to engage in new work activities".[68] 'Twist' was "an addictive American commercial product consisting of cured tobacco twisted into 'sticks' and often soaked in molasses".[69] These sticks became a currency that could be exchanged for pretty much anything one wanted, such as coconuts, labour, or land. At a German trading outstation on New Ireland in 1897, a stick of tobacco could secure ten pineapples.[70] An early Australian explorer visiting British New Guinea in 1884 found a stick of tobacco bought more items than a nugget of gold.[71]

The missionaries were delighted. The London Missionary Society (LMS) obtained sago from Puraru Delta people at the rate of one stick of trade tobacco for a bundle of sago or 25-30 pounds of taro or yams.[72] Two or three tobacco sticks would secure a wallaby, four or five sticks a turtle.[73] On exchanging a stick of tobacco for 28 coconuts, William MacGregor remarked: "It is wonderful that they care to take so much trouble for such poor returns".[74] Labour could also be secured with tobacco. In 1891, another missionary was trying to get a mission house built on top of a hill. He wrote "some of the posts...are twelve feet long and very heavy, and it is with difficulty that we are getting them taken up the hill. I gave five sticks of tobacco for every post taken to the top, and we have twenty up already".[75] Tobacco was used as a performance enhancer rather than reserved for times of relaxation. One missionary on Goodenough Island wrote of the native: "Tobacco really does appear to stimulate him, much more than it does us. Every now and then a native will pause in his task to inhale a whiff or two from his cigarette or a mouthful of smoke from his pipe. A whale-boat crew with a stick of tobacco will row twice as far in the same time as a crew with none".[76]

While the LMS missionaries forswore offering tobacco as a means of tempting people to come to their services, the Roman Catholic priests at the Sacred Heart Mission had no such scruples. This partly reflected their greater proclivity for smoking. According to one account,

In the Anglican and LMS missions some individuals indulged in a pipe or even a cigarette, but in the Sacred Heart Mission smoking was almost a universal habit amongst the male missionaries. The ascetic Father Chabot, at first nauseated by his companions' smoking became a devotee of the pipe. Brother Lainé smoked a long tube of newspaper containing native tobacco, Father Guilbaud a bamboo pipe which stained his white beard orange, and Father Norin was always remembered after his death with an "eternal cigarette". In a revealing comment made in a letter to his sisters, de Boismenu wrote: "I must chat a little with you, a humble cigarette on the corner of the table. Don't open your eyes wide. It substitutes for so many things".[77]

One of the priests would "go through the village on Sunday morning with a basket containing a supply of tobacco. He promised a piece of tobacco to every man who attended service, and, in consequence, his ministrations were greatly esteemed by a considerable number of the heathen".[78] This made things difficult for the LMS workers who

> continued to report "indifference" and "irregular attendance" among the people. "They were frank with us to the point of cruelty", wrote one missionary. "They told us that if we did not pay them in tobacco to listen to our Message, they did not want us in their villages".[79]

Thomson opined that "the success of the Mission in many places is in proportion to the amount of tobacco distributed".[80] Local people around Port Moresby "received their entire supply of tobacco through the Mission, and their name for the Mission vessel was the 'Tobacco Ship'".[81] Not everyone was sanguine about tobacco's presence, however. An Assistant Resident Magistrate described trade tobacco as "one of the greatest curses to the native...with the tobacco he buys the best of food and luxuries, and leads a most immoral, lazy, and sluggish life".[82] In another part of Papua, the government anthropologist F.E. Williams related the local people's explanation for more people dying as being due to tobacco. One old man described a stick of trade twist as the ruin of women's virtue: "in his youth women's favours were not easily obtained [but now]...for a stick of trade twist, tobacco led to adultery, and adultery to death by sorcery".[83]

Objecting to tobacco

Despite the vogue for tobacco amongst male elites in London and elsewhere, opposition to it continued apace in the 19th century. Some descriptions of smoking habits at that time are reminiscent of rules about smoking in the 21st century (Chapter 10). In one account men had either to indulge in the practice out of doors, or else...sneak away into the kitchen when the servants had gone to bed, and puff up the chimney...It was only in large houses that a billiard room could be found...smoking rooms could no more be found in middle class houses than bathrooms".[84]

The tropes of objection to tobacco continued to diversify and became more complex in tandem with and in response to the changing nature of people's entanglements with it. I present three examples – an account of tobacco addiction embedded in Charles Lamb's essay 'Confessions of a Drunkard', the development of the British Anti-Tobacco Society and what became known as the 'Great Tobacco Controversy', and the continuing gendered objections to tobacco exemplified by Rudyard Kipling's jocular poem 'The Betrothed'.

Lamb's 'Confessions'

In 1822, Charles Lamb, essayist and employee of the East India Company in London, published 'Confessions of a Drunkard'. It portrays the author's enjoyment and subsequent regret of time spent with a group of men who were "of boisterous spirits, sitters up a-nights, disputants, drunken; yet seemed to have something noble about them"[85] once he realized "time has a sure strike at dissolving all connections which have no solider fastening that this liquid cement" (i.e. alcohol). Instead, he fell in with a different set, two of whom smoked tobacco. "The devil could not have devised a more subtle trap to re-take a backsliding penitent", he writes, since "the transition, from gulping down draughts of liquid fire [i.e. spirits] to puffing out innocuous blasts of dry smoke [i.e. smoking tobacco], was so like cheating him". Apart from the "white devil" (as he calls it) leading him back to increasingly spirituous beverages, he laments the "drudging service" he has paid,

> the slavery which I have vowed to it. How, when I have resolved to quit it, a feeling of ingratitude has started up; how it has put on personal claims and made the demands of a friend upon me...I feel myself linked to it beyond the power of revocation. Bone of my bone.[86]

Lamb's is a reflective, complex piece of work. It is indicative of the increasing sophistication with which some intellectuals at least were coming to regard "the countless nails that rivet the chains of habit",[87] and articulates a sense of people and tobacco inexorably entwined physiologically, psychologically and socially. Its structure – tobacco embedded within an essay ostensibly about alcohol – reflects the 'hidden in plain sight' qualities of tobacco, and the way in which drinking was regarded as much the more serious problem in Victorian England, and indeed by Lamb himself.

The British Anti-Tobacco Society and the 'Great Tobacco Controversy'

The anti-tobacco movements in Britain or North America were a discordant mix of "old-time temperance advocates, self-fashioned modern critics of waste in an age of efficiency, social reformers who perceived a link between tobacco and delinquency, physician reformers anxious about the health implications of smoking, and eugenicists who believed...use was associated with degeneracy".[88] Some people's criticisms of tobacco took a decidedly religious tack. One campaigner dreamt:

> I was smoking a cigar and it broke in the centre, and out of it came a fearful looking bug which swelled to a large size, and had the head of *Satan* on it, and after grinning horribly at me, it reduced its size, and while I was wondering at it, suddenly it leaped down my throat, and the gnawing pain woke me up.[89]

The British Anti-Tobacco Society (BATS) was established by Thomas Reynolds in 1853, although he was at times its only campaigner.[90] There were 146 promoters initially, 38 of them active scientists and the rest "moralists, evangelicals and social critics".[91] The following year Professor John Lizars published a book *Practical Observations on the Use and Abuse of Tobacco* in which he attempted to summarize what was then known or surmised about the health problems associated with tobacco use. A dispute over the merits and demerits of smoking arose in the pages of *The Lancet* in 1856 when Samuel Solly ascribed the more frequent reporting of cases of "general paralysis" to the upsurge in tobacco smoking. A flurry of letters ensued, which led to the publication of two editorials "in the hope of ending the controversy until an extensive investigation had been made".[92] Meanwhile, the debate had spilled out into other journals and the popular press and became known as the 'Great Tobacco Controversy'.

An approach to smoking epitomized by *The Lancet* editorials around this time argued for distinguishing between 'moderation' and 'excess' (or 'use' and 'abuse'). For *The Lancet* editors, 'excess' was constituted by one or more of the following: smoking before breakfast, 'slavery to the habit', 'premeditated sensuality' and more than two pipes or cigars a day. Smoking by children or youths was also regarded as excessive. "The influence of immoral associations, and the solicitations to, and opportunities of, vice...are hardly to be resisted by the feeble will, the plastic temper, and the warm passions of juvenescence", they wrote.[93] It was not so much any direct dangers from tobacco per se and the immoral associations, solicitations and opportunities it offered for 'vice' that were seen as the greatest danger to children and young people. Moderate use was acceptable, the implication went. It was the different categories of excess that constituted abuse.

Others were concerned with what the working classes might be spending on tobacco. For one Professor, "in working men, the expense of smoking, as of drinking, is a grave deduction from the slender funds which are to support and wife and rear children; a mere sensual and pernicious indulgence of the 'head' of the family at the expense of the 'rest'".[94] However, the mix of moral and medical arguments against tobacco at this time won tobacco control relatively few friends, and the BATS was ribbed mercilessly in the pages of *Cope's Tobacco Plant*, with the manufacturers at one point, in view of the society's dire financial circumstances, "cheekily offering Reynolds a £1,000 testimonial if he would stop publishing the *Anti-Tobacco Journal*".[95] Later, *Cope's Tobacco Plant* offered the hapless Reynolds a page in each issue devoted to the anti-smoking cause.

Temperance was generally a stronger force in North America than Europe, although I disagree with Hilton that it should be regarded as "a minority fringe element of those other medico-moral campaigns against the perceived vices of drinking, opium taking and gambling" on either continent.[96] There was a diversity of viewpoints and positions to acknowledge. Many maintained that tobacco use was a private matter and refused to discuss it. Some were quite willing to argue against tobacco on, say, health grounds – there was general agreement on the link between pipe use and lip, mouth and throat cancer, for example – but eschewed the dramatic claims about "the more apocalyptic illnesses few medics or smokers would have witnessed: deafness, blindness, and physical, mental and moral paralysis"[97] that were made by some of the more extreme temperance campaigners. It is worth remembering that there were an estimated 1 million teetotallers in the UK in 1860.[98] Some non-teetotallers (such as Ruskin, above, and Gladstone) opposed smoking, but the temperance movement against alcohol was always much larger than that against tobacco. While not all teetotallers opposed tobacco, some groups such as the Good Templars made their juvenile auxiliary take an anti-smoking pledge, and others such as the Band of Hope prohibited tobacco altogether.[99]

Gendered responses to tobacco

The case of 24 year-old Maggie Dochead Watson and William Kirkland, concerning a £500 'breach of promise' three years after their betrothal, indicates some of the stresses and strains tobacco led to in gendered and domestic relationships. Watson claimed she accepted Kirkland's proposal of marriage on condition that he gave up smoking. Kirkland, a warehouseman in Glasgow, Scotland, was already a teetotaller. According to the report in the *Oamaru Mail* earlier that year Watson became concerned that her fiancé had started "indulging in cigars" and visiting his betrothed less frequently. Challenged by letter with the accusation that "you seem to put my happiness on a level with a cigar", the warehouseman replied "I do not intend to give up smoking...There is just a little too much coercion in your letter and I won't be coerced".[100]

This case inspired Rudyard Kipling's poem 'The Betrothed'. Kipling had started smoking in his schooldays, though in later years he was obliged to give up his dedication to the practice on medical grounds. Kipling's poem places women and cigars on the same comparative plane. The narrator is Kirkland, who finds cigars are always there to do his bidding, whereas Maggie "is exacting". He asks, in a misogynistic way, "Which is the better portion – bondage bought with a ring,/Or a harem of dusky beauties, fifty tied in a string?" The different temporalities of women and cigars are likewise compared and the former found wanting. While a woman "is pretty to look at...the prettiest cheeks must wrinkle, the truest of loves must pass", a finished cigar, by contrast, can be "thrown away for another as perfect and ripe and brown". The cigars are subaltern "servants" offering a diversity of psychological services ("counsellors cunning and silent – comforters true and tried...Thought in the early morning, solace in time of woes, Peace in the hush of the twilight, balm 'ere my eyelids close") and "asking nought in return,/With only a Suttee's passion—to do their duty and burn".[101] The narrator concludes "a woman is only a woman, but a good Cigar is a Smoke...If Maggie will have no rival, I'll have no Maggie for Spouse!"

An even more dastardly rendition of similar sentiments is presented by cavalier aristocrat Franklin Blake in Wilkie Collins' *The Moonstone*. "Is it conceivable that a man can have smoked as long as I have without discovering that there is a complete system for the treatment of women at the bottom of his cigar case?...You choose a cigar, you try it and it disappoints you. What do you do upon that? You throw it away and try another. Now observe the application! You choose a woman, you try her and she breaks your heart. Fool! Take a lesson from your cigar case. Throw her away and try another!"[102] Here is tobacco offering a misogynistic breeding ground transecting and challenging gender relationships more widely.

Overall, however, while there were multiple objections to tobacco being voiced at this time, they were disparate, linked to other things (temperance, patriarchy) and lacking the binding threads of knowledge and experience regarding dangers to the health of self and others that emerged during the following century. There was also, more than likely, less ill-health linked specifically to tobacco than can be identified today, both because people were generally dying earlier, of many more preventable illnesses, and the modes of consuming tobacco were more diverse and, possibly, less harmful. There is a sense of 'the calm before the storm' when we trace the history of objections to tobacco in the 19th century. The Bonsack cigarette machine was about to become the object around which so many of the subsequent concerns, and developments that crystallized into a more formal movement for tobacco control, were to coalesce.

All hail the Bonsack machine

The Bonsack cigarette machine was to have "truly revolutionary effects on the subsequent development of the industry",[103] and marked the real triumph of tobacco's diversification and commodification. As well as having a profound effect on the organization of the tobacco industry, particularly the rise of the tobacco corporation, it also enhanced tobacco's ability to be central to the experience of many soldiers in the First World War (Chapter 7).

The earliest recorded cigarette machine was displayed at the Paris Universal Exhibition in 1867, although its mechanism was extremely complicated. Several different machines were developed in a process described as "multiple, simultaneous invention".[104] In 1881, James Bonsack of Salem, Virginia, patented a much improved machine offering significant advantages over anything else available at the time (Fig. 6.1), distinctive because of a new kind of feeding mechanism, the cigarette former, and a knife (the "cut-off"). The Bonsack Machine Company came to Paris in 1883, something of a hub for international exhibitions. Bonsack was invited to visit the Bristol works of the Wills Company where he set up a prototype machine for close scrutiny. The consultant engineer called in to inspect it found faults with its major operations, particularly what happened at the end. He felt the machine terminated too soon, suggesting "it should be extended so as to present the cigarettes in a convenient position and without jars or jerks to the girls who pack them".[105] However, he recorded that the best continuous run managed to produce 133 cigarettes a minute, around 8,000 in an hour, in other words, an almost sixty-fold increase on the production rates achievable by human subjects. Moreover he found the finished product more pleasant and easier to smoke than handmade cigarettes – "free from the usual tendency to transfer some of the tobacco to the lips or into the mouth", for example. However, cigarettes only accounted for a fraction of one per cent of total tobacco consumption at that time and machine-made cigarettes were still twice the price, ounce for ounce, of pipe tobacco.

There was also considerable scepticism about the cigarette itself. An article appearing in the London trade journal *Tobacco* in 1889, 'The Future of Cigarettes', concluded "the smoking of cigarettes savours of the effeminate, and is not suited to the English nation. If this is a correct assumption, it follows that the practice is but a passing fancy, which may hardly last out the present generation".[106] Wills' directors shared this view – their decision to buy exclusive UK use rights for the Bonsack machine was purely a precaution.

> Although the fashion of cigarette smoking was obviously spreading, none of them believed cigarettes would ever offer a serious challenge to pipe smoking. Even the most optimistic among them, when the Firm went into machine-made cigarette production, were astounded by the success that this quite soon led to.[107]

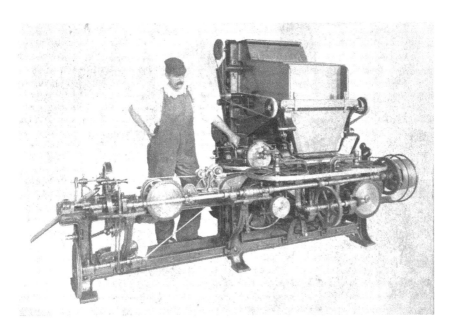

Fig. 6.1 The Bonsack cigarette-making machine, 1880s
Source: Courtesy of the State Archives of North Carolina

The Bonsack was not the only cigarette machine to be developed. The French had the Decouflé. Gallaher and Co. started using a Luddington, a machine which could manufacture cigarettes of different sizes but which the trade magazine criticized for requiring the attention of an engineer "almost daily". Retail tobacconists, Salmon and Gluckstein, started using another machine, the Munson, for the manufacture of their cheap brands. In the USA, the Elliot was developed by Bernhard Baron to rival the Bonsack, and was adopted by the Nottingham-based John Player and Sons. By 1899, both Players and Stephen Mitchell and Son in Glasgow were operating 34 Elliot machines between them.[108]

Cigarette sales growth in Britain obviously depended on the phenomenal increase in production capacity afforded by the new machines, but they were backed up by Wills' marketing strategies for selling its 'Wills Woodbine' and 'Cinderella' at the extremely low retail price of five for one penny.[109] Wills supported this by increased discounts to retailers and new packaging. The latter included card 'stiffeners' that quickly became decorated initially by prints of the Kings and Queens of England. In the ten years from 1889 (when these cigarettes were first marketed), sales increased 35-fold from 137,709 lbs to 4,933,352 lbs, with cigarettes as a proportion of Wills total tobacco sales increasing from 3.0 to 53.3 per cent, more than doubling their total sales of tobacco during this time. By 1905, cigarettes accounted for 25 per cent of all British tobacco sales by weight. The export trade in cigarettes went up by a similar proportion, as British consumers migrated to the settler colonies. The popularity of cut-price cigarettes allowed non-specialist retailers to use them as a means of attracting extra customers. These tactics seriously undermined specialist tobacconists; through its brands and industrial-scale production methods, tobacco had developed as a commercial force that took on a momentum of its own – supported by an increasingly corporate style of business practice.

Tobacco turns corporate

Described by one historian as "aggressive and untethered" (except to tobacco), James ('Buck') Duke in the USA was responsible for pushing through the technological, marketing and organizational innovations that were not only to revolutionize the tobacco industry but would help "define the coming new age of consumption".[110] Duke's father, a former subsistence farmer from Durham, North Carolina,[111] returned from Yankee imprisonment at the end of the American Civil War and started selling Bright leaf smoking tobacco that he had hidden in an outhouse to evade looters. He called it *Pro Bono Publico* ('For the Public Good').[112] Facing strong competition from Bull Durham, a popular rival brand, however, Buck Duke decided to move into the cigarette business on taking up a controlling interest in the family firm in 1887. He initially employed ten workers hand rolling cigarettes, but took advantage of a strike at Goodwin and Company in New York to encourage 125 young Polish, Jewish men to move south and expand his labour force, enticed by the offer of moving expenses and a wage of 70 cents per 1,000 cigarettes. A dedicated worker could earn more than $2.00 in a typical 12 hour day, an exceptional amount in those days.[113]

The manufacturing process adopted was similar to that of W.D. and H.O. Wills in their pre-machine days, involving a smooth piece of wood or a marble slab, sheets of thin paper attached with flour and water paste to the top of the slab to prevent slipping, and the exact amount of tobacco needed for a cigarette.

> A careful account is kept with each operative. Enough prepared tobacco and paper is weighed out for a day's work, and when returned, the cigarettes are again weighed, carefully inspected, and all the imperfect ones thrown out. By a system of charges and credits, good and bad workmanship is discovered and recorded and a thorough discipline preserved,

wrote one admiring visitor.[114] However, employee relations were not sanguine. Duke's father later reminisced that they had never had any unrest "except when 125 Polish Jews were hired to come down to Durham and work in the factory. They gave us no end of trouble. We worked out of that and we now employ our own people".[115] By this he meant "native white girls, a cheaper, more tractable class of employees".[116]

Duke secured a secret leasing contract on very favourable terms with Bonsack,[117] much as W.D. and H.O. Wills had done in the UK, and bought exclusive American rights to the French Decouflé machine to stop his competitors adopting it. These measures gave his company a competitive advantage. "The installation of Bonsack's machines at the Duke factory was an unwelcome sight to his employees. For Duke, it marked a new form of control over the vicissitudes of human capital".[118] Duke spent much more on advertising and marketing than rival firms since, given the high production volumes of which the new Bonsack machines were capable, a serious risk of overcapacity meant consumption had to increase. In 1886, dissatisfied with the rate at which customers were shifting to cigarettes, Duke offered every dealer who ordered 1,000 cigarettes a pound of Duke's Mixture smoking tobacco – free. He installed a colour lithography print shop in his Durham factory to increase the appeal of his packaging, enabling the insertion of attractive, collectable cards similar to those used by Wills in the UK. But where Wills had used kings and queens of England as their draw, Duke offered lascivious photos of scantily clad actresses to appeal to the young male clientele who were the main target for his wares. Lithograph albums were made available to card collectors in exchange for vouchers indicating the applicant had purchased so many hundred cigarettes. According to a *New York Times* reporter writing in 1888: "Twelve different albums are now offered as prizes for smoking certain brands of cigarettes. Many a boy under 12 is striving for the entire collection, which necessitates the consumption of nearly 12,000 cigarettes...He will become demoralized, and possibly dishonest, to accomplish his purpose".[119] By the end of that year, Duke claimed to be the largest cigarette manufacturer in the world. Duke senior began a philanthropic programme endowing local Methodist churches and Trinity College, latterly insisting that the College (which was eventually renamed Duke University after his son) should "open its doors to women, placing them on equal footing with men".[120]

The radical organizational innovation that Duke instigated was the creation of a consortium, the American Tobacco Company (ATC), in 1890. Large sections of the American industrial economy restructured to form big corporations during the second half of the nineteenth century. They sought to integrate "both forwards, into distribution, and backwards, into the acquisition of raw material supplies".[121] The ATC had a virtual monopoly on cigarette sales across the nation. It bought out independent rivals, closed their plants, and consolidated their machinery and materials. The Tobacco Trust, as it came to be known, achieved economies of scale and vertical integration that sought, as Wills had done with its branded products in the UK, to phase out middlemen. In addition, however, the ATC aimed to monopolize every point in the supply chain – both the acquisition of tobacco as commodity and its distribution as manufactured brand. Interestingly, though, while it purchased subsidiaries making boxes, foil and pipes, the ATC made no concerted efforts to take over ownership of the tobacco fields. "Most likely there was no need to control supply directly because the company already had all of the bargaining power it needed...it acted virtually as a single buyer, while most farmers...produced too little to affect the market price", suggests Goodman.[122] Another reason, as Duke knew from his childhood, was that "capital investment did not generate the same economies of scale on farms as in factories".[123] Instead, the ATC created a 'Leaf Department' that put an end to competitive bidding in the tobacco auctions,[124] in the process reinforcing "the enormously inequitable division of power between cultivators, on the one hand, and distributors and manufacturers on the other, that characterized tobacco culture from the beginning, and continues to do so even now".[125] This was but a prelude to what was to come in the 20th century, however, which will be the subject of the next two chapters.

Conclusion

Tobacco in the 19th century diversified into a number of different forms and diverse brands spanning a range of material, geographical, colonial and anti-tobacco worlds. The appropriation of eulogies about smoking by literary 'greats' and their transformation into brands such as 'Three Castles' and 'Westward Ho!' contributed to the increasing allure and reach of tobacco products marketed by manufacturers such as W.D. and H.O. Wills direct to consumers. Technical innovations such as safety matches, packaging, cutting and flue curing were also significant and essential for tobacco to maintain its ascendancy. So was its use as a 'drug food'; a means of incorporating colonized peoples into the commercial and spiritual realms of the colonial endeavour.

All these, however, were but a precursor to the Bonsack cigarette-making machine, probably the most important innovation in the history of tobacco since its escape from the Americas at the end of the 15th century. Its industrially produced output, the cigarette, was the mediator for a number of ensuing, more-than-human worlds. In this chapter I have tracked the paths taken by cigarettes from their technological progenitor to the rise of the tobacco corporations. However, there were continued misgivings about the role and purpose of cigarettes. How these concerns developed, but how power and circumstance prevented them being acted upon until relatively late into the 20th century, are the subject of Chapter 7.

Notes

1 Ortiz (1995: 309).
2 Wilbert (1987: 10).
3 Ortiz (1995: 77).
4 Peninsular War 1807–14.
5 Stubbs (2012: 7).
6 See, for example, Browne (1842).
7 Dickens (1842: 141).
8 Gately (2001: 174).
9 Dickens (1842: 141–2).
10 Ibid. (142).
11 Alford (1973: 110).
12 Ibid. (Chapter 5).
13 Women were the producers of cigarettes, men the consumers. Wills employed a Polish immigrant, Bogosoff, to teach women in London and Bristol how to make cigarettes in their factories. A skilled woman could produce about 1500 a day.
14 Alford (1973: 123) describes one of them as "Theodoridi, a Greek from Odessa, who began to produce cigarettes in England in 1857".
15 Best Birds Eye was so called because it contained small quantities of finely chopped stem which were similar to actual birds' eyes. Bishop Blaze (a pun on his written name, Blaise) was an early Christian martyr whose flesh was cut with combs.
16 Horniman's tea had similarly been sealed in labelled packets since 1826 to preserve its quality.
17 Alford (1973: 97).
18 Hilton (2000: 43–4).
19 Hilton (1998: 116).
20 Ibid. (131).
21 Hilton (2000: 92).
22 Alford (1973).
23 Three Castles tobacco was introduced in 1877; Three Castles cigarettes in 1878.
24 Watry (2002).
25 Ibid. Thomson was also plagued by insomnia, alcoholism and chronic depression and died in London at the age of 47.
26 A few writers, like Goethe and Heine, abhorred tobacco and its smoke (Kiernan 1991: 198).
27 Kiernan (1991: 175).
28 Trench (1978: 142) quoted in Kiernan (1991: 176).
29 Kiernan (1991: 176).
30 Reported in Kiernan (1991: 185).
31 Ibid. (184).
32 Marx (1977: 163).
33 Ibid. (163–4).
34 Brookhenkel (2009).
35 Willburn (2006: 100).
36 Kiernan (1991: 184).
37 Coleridge (1966: 462–3).
38 In Klein (1993).
39 Baudelaire (1993: 136, 138), my translation.
40 Prettejohn (2012): 80) describes their focus on both mind and life as involving "the mind and the mind's workings, not the remains of earnest thought which

has been frittered away by a long dreary course of preparatory study, by which all life has been evaporated".

41 Tupper (1849), original emphasis.
42 Maitland (1871: 349). Maitland is a pseudonym disguising the writer Robert Buchanan. Buchanan's own tobacco proclivities are reflected in the story that on a pilgrimage to the home of Thomas Love Peacock he was dismayed to find his host abhorred tobacco. Buchanan, forced to make a solemn promise that he would not smoke within five hundred yards of the house, "violated the arrangement" and "well remembers one night stealthily opening the bedroom window in the house at Halliford and 'blowing a cloud' out into the summer night" (Anon, 1875: 416).
43 Rossetti (2013: 251). Tennyson was so addicted (and fastidious) that Rossetti narrates a story about him in Italy, unable to find a shop which could sell him his favourite tobacco – Bristol Bird's Eye. "To his dismay, no such thing was to be found; *some* tobacco there was – but not *his* tobacco. What was to be done in this woeful penury of the right sort to smoke? Tennyson packed up his luggage, abandoned all his Italian interests and desires, and returned to London" (Rossetti, 2013: 257).
44 Buckley (2012: 166).
45 Anon. (1858: 71, 72, 72-73).
46 Hilton (2000: 23).
47 Ibid. (22).
48 Anon. (1858: 73).
49 Hilton (2000: 22).
50 Lowell (1904).
51 Alford (1973: 111).
52 Hilton (2000: 43).
53 Barrie (1925: 20).
54 Ibid. (21).
55 Ibid.
56 Hilton (2000: 19).
57 Zieger (2014: 24).
58 Hilton (2000: 19).
59 Bratby (2014), drawing on Northrop Moore (1984).
60 Goodman (1993: 164).
61 Livingstone (1866: 256-7).
62 Hilton (2000: 41).
63 Stone (1880: 89), quoted in Hays (1991: 93).
64 Jankowiak and Bradburd (1996).
65 Brady (2002) provides a good example of the central role tobacco played in the colonial encounter in Australia.
66 Brady (2013).
67 See for example Feinhandler et al. (1979). Such myths have the merit of novelty and foster confusion about the true origins and distribution patterns of tobacco: Feinhandler, for example, when a lecturer in cultural anthropology at Harvard Medical School, "received more than a quarter million dollars between 1977 and 1980 to carry out research on smoking customs" designed to "produce knowledge-diverting attention from the dangers of tobacco" (Kohrman and Benson 2011: 337).
68 Hays (2003: 59).
69 Ibid.
70 Ibid. (2003: 61).

71 Bevan (1890), cited in Hays (1991: 93).
72 Hays (1991: 94, 95).
73 Chignell (1915: 133) quoted in Hays (1991: 95).
74 MacGregor (1892: 32) quoted in Hays (1991: 95). The use of tobacco as a form of currency continues today in Papua New Guinea's main prison, outside Port Moresby, where "new prisoners are amazed to discover that cigarettes have taken on the role and function of currency. Any informal transactions in the gaol are conducted with 'cigarette money'" (Reed 2007: 37).
75 Albert Maclaren, quoted in Synge (1908: 140).
76 Jenness and Ballantyne (1920: 163), quoted in Hays (2003: 62).
77 Langmore (1981: 145).
78 Thompson (1900: 76) quoted in Hays (1991: 96).
79 Langmore (1981: 218).
80 Thomson (1889: 528), quoted in Hays (1991: 97).
81 Hays (1991: 99).
82 English (1905: 23), quoted in Hays (1991: 97).
83 Hays (1991: 97).
84 Apperson (1914: 164).
85 Lamb (1985: 156) I am indebted to Prof. David Fuller for alerting me to the presence of tobacco within Lamb's autobiographical account.
86 Ibid. (158).
87 Ibid.
88 Brandt (2007: 47).
89 Hilton (2000: 69).
90 Walker (1980).
91 Berridge (2013: 53); Hilton (2000: 63).
92 Hilton (2000: 63).
93 *The Lancet* (1857: 354), cited in Hilton (2000: 69).
94 Cited in Hilton (2000: 70).
95 Hilton (2000: 66).
96 Ibid. (63).
97 Ibid. (65).
98 Gregory (2003: 633).
99 Ibid.
100 Anon. (1888a: 4). The fact this story was being discussed in the antipodes points to the extent of global communications at this time, as well as the intrinsic interest in the story of tobacco-person men choosing tobacco over female company.
101 Kipling (1994) The "Suttee's passion" is the ritual immolation of Hindu widows on the funeral pyres of their husbands (see Spivak 1988).
102 Collins (1874: 194).
103 Alford (1973: 139).
104 Hannah (2006: 64), quoted in Hahn (2011: 93).
105 Alford (1973: 145).
106 *Tobacco* (London) 9 (103): 198, quoted in Cox (2000: 47).
107 Alford (1973: 155).
108 See Cox (2000: 53).
109 Hahn cautions against assuming technologies can account for the rise of big business. "Human choices dictate the course of history...human decisions cause human history" (2011: 4). However in this case, like Latour's gun (Introduction), it is hard to dismiss the view that the machine had something to do with it.
110 Brandt (2007: 27).

111 Work was undoubtedly hard on the farm: "I have made more furrows in God's earth than any man of forty years of age in North Carolina" Washington Duke is reported to have said in 1890 (Robert 1949: 138), but Hahn (2011: 92) suggests the fact Duke senior was able to seek credit in New York in 1856 complicates the myth of the poor yeoman farmer somewhat.
112 Hahn (2011: 92).
113 Roberts and Knapp (1992: 260).
114 Described in Roberts and Knapp (1992: 260, 262).
115 Cited in Roberts and Knapp (1992: 273).
116 Roberts and Knapp (1992: 260).
117 Despite having offered a prize of $75,000 for a cigarette-making machine that worked, a rival company, loathed to part with the money, had rejected the Bonsack machine.
118 Brandt (2007: 30).
119 Anon. (1888) cited in Brandt (2007: 32). Note the omission of any health risks in this report.
120 Durden (1975: 110).
121 Goodman (1993: 232).
122 Ibid.
123 Benson (2012: 73).
124 Campbell (2005).
125 Goodman (1993: 232).

Chapter 7

Enchantment and risk: tobacco, 1900–1950

Introduction: two world wars

Cigarettes transculturated well, like other tobacco products before them.[1] Many people forget that the history of machine-made cigarettes is so recent. They are easy to use and easy to share. So normal and unremarkable did they quickly become that soon it was hard to remember (or imagine) life without them. How humble, in Miller's terms, how ill-apparent and peripheral, yet so strongly determinant of action and identity.[2] In this chapter, I shall describe the increasingly global assemblages this transculturation made possible – the rise of the tobacco corporations and the resistance they engendered from both small tobacco farmers in the USA and the growing tobacco temperance movement. These oppositional voices were silenced, at least temporarily, by the onset of the First World War. Tobacco played a central role in this conflict. The interwar period saw tobacco further in the ascendant, changing behaviours around inhalation and with increasingly powerful, confident, and creative corporations promoting cigarettes as objects/subjects of glamorous and freedom-loving relationships. Resistance to women smoking was countered by marketing them first to male-female couples, complemented by clever strategies employed by workers in the emergent field of public relations (PR) to manipulate the attitudes towards women smoking amongst the public at large.

Yet clouds were building on the horizon even as a tobacco nirvana beckoned. Scientists in the German Weimar Republic were developing compelling scientific evidence about the health harms of cigarettes – evidence, however, that became obscured and tainted by the rise of the National Socialist (Nazi) party. Hitler's attempts to further tobacco research and develop tobacco control policies were remarkable but largely ineffectual and, in the war's aftermath and the division of Germany, counter-productive. Irrespective of what scientists knew, however, the relationship between tobacco and its users, reflected in the experience of many 20th century European artists and intellectuals, became increasingly troubled, or at least defensive. The chapter ends with a consideration of why it took so long for the increasingly clear (but 'hidden in plain sight') dangers of tobacco to be recognized and then enacted in public health policies and legislation. Why, following the debacle of the Second World War, were non-German scientists who picked up the baton of research into tobacco and health so slow at recognizing the significance of their findings? Were they subject to a form of narcotic enchantment that dulled their perspective?

Corporate expansion and resistance

In 1900, 44 per cent of US tobacco consumption was still in the form of chewing tobacco,[3] but by 1910, the American Tobacco Company (ATC) had swallowed so many rivals it accounted for 75 per cent of the USA's total manufactured tobacco output. Buck Duke continued his expansive global aspirations, however, establishing subsidiaries and controlling interests in Canada, Australia, Japan, and China. By 1902, the Chinese market alone comprised more than half a billion cigarettes.[4] One year earlier, Duke had crossed the Atlantic with the intention of buying Ogden Ltd, a British firm. In response, the 13 largest British tobacco manufacturers combined into a new company, Imperial Tobacco. In a partnership deal, each side agreed not to operate in the other's domestic market, while tobacco products for the rest of the world would be supplied by a new joint venture: the British American Tobacco Company (BAT). China was a major target – BAT built two new factories, adding to one that had been opened by the ATC in Shanghai in 1891. By 1916, BAT was selling more than nine billion cigarettes annually in China,[5] nearly half of which were manufactured in China itself. Similar opportunities were exploited in India, Malaya, the Dutch East Indies, and Egypt. The only country where Duke's plans were unsuccessful was Japan. Calling him a "capitalist...intending to monopolize the whole world", the Japanese government forced Duke out by nationalizing its tobacco industry in 1904.[6]

In its home territory, the way the ATC used its monopoly to drive down prices fanned simmering resentment amongst tobacco farmers themselves. The 'Black Patch' was an area in south-west Kentucky and north-west Tennessee that was a leading producer of dark fired tobacco for snuff, chewing and pipes. Between 1904 and 1909, resentment turned to despair and erupted into what became known as the Black Patch Tobacco Wars,[7] precipitated when local farmers attempted to form themselves into a cooperative to 'pool' and withhold their tobacco crop until the ATC agreed to pay higher prices. Some of the farmers formed groups – called 'Possum Hunters' – that were vigilante night patrols aimed at 'encouraging' farmers and tobacco buyers to join the association. Confrontations escalated to beatings and whippings, and the destruction or choking of non-members' tobacco fields and plant beds by scrapers, salt or grass seed.

Then the 'Night Riders of the Silent Brigade' were formed, a group named because of their practice of muffling their horses' and mules' hooves during a mission. They started night attacks on ATC warehouses where auctioned tobacco was stored. The first mission occurred at Trenton and Elkton, followed by Princeton, Hopkinsville, Russellville and Dycusburg, Kentucky where tobacco factories and warehouses were burnt to the ground. Equally momentous events were going on in the burley region of Kentucky.[8] The Night Riders would drift into town in small groups during the day, then at a pre-arranged time occupy the police station and other key municipal buildings. Any householders trying to look out or come outside were liable to be met with a shower of bullets through their windows and doors. In some ways, the Night Riders achieved their demands. The USA's colonial past had left it with a "political culture with a deep historical antipathy to monopoly and 'restraint of trade'".[9] The Sherman Antitrust Act, passed by Congress in 1890, had the intention of limiting the consolidation of corporate power and promoting competition. In 1911, the US Supreme Court ruled that the ATC was indeed a monopoly and dissolved it. The 'Tobacco Trust' was reconstituted as four new firms – the ATC, Liggett and Myers, R.J. Reynolds, and P. Lorillard. However, according to Brandt, the monopoly was simply replaced by an oligopoly, a small number of large companies.[10]

The temperance movement was also coalescing against the power of tobacco capitalism, with a particular focus on cigarettes. Three US states had banned the sale of cigarettes by 1900 and four more were to do so by 1909.[11] Three Canadian provinces banned sales to minors in 1900, and three years later the Canadian Parliament passed a resolution prohibiting the manufacture, importation, and sale of all cigarettes.[12] Adams Henry's book *The Deadly Cigarette*, dedicated "To My Son, William Mellors Henry, who is pledged against smoking, drinking, gambling and swearing", was co-published with the British Lads' Anti-Smoking Union in London in 1906 with material assembled in the USA. In a wonderful illustration of the power of hybridity, women armed with tomahawks are pictured chasing anthropomorphized cigarettes off cliffs (Fig. 7.1). In the midst of rants like "tens of thousands of innocent little ones are annually crippled, maimed, and slain by the fatal fumes of the poisonous cigarette",[13] prescient comments include "the prevalence of the cigarette custom indicates that a bitter harvest will soon be reaped".[14] Referring obliquely to Buck Duke, Adams commented "the cigarette manufacturer may endow colleges, but…An economic system that coins from the child's life blood, the profits that enrich the capitalist, cannot promote the sobriety and moral power of citizenship".[15]

Like their 19th century forbears, these campaigners were more than "a few crackpots firing from the lunatic fringe".[16] The legislative record alone shows that the temperance movement was far more important politically than has been recognized. According to one analyst, "in promoting their cause, the first generation of anti-cigarette crusaders articulated virtually every issue that is still being debated about smoking today. Theirs was not a failure of rhetoric or determination, but of timing".[17] In the UK, the rejection of many working-class recruits deemed too physically feeble to fight in the second Boer War

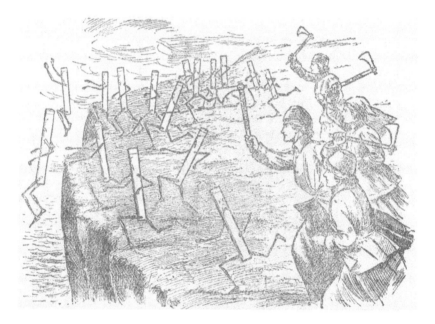

Fig. 7.1 Tomahawking the cigarette
Source: Henry, 1906: 44

(1899–1902) caused much national soul-searching, with tobacco, especially cigarettes, spotlighted amongst potential causes. The 1908 Children's Act, as well as prohibiting children from pubs and the sale of alcohol to them, also made it illegal to sell tobacco to children, or to sell it in sweetshops.[18] The latter two clauses were a small victory for the anti-tobacco movement, although it "largely collapsed" after the introduction of the Act.[19] With legislation about selling tobacco to children in place there was a sense of 'job done', and things were soon to become complicated by the onset of the First World War.

Tobacco shapes the First World War

The ubiquity of the cigarette and the invention of the cigarette lighter reinstated "the intimate connexion between war and tobacco".[20] The cigarette, until then "a popular, if marginal, product",[21] really came into its own during the time of the First World War, offering several practical advantages over pipe smoking in the diabolical conditions of trench warfare. The war effectively silenced the objections to tobacco being voiced by non-users and anti-tobacco groups. After all, or so the argument went, how could young men who were risking their lives for their country be restricted in their use of tobacco? "The men who for us have so long breathed the battle-smoke are to be defended from the dangers of tobacco smoke",[22] wrote G.K. Chesterton disparagingly in 1917, in opposition to a eugenicist, Dr Caleb Saleeby, who argued smoking was sapping the fibre of manhood. 'Battle-smoke' had new connotations in the First World War, since it was the first time poison gases had been widely used, and a gas mask had become an essential item of apparel. In an era characterized by "terror from the air",[23] requiring men to breathe through a piece of technology ('kit') in order to protect their lungs from harm, might there not have been a subliminal thought that cigarettes, another form of mediating technology between man and air, were possibly less dangerous? Chesterton argued for the "poor, plain, exhausted fellow, who may be in torments in ten minutes, tortured in the green fumes of the modern witchcraft, stolidly puffing at a stale cigarette, that has wandered his way for once in a hundred times".[24] How, he wondered, could anyone go up to such a man and tell him he was doing something that might reduce his longevity?

Thus the brutality of war distracted from arguments over the risks of smoking. Indeed, for large proportions of the medical profession, cigarettes were a positive balm. A *Lancet* commentary in 1915 argued that "[T]he significance of the demand from men in the trenches for cigarettes cannot lightly be ignored...[smoking] undoubtedly affords relief and diversion in all nerve-straining tasks".[25] And cigarettes were indeed in high demand in the trenches. The YMCA (Young Men's Christian Association) and the Salvation Army, organizations which had been at the forefront of opposition to cigarettes, "found themselves eagerly distributing them near the front and basking in the popularity of this largesse".[26] Volunteers in the UK, USA and Canada demonstrated their support for frontline troops by collecting donations to ensure them an adequate supply. In the USA, a National Cigarette Service Committee was formed to ensure soldiers without families were not disadvantaged, and the US War Department initiated a rationing system to ensure everyone had a fair opportunity to smoke.[27] Subscribers in the UK raised enough to supply over 232 million cigarettes for this purpose.[28] According to one historian, "cheap cigarettes ('fags')...were as much a part of the life of the trenches as the barbed wire".[29] Complaints about locally available varieties were rife. Wilfred Owen complained "the stuff sold out here is abominable, except Turkish, which are cheap and good".[30] For the author Jerome K. Jerome, working as an ambulance driver,

> The parcel from home was the great event of the week. Often, it had been opened. We had to thank God for what was left. Out of every three boxes of cigarettes that my wife sent me, I reckon I got one. The French cigarettes, that one bought at the canteens, were ten per cent poison and the rest dirt. The pain would go out of a wounded soldier's face when you showed him an English cigarette.[31]

Tobacco (at least, good quality stuff) in the First World War was thus part of the 'great event' in more ways than one. Siegfried Sassoon adopts a jocular tone to describe finding himself next to a muddy shell crater on a night patrol with enemy guns nearby. He was "miserably wondering whether my number was up; then I remembered that I was wearing my pre-war raincoat; I could feel the pipe and tobacco pouch in my pocket and somehow this made me less forlorn".[32] An advertisement that appeared in the *Toronto Daily News* in 1915 sports a generic 'Tommy Atkins' lighting his pipe saying "Arf a Mo, Kaiser" (recycled as "Arf a Mo, 'Itler!" in the Second World War). It reflects both the play-acting and attitudinizing that had to happen to keep the war going "in the right spirit",[33] and the centrality of tobacco in the conflict.

Tobacco also offered solace for those who remained. Kipling wrote a sombre, tobacco-themed tale titled 'In the interests of the brethren' towards the end of the First World War that included a rich description of the contents of an old-fashioned tobacconist's shop:

> It had been established by his grandfather in 1827, but the fittings and appointments must have been at least half a century older. The brown and red tobacco- and snuff-jars, with Crowns, Garters, and names of forgotten mixtures in gold leaf; the polished 'Oronoque' tobacco-barrels on which favoured customers sat; the cherry-black mahogany counter, the delicately moulded shelves, the reeded cigar-cabinets, the German-silver-mounted scales, and the Dutch brass roll- and cake-cutter, were things to covet.

The tobacconist offers to induct the narrator into a Masonic Lodge. Kipling was a Mason himself (he joined a mixed Lodge in Lahore when he was 20 years old), and the piece expresses the author's pleasure in Masonic rituals and materials. It is perhaps significant that it is a tobacconist who leads the Lodge, a giver of life, camaraderie and some hope, in this tale.[34] Kipling was attracted by the easy male comradeship Lodges provided, the social mix and the chance to exchange opinions between men who would otherwise have been unlikely to ever meet, sentiments strongly redolent of the sociability found in a 17th century coffee shop (Chapter 4). There is also a thinly veiled argument that it would be in the interests of the London Lodges of the time to relax their usual rules and welcome visiting soldiers with Masonic credentials, particularly those on leave or convalescing from wounds. A deep sense of the need for healing and new beginnings pervades the piece; Kipling's son had died in the trenches of the First World War and Kipling held great store in the solace to be found in the 'Arcadia Mixture'.

Learning to inhale

Whatever its ghastly costs in terms of human destruction, the First World War overturned any misgivings that may have remained about the relationship of cigarettes and manliness.[35] There was still a lag time in people discovering how to use them appropriately, however. Christopher Isherwood was sitting in a tent on a Greek island in 1933 trying to write a novel, but the "heat, dirt, bad food and worse water, stinging flies and yelling Greeks" were making it difficult. Writing in the third person, Isherwood recounts how, at one particularly stressful juncture, he

> was suddenly possessed by the hysteria of the scene. He had a cigarette in his mouth and, involuntarily, he inhaled its smoke. This was the first time he had ever inhaled – he didn't know how to – although he had been a smoker for ten years. The lift of the intoxication made him feel as though he were levitating; for an instant, he almost lost consciousness. After this, he began to inhale regularly and thus became a nicotine addict for the next thirty years.[36]

Simon Gray started to smoke from a much earlier age, in a communal setting during the Second World War. He was seven years old:

> [O]ur smoking was exhilaratingly furtive, the deep, dark, swirling pleasures of the smoke being sucked into fresh, pink, welcoming lungs, it took me just three or four cigarettes to acquire the habit and you know there are still moments now when I catch more than a memory of the first suckings-in, the slow leakings-out when the smoke seems to fill the nostrils with far more than the experience of itself.[37]

Not all first experiences were as delectable as Gray's, however. The fictional Zeno Costini's first encounter with tobacco smoke – through cigars stolen from his father – was less salubrious:

> At the very moment I grabbed them I was overcome with a shudder of revulsion, knowing how sick they would make me. Then I smoked them until my brow was drenched in cold sweat and my stomach was in knots.[38]

Clearly there was a lot more going on than just 'the experience of itself', to paraphrase Gray. For a lot of people, cigarette smoking commenced (and continues to begin) as a form of youthful rebellion, furtive and exhilarating in Gray's case. However, the ease with which machine-produced cigarettes can be obtained and consumed, and the associated changes in behaviour they precipitate – the 'easy rituals' and changing identities associated with their use, as well as the inhalation of tobacco smoke deep into the lungs – constituted a fundamental change in the practice of smoking. The word 'inspiration' has a double meaning – the literal action of breathing in or inhaling, and the figurative meaning with its spiritual overtones that implies having reached some kind of exalted state, usually because of some kind of frequently mysterious external influence. However, tobacco – not necessarily inhaled – still had plenty of champions who attributed many of their most famous pieces to its influence on their work.

Davis calls crack cocaine "the narcotic equivalent of fast food",[39] but it is a term that could be, and has been, as easily applied to the cigarette.[40] In what has been called the "cigarette century",[41] cigarettes took an increasingly large share of the tobacco market worldwide. Smoking rates reached their peak in Britain in 1948 at around 60 per cent overall;[42] in the USA tobacco use per capita peaked in 1954.[43] However, such blanket figures mask significant differences. Rates for women, unlike men, did not peak until 1966 in England, at a lower rate (50 per cent, compared to an estimated 81 per cent for men in 1949). The reasons for these differences are not random movements in fashion. After the First World War had helped (temporarily for some, permanently for many) to ensconce tobacco firmly in the male behavioural repertoire, tobacco corporations, having established cigarettes in couples' relationships through their advertising, aimed to expand the human–non-human bond in a different direction, by commencing a powerful marketing drive aimed at women.

Corporate arts: marketing cigarettes to women

The heavy marketing of cigarettes intersected with the First World War to secure the strong presence of cigarettes in men's lives in the UK during the period 1890-1920, but women were not subject to such marketing strategies until the 1920s.[44] In the USA, like many societies in the early 20th century, the idea either of a woman smoking, whether privately or in public, was widely regarded as sinful or a symbol of harlotry. In New York City, a woman was arrested for smoking in public in 1913. Some of the earliest advertising work in this direction emphasized 'couples' situations in which men smoked and the women did not, such as in a striking image of two couples dancing, maypole-like, round a giant Murad Turkish cigarette in a 1919 advertisement.[45] That this situation was amenable to change was in no small part due to the development of the PR field, in which Freud's US nephew, Eddie Bernays, had become a leading light. He was determined to put his uncle's insights about the power of the unconscious to corporate use in 'spinning' public opinion without moral scruple beyond furthering the 'bottom line', and would sell his expertise to whoever was the highest bidder.

In a seminal book, *Crystallising Public Opinion*, Bernays argued that PR should create news "in order to appeal to the instincts and fundamental emotions of the public".[46] His particular skill was in 'engineering consent', a deeply ironic phrase in which 'consent' meant nurturing an illusion of human autonomy and choice in the face of the manipulative power of the tobacco corporations. This, Brandt suggests, "was a critical component of the consumer culture and a central element of the promotion of cigarette smoking".[47]

However, to attribute everything to the growing power and sophistication of the corporate machine is to deny the importance of the substance at the heart of it all. It is unlikely such an illusion would have had to be maintained in the case of soap powder or a pickled onion, for example.

Bernays put his 'engineering consent' ideas into practice in 1928 when he entered into a contract with the ATC to get more women smoking its 'Lucky Strike' brand. For the chairman of the ATC, cracking the female market was "like opening a new goldmine right in our front yard".[48] The ATC first decided to appeal to women by focusing on their waistlines. "Reach for a Lucky instead of a sweet" was the slogan, and Bernays was employed to turn this exhortation into reality. Then came the notion of manipulating public opinion so that women's smoking became a symbol of women's rights.[49] Following the arrest of women for smoking in public at the turn of the century, women were still afraid to smoke in public view. Bernays organized a 1929 Easter Sunday parade in which ten women sauntered down Fifth Avenue, New York, flagrantly smoking cigarettes. This 'Torches of Freedom' campaign, as it came to be known, tapped into a variety of contemporary gender issues such as an increasing urge for equality and the right of women to be more like men. Tobacco, in the form of cigarettes, was the substance at the heart of this campaign, the means whereby women could succeed in the symbolic achievement of such aspirations. Bernays' campaign involved more than the crystallization of public opinion – its outcome was the more-than-human conglomeration of women and cigarettes to form a new world of non-human agency.

The issue of inhaling continued through the 1930s and 40s, with Lucky Strike running a short-lived campaign "Do You Inhale?" between 1931 and 1932, with follow-ons such as "A frank discussion at last on a subject that has long been 'taboo'", "Everybody's doing it", and "Luckies 'make no bones' about this vital question". Examples continued into 1942, when Philip Morris introduced a "little Johnny", bellboy character who wisecracked "Sure you inhale – so play safe with your throat!" By 1949, Lorillard's Embassy Cigarettes were able to cry triumphantly "Inhale to your heart's content".[50]

The cigarette speaks

Bernays was cautious about the use of advertising, which he saw as making the interest of the advertiser too open. He preferred the hidden approach to engineering 'consent', a carefully constructed myth that the consumer was in control. Yet advertising also had its place in the manipulation of public opinion.

A clever Lucky Strike advert[51] effectively marries the two in featuring a speaking cigarette. A man and woman, clearly on an ocean liner, are standing by a porthole, smoking. In front of them, a cigarette communicates direct to its public via a white speech bubble. "When two is company I don't make a crowd", it says (i.e. it knows how to remain discretely 'hidden in plain sight'). The cigarette then makes a stronger claim to human–non-human communitarianism: "I'm your best friend – I am your Lucky Strike". Yet in case one might be thinking this was friendship, either on a par with or possibly challenging the intense relationship being enjoyed by the couple behind the cigarette's speech bubble, the cigarette's further references are all purely botanical.

> You wonder what makes me a better friend. It's center leaves. I spurn the sticky, bitter little top leaves. I scorn the coarse, grimy bottom leaves. I am made only of the mild, fragrant, expensive center leaves.[52]

Here is a cigarette speaking, but clearly about plant rather than human matters. Its conversation hardly makes it likely to captivate guests at the unspecified but clearly elegant evening engagement to which the couple appear to be going. Finally, playing to the most pressing health problem any advertiser was willing to own up to at that time, the cigarette's soliloquy ends with the assurance "I do not irritate your throat".

Tobacco tested

The German Weimar Republic, in the years between the First and the Second World Wars, had some of the highest smoking rates in the world.[53] Chemnitz (near Dresden) was the city with the highest lung cancer rates in the country, and it was here in 1928 that a curious physician conducted what is now known as a 'case series' study of the smoking habits of a series of lung cancer patients. He noticed the high proportion of patients who smoked cigarettes and even hypothesized a second-hand smoking risk for women married to men who smoked.[54] A year later, a Dresden doctor, Fritz Lickint, published another piece of statistical evidence connecting lung cancer to cigarettes. However, his masterwork went much further. *Tabak und Organismus* ('Tobacco and the Organism'), published in 1939 in collaboration with the Reich Committee for the Struggle Against Addictive Drugs and the German Antitobacco Association, is a 1,200 page indictment of tobacco as a public health menace. Illnesses attributed to the *Rauchstrasse* ('smoke pathway') included cancers of the lips, tongue, mouth, jaw, oesophagus and lungs. In addition, tobacco was seen as the cause of arteriosclerosis, infant mortality and stomach ulcers, not to mention the less life-threatening problem of halitosis. Lickint identified the powerfully addictive properties of tobacco and coined the term *Passivrauchen* ('passive smoking') as a threat to non-smokers living with people who smoke. In 1939, another physician, Franz conducted the first case-controlled study of lung cancer, in which he compared the smoking history of 86 male lung cancer cases with 86 'control' subjects. All but three of his lung cancer patients were smokers.

The climate of scientific advance and political ideology proved fertile for this research. Hitler had reportedly smoked between 25 and 40 cigarettes a day in his younger adult life. In a fit of willpower in 1919, however, he threw his cigarettes into the Danube, calling them "a waste of money".[55] He never again smoked (so he claimed). Some of Hitler's pronouncements resonate with those of James I over 300 years earlier in his preoccupation with the tainted associations of a substance both originating and widely used in the lands of black and Amerindian peoples. Hitler saw tobacco as "the wrath of the Red Man against the White Man for having been given hard liquor". He even went so far as to attribute the success of Nazism to his decision to give up smoking. "Our Führer Adolf Hitler drinks no alcohol and does not smoke...His performance at work is incredible" wrote one sycophantic commentator in 1937.[56]

Health was much more than a lifestyle choice for the Nazis – it was the very foundation of the national and racial strength of the Third Reich, the combined product of individual self-discipline and coercion by the state. Women and young people were seen as particularly vulnerable to tobacco as a 'racial poison' and were especially targeted by anti-smoking propaganda in consequence. Cigarettes were seen as grave threats to both the strength and reproductive potential of the Aryan race. *'Die deutsche Frau raucht nicht!'* ('The German woman does not smoke!') became a particularly famous party slogan.[57] Pregnant women (and all women under the age of 25) were denied wartime tobacco rationing coupons, and rules prevented restaurants and bars from selling cigarettes to any women. In similar vein, a 1941 guide for Hitler Youth members and their parents told them that "your body belongs to your nation", and that the pursuit of hedonistic pleasures such as smoking was nothing but the flagrant exhibition of Marxist tendencies.[58] From July 1943 it was made illegal for anyone under the age of 18 to smoke in public.[59]

Further research into the dangers of tobacco was taking place in Germany at that time. The *Wissenschaftliches Institut zur Erforschung der Tabakgefahren* ('Institute for Tobacco Hazards Research') opened with much fanfare at Friedrich Schiller University in Jena, Thuringia, in 1941. The Foundation of the Institute was supported by 100,000 Reichsmarks (the equivalent of more than 1 million US dollars today) ordered directly by Hitler from the Reich Chancellery. "Best of luck in your work to free humanity from one of its most dangerous poisons" Hitler wished participants in a telegram he sent to the Institute's opening conference.[60] Institute head was Karl Astel, leader of the Thuringia Office of Racial Affairs and, amongst other things, a keen proponent of involuntary euthanasia for the mentally ill. The Institute was to become the most significant anti-tobacco organ in Nazi Germany. Fritz Sauckel, author of the original proposal for an Institute, made non-smoker status an employment requirement "as important as Aryan ancestry". His argument was that tobacco addiction would jeopardize the "independence" and "impartiality" of the science produced.[61]

The Nazi government introduced further policy measures, partly as a result of the Institute's work. They included a ban on smoking in many workplaces, government offices, hospitals and rest homes. Police and SS officers were banned from smoking while in uniform and on duty, and soldiers were prohibited from smoking while on the streets, while marching, or during brief off-duty periods. Sixty cities banned smoking on trams in 1941, and trains and buses in every city followed in 1944. This latter directive came from Hitler himself, who was worried about young female conductors being exposed to tobacco smoke.

At one level, these actions are easily dismissed as the misguided efforts of fascist lunatics. At another, however, they derive from a strong thread of anti-tobacco sentiment in Germany going back to the Archbishop of Cologne's preachings in the 17th century,[62] and continuing with Frederick the Great of Prussia, whose concern for the effects of tobacco on young people and society led to a public smoking ban in 1764. Whatever the misguided premises of much Nazi tobacco control, it had no lack of respect for the power and agency of the cigarette, as the somewhat alarming depiction of a cigarette gobbling up a smoker in *Der Kettenraucher* ("The Chain Smoker – he doesn't eat *it*, it eats *him*!") graphically demonstrates (Fig. 7.2).

For all the rhetoric, however, Nazi approaches to tobacco control were complex, ambivalent and poorly enforced.[63] Cigarette consumption continued to increase during the first eight years of the Third Reich, even doubling between 1930 and 1940, although at a lower rate than smoking rates in the USA, for example.[64] Other members of the high Nazi leadership were strong tobacco advocates. Martin Bormann and Hermann Göring, for example, continued to smoke, while Hitler's campaigns against women's tobacco use were somewhat undermined by the notorious smoking habits of his mistress, Eva Braun, and by Goebbels' wife Magda, who liked to smoke her cigarettes through a gold-tipped mouthpiece.[65] Some powerful German tobacco companies, such as the Reemstma Cigarette Company, supported them. Reemstma was careful to express its support for the regime, as various series of patriotic cigarette cards with titles like 'The German Army', and 'The 1936 Olympics' demonstrate.[66] It subsequently produced about 2.3 million copies of an album *Adolf Hitler: Pictures from the Life of the Führer*, that required consumers to collect coupons in their cigarette packets that they could submit for photographs sent by mail.[67] Reemstma had run into conflict with the Nazi Party in the early 1930s, not only because one member of its governing board was Jewish,[68] but also because it was a competitor for the Stormtroopers (SA)s' own cigarette brand 'Sturmzigaretten', produced by Trommler, a rival Dresden company.[69] It is an ironic commentary on the ambivalence of the Nazi views on tobacco that the SA derived half their income from this brand. After the war, a former Gestapo leader recounted:

SA men were supposed to smoke only Trommler cigarettes. Retailers of Reemtsma brands were beaten, their display windows smashed...In

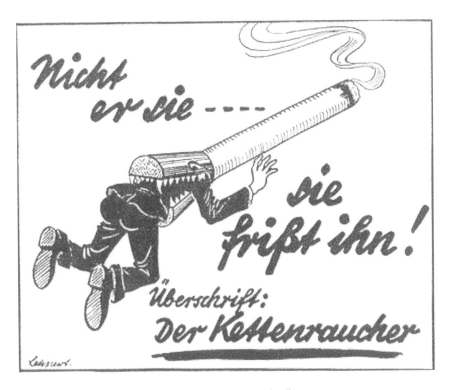

Fig. 7.2 'The Chain Smoker – he doesn't eat *it*, it eats *him*!'
Source: *Reine Luft* (1941 23: 90)

August [of 1933] a meeting was arranged between Reemtsma and Göring...Göring had no desire to kill the hen that laid the golden eggs. He proposed a truce – actually a deal – and Reemtsma accepted. Göring needed sponsors for his art addiction, for the Berlin Opera, and for his project to breed bison and elk. [70]

There was resistance to the anti-smoking propaganda amongst the public too. The 'Edelweiss Pirates', a loose association of youth groups opposed to the Nazi regime, used tobacco smoking as a form of resistance.[71] A 'Hitler Youth' surveillance team that infiltrated a party by a Pirates' affiliate group, the 'Hamburg Swing Youth', were shocked by the "appalling sight" of various kinds of wanton dancing, culminating in everyone jitterbugging on stage "like wild creatures. Several boys could be observed dancing together, always with two cigarettes in the mouth, one in each corner".[72]

The German government was also concerned about the effects of limiting tobacco's availability on both civilian morale and treasury revenues. Tobacco accounted for about a twelfth of the Reichstag's entire income in 1941. There were also 60,000 tobacco growers in Germany. Despite Hitler's regret that German troops had been given daily tobacco rations since the beginning of the war,[73] soldiers continued to receive six cigarettes a day, with additional tobacco benefits for military personnel involved in extermination activities on the Eastern front and in the death camps, the latter a sardonic commentary on a regime that claimed tobacco was one of the most dangerous racial poisons in existence. That smoking rates began to decline in Germany from 1942 onwards appears to have had as much to do with the deprivations of war as with Nazi efforts to become "masters of death"[74] in more ways than one.

Tobacco meetings in post-war Germany – politics and experience

On April 25th, 1945, the Russian and American forces, advancing across Europe from different directions, met at Torgau on the River Elbe.[75] The following day, unit commanders met for an official handshake under a hastily prepared sign "East Meets West". What did they do at this pivotal moment in world history? The picture of this historic occasion held in the National Archives and Records Administration in the USA is captioned 'They battled across Europe for a Camel' (Fig. 7.3).

This striking image, in which the cigarette plays a central role,[76] was destined to become a nostalgic record of east-west camaraderie in the subsequent Cold War years, reminiscent of how hostilities stopped for a Christmas game of football and exchange of cigarettes during the First World War. Similarly symbolic was the camaraderie fostered by the dispensing of American coffee and cigarettes to German civilians by military government officials, something they were encouraged to do as an exhibition of "American and democratic values".[77] Alarmed that Russian cigarettes in Berlin appeared more popular than their American counterparts, US military magazines ran articles criticizing Russian infiltration of the black market and suggested that the cigarettes supplied by the Soviet Rasno Export Agency were full of sulphur and hence harmed the throat and lungs.[78] The battle for consumer confidence was political as much as it was economic.[79] For the Americans, success in the developing Cold War required them to prove the superiority of consumer capitalism amongst the occupied. This in turn, they felt, would lead to the adoption of democratic values through a process known as "occupation mimicry".[80] Their cigarettes offered a way of reorienting Germans politically and economically towards the West, shifting German preferences away from their pre-war preferences for Balkan tobaccos as they did so. For some diplomats and tobacco industry authorities, even "GIs represented walking billboards, popularizing the American style cigarette among German citizens".[81]

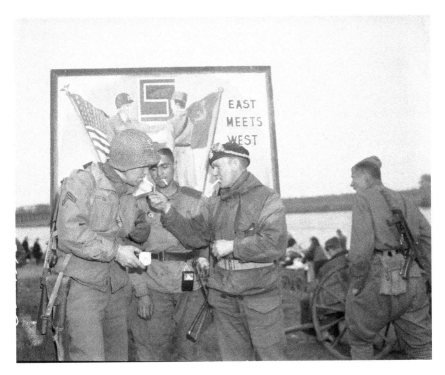

Fig. 7.3 'They battled across Europe for a Camel'
Source: National Archives and Records Administration, Maryland: 111-SC-205353

In the immediate aftermath of the Allied occupation of West Germany, cigarettes became the main medium of exchange in the all-important black economy. The British and American military governments maintained the rationing scheme introduced by the Nazi government in the latter years of the war. This gave every man over the age of 18 forty cigarettes a month; every woman over the age of 25 received twenty. The ration interval was extended in May 1946 from four to six weeks, increasing the general sense of misery and demoralization amongst the populace. Meanwhile, some GIs and civilians had become heavily involved in the creation and maintenance of a black market which was hard to police. One of these was Benno Mattel, son-in-law of the composer Anton Webern. Webern was a member of the 'Second Viennese School', which included Arnold Schoenberg and Alban Berg. They were all heavy smokers.[82] Webern's death in 1945 was a sorry consequence of his smoking habit.[83] Mattel, formerly an SS officer, had gone into partnership with soldiers of the US 42nd division as a black market trader in the village of Mittersill, near Salzburg. He invited the Weberns to a dinner party with the temptation of a major tobacco 'carrot'. "Do you know by any chance what an historic day it is today?" Webern asked his daughter. His son-in-law had secured him what was to be his first ever American cigar. However, two American soldiers had been authorized to undertake a 'sting' operation to catch Mattell in his black market dealings. The Weberns needed to leave their son-in-law's house at 9.45 p.m. in order to get back to their quarters before a 10.30 p.m. civilian curfew. Webern tiptoed outside (so as not to disturb his sleeping granddaughters) with the intention of partly smoking the cigar before he and his wife left. Stepping out onto the balcony, however, he disturbed one of the soldiers, who shot him "in self defence".[84]

Tobacco desperation in post-war Germany

Larkin relates a *Reader's Digest* story, 'The Trail of a GI Cigarette', in which a 1947 cigarette takes a journey from an American GI via a cobbler, coal dealer, butcher, and plumber to a farmer.[85] Only the farmer can afford the luxury of actually smoking it. By becoming a currency, cigarettes had moved into a sphere of exchange where they were too valuable for most people to be smoked, except in desperation or if you had alternative ways of accessing the things you were seeking to exchange (such as the farmer, who could grow and sell his own food). Non-smokers in receipt of rations had a decided advantage over smokers, since they could barter their ration for other things. The cigarette assumed the role of medicine rather than pleasure, with those who could not resist the urge to consume their ration themselves tending to schedule their consumption at times that would quell their hunger pangs. The use of substitutes and additives became common, while home cultivation of tobacco was an option for those lucky enough to have the land available.

All this reflected the abject state of the much of the populace forced to scratch a living in bombed-out cities. In this environment, *Stummeling* or *Kippensammlung*, the abject practice of collecting tobacco from used cigarette butts to make new ones, became common. Children became attuned to the different smoking habits of American, French and British soldiers and the likelihood of obtaining discarded butts from them. The French typically "smoked cigarettes down to nothing", inserting a needle into the remainder so they could use up the final bit until nothing remained. The Americans, on the other hand "took a few puffs and then threw away their cigarettes".[86] Thus "in cities and towns with significant GI populations...Stories of tram conductors stopping their vehicles to gather a 'Gross Stomp' from the gutter and physical altercations between Germans, old and young alike, over cigarette butts illustrated the depths of Germany's decline".[87]

American tobacco growers saw the scarcity of tobacco in West Germany as a prime opportunity to develop a potentially lucrative new market. However, Greek and Turkish suppliers were keen to be allowed to resume the trade with Germany that had been severed by the war and the tense post-war political situation. With many Balkan states falling to communism, it behoved the Americans to take the pleas of Cold War allies such as Greece and Turkey seriously. Regardless of these concerns, the first consignment of US leaf arrived in Germany on the SS Flying Independent in December 1948 after pressure from the US Department of Agriculture and the US tobacco lobby. Here was tobacco described as an import to "'brighten' the faces of long-suffering smokers and contribute to the 'rebuilding of Europe in the sense of the Marshall Plan'".[88] Its arrival, at much the same time as the airlifting of supplies by British and American pilots into blockaded Berlin, was an event of huge symbolism in the geopolitical arena. By 1949, despite the concerns of Greek and Turkish suppliers, more than half of tobacco imports into West Germany were from the USA.[89] The nature of the tobacco consumed altered radically as well. During the 1930s, around 95 per cent of the cigarettes consumed in Germany were manufactured from Oriental tobaccos imported from places like Turkey, Greece and Bulgaria. By 1949, 90 per cent of German cigarettes were a blend of US and Oriental tobaccos.

American officials on both sides of the Atlantic anticipated German tastes reverting to their pre-war preference for Oriental tobaccos from the Balkans. Thus, it was important to educate the palate of the German consumer as quickly as possible (Fig. 7.4). The Reemtsma advertisement for 'Ova' cigarettes acts both as publicity for its relaunched brand and education for consumers in how the product had changed.

The advertisement for 'Fox' cigarettes, from the same period, attempts to educate the consumer in a subtly different way (Fig. 7.5). Reemtsma introduced the Fox brand in 1948, again with a blend of Virginia and Oriental tobaccos. In their 1950 advertisement, the heading 'America, you do not smoke better' alludes to a poem by Goethe which stated 'America, you have it better than our old continent'. Consider the 'speed and rhythm' of the American harbour with its busy stevedores and impatient tug boat, funnel smoking, against a backdrop of skyscrapers and a suspension bridge: no bombed-out buildings or ruined bridges here. The upper scene contrasts with the 'calm' (but also ancient) allusions in the depiction of the Oriental shoreline below, with its sailing boat and oar-propelled cutter, and a nondescript shed across the bay. Note the sleeping figure portrayed in the right of the picture, and the archaeological ruins atop a rocky promontory. For which was the German consumer supposed to feel more affinity? Furthermore, the American scene is quasi-photographic (as is the cigarette packet itself), whereas the Oriental is a pre-modern line drawing. Who in the circumstances of post-war reconstruction could resist the modernist attractions of the former with its superiority implicitly fashioned in the very layout of the advert?

Neither of these Reemtsma advertisements show German people actually smoking.[90] Given the recent past, in which cigarettes had become objects of

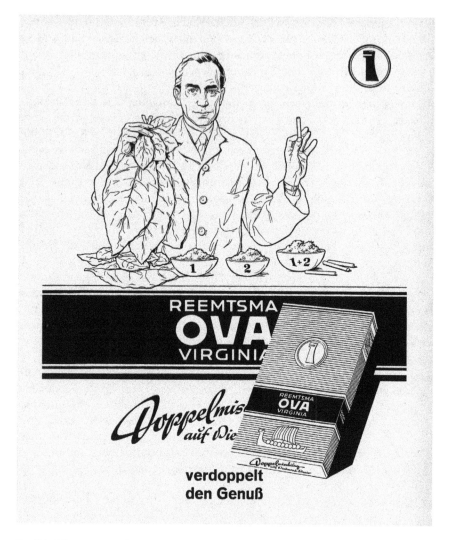

Fig. 7.4 Advertisement for a relaunched 'Ova' cigarette, a blend of American and Oriental tobaccos

Source: Museum der Arbeit (Hamburg), Reemtsma-Archive

currency rather than consumption and "observers frequently insisted German smokers who could afford to smoke cigarettes came from the upper class or secured a lucrative lifestyle through illicit or immoral behavior",[91] this is perhaps understandable. It is the product that forms the essential core of these advertisements.

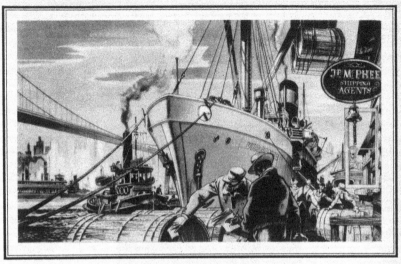

AMERIKA *du rauchst nicht besser...*

Wir alle schätzen den würzig-kraftvollen Geschmack des amerikanischen Virginia-Tabaks; kein rechter Raucher möchte seine belebende, anregende Wirkung mehr missen. Ebenso aber schätzen und lieben wir Deutsche von jeher den Duft und das unvergleichliche Aroma echten, edlen Orient-Tabaks.

Wer tätig-strebend sein Leben meistern will und sich den Sinn für verfeinerten Lebensgenuß bewahrt hat, wird sich daher - bewußt oder unbewußt - stets für eine Cigarette entscheiden, in der sich das Kraftvoll-Belebende des Virginia-Tabaks mit der genießerischen Delikatesse des Orient-Tabaks verbindet.

Beide Elemente aber machen das Besondere der ℱℴℰ aus.

TABAKLAND VIRGINIA und TABAKLAND ORIENT geben ihr Bestes zum Besten der ℱℴℰ

mild und süß

Fig. 7.5 'America, you do not smoke better...'

Source: Museum der Arbeit (Hamburg), Reemtsma-Archive

Smoking and lung cancer in Britain and the USA – what took so long?

Considering how clearly scientists in the Weimar Republic, and, subsequently, the Third Reich, had identified the dangers of cigarette smoking, it is amazing how long it took their counterparts in Britain and the USA to follow suit. The slang terms by which cigarettes became known in Britain – 'little white slavers', 'coffin nails', 'fags' – reflect a knowing if sublimated lay appreciation of the dangers inherent in their use. Britain was experiencing a similar increase in lung cancer rates amongst men over 45 years, consequential of the uptake of smoking during the First World War: there was a six-fold increase in the figures between 1930 and 1945. Similar trends could be observed in the USA, where lung cancer rates exploded from one per 100,000 deaths in 1920 to 13 per 100,000 deaths in 1950.[92] In fact, the US pathologist Isaac Adler had suggested as early as 1912 that the newly fashionable cigarette might be the cause of a discernible increase in lung cancer rates, while still being able to state at that time that "primary malignant neoplasms of the lung are among the rarest forms of disease".[93] In 1938, Raymond Pearl, a biology professor at Johns Hopkins University, conducted a study for the insurance industry in which he divided a sample of 6813 subjects into non-smokers, moderate smokers and heavy smokers. Sixty-seven per cent of the non-smokers lived to beyond 60 years of age compared to 61 per cent of moderate and 46 per cent of heavy smokers. Despite *Time* magazine saying "the results should make tobacco users' flesh creep", the main message taken from the study was that moderate smokers had little to worry about (since their longevity appeared from these figures to be only a few points behind those of their non-smoking compatriots).[94] It is as if some kind of distorting, perspectival lens made it impossible to take on board the more serious figure for the heavy smokers.

Yet despite the patterns that were emerging, there was a curious lack of momentum amongst scientists to acknowledge a problem, let alone its cause. It was as if the pre-war research in Germany and the USA had not taken place. In the case of Germany, a simple language barrier may have played a part, as it does in science to this day. However, the practical and ideological consequences of the unravelling of the Nazi regime also played a role. Many of the key German scientists responsible for investigating the relationship between smoking, lung cancer, and other diseases were either dead or had disappeared into obscurity. Astel committed suicide in his office on the night of 3rd–4th April 1945; Sauckel was executed on 1st October 1946 for crimes against humanity. There was also a more general antipathy to all things Nazi. Thus, "much of the wind was taken out of the sails of Germany's anti-tobacco movement".[95] This does not explain the failure to acknowledge the evidence that had accumulated in the USA, though.

Starting afresh, in 1948, Bradford Hill and Richard Doll send out letters to 60,000 British doctors asking them to take part in a prospective study of possible links between smoking and lung cancer; 34,000 men and 6,000 women agreed to take part. The results, published five years later, made it clear that death from lung cancer was much more common amongst doctors who smoked than amongst those who did not. Moreover, those who smoked more were more likely to die prematurely than those who smoked less. Yet the many changes and technological innovations that British society had seen during the preceding half century meant that the precise reason for the increase remained elusive. With the wisdom of hindsight, Doll expressed complete surprise at their findings, claiming, "I suspected that if we could find a cause it was most likely to have something to do with motor cars and the tarring of the roads".[96] In a statement to a UK House of Commons Select Committee some 50 years later, he talked of "the ubiquity of the habit [smoking], which was entrenched among male doctors and scientists". This, he suggested, "had dulled the sense that tobacco might be a major threat to health".[97] This is a remarkable statement for someone as schooled in scientific methods as Doll. More than a simple oversight, an enchantment appears to have settled over the scientific community, a trance-like state of inertia that "dulled the sense" of the significance of the arrival of machine-produced cigarettes, their mass consumption and deep inhalation practices, and the dire consequences of these long term.

The smoking status of both authors may have led to the lack of further activity deriving from their findings at the policy level. Hill and Doll were both smokers at the start of their study. Perhaps their addiction to tobacco made it hard to admit the implications of their results. In the words of one commentator on the relationship between 'evidence' and 'policy', "resistances erect their own barricades of perception and knowing".[98] Yet as these figures filtered back into population consciousness and experience, many users came to recognize that long-term use of tobacco involved risk of some kind of significant future payback. Publication of Hill and Doll's results led doctors to become the first professional group in the UK to give up smoking in large numbers.

While the relationship between tobacco and people was undoubtedly souring, another reason this did not lead to immediate tobacco control measures was the stringency of the proofs epidemiological science felt it needed to confirm the long-term effects of particular substances on health. The scientific study of the distribution and causes of disease very much relied on the postulates (criteria) of German physician Robert Koch. These worked well in studying acute infectious diseases, such as cholera and tuberculosis, but with the longer timescales that are usually involved in non-communicable diseases, asserting causality is often much more difficult. Koch's postulates, developed in the last quarter of the 19th century, insisted that the causative agent (in his case, bacteria) must be present in every case of disease, that it could be isolated from the host with the disease and grown in pure culture, that inoculation by a pure culture of bacteria into a healthy susceptible host should reproduce the disease, and that the bacteria must be recoverable from the experimentally infected host.[99] Even with bacterial diseases, meeting all Koch's postulates without exception can be tricky; not all bacteria can be cultured externally, for example. It is much more difficult to achieve this level of proof in the case of a substance like tobacco.

The powers of enchantment and rigours of Koch's postulates notwithstanding, a dissonant recognition of the dangers of tobacco (particularly its inhaled smoke) alongside a widespread acceptance of tobacco use amongst the adult population was developing – tobacco resplendent and tobacco risky miring their human hosts in a smoky cloud of confusion. The tobacco industry – corporate tobacco – did nothing to clear the air on this score. In fact, as we shall see in the next chapter, its response to the growing evidence of harm was to increase the controversy, not defuse it.

Conclusion

The First World War, with its reinstatement of the connection between tobacco and military service, marked the start of what has been called the 'cigarette century'. Two World Wars proved something of a lifeline for the increasingly powerful tobacco corporations, who otherwise faced challenges to their ways of operating from producers and public alike. A major block to tobacco's global expansion was the recalcitrance of many women to the idea of smoking, and in the interwar years, using some of the insights of Freudian psychology, the industry used the emergent PR field in order to change public opinion in the USA and the UK in this regard. The industry – largely through its advertising – was also adept at developing an illusion of human agency, of tobacco consumption being about glamour and freedom rather than abjection and dependency. The desperate circumstances of post-war Germany, a desire to sublimate its recent political history, and the influx of American tobacco as part of the Marshall plan, led to West Germany turning its back on its tobacco control past. It is in many ways unfortunate that Hitler not only existed but should have been the first major 20th century leader to follow the trend of autocrats since the 17th century in finding tobacco detestable. However, this cannot fully explain the time it took for post-war researchers on both sides of the Atlantic to pick up the research baton once more and identify what was going on with regard to cigarettes and lung cancer. A model of enchantment, I have argued, helps explain why it took researchers in the UK and the USA such a long time to recognize the link between smoking and lung cancer and, more importantly, for this realization to be acted upon.

Notes

1 See Chapters 2 and 4.
2 Miller (2005: 5).
3 Rogoziński (1990: 111), cited in Goodman (1993: 92).
4 Cox (2000: Table 6.1) Goodman, (1993: 234).
5 Cox (2000: Table 6.1) Goodman's figures for Chinese sales (1993: 234-5) are somewhat different, but similarly astronomical in extent.
6 Goodman (1993: 235).
7 Campbell (2005).
8 Campbell (2005: 215). Burley is a form of tobacco leaf characteristic of Kentucky although Hahn (2011) cautions that much of the apparent distinctiveness of leaf types is constructed through companies' need for branding.
9 Brandt (2007: 34).
10 Brandt (2007: 41). It is ironic to note that in 2017, BAT was reunited with R.J. Reynolds once again (Kollewe and Glenza 2017).
11 Brandt (2007: 47).
12 Alston et al. (2002).
13 Henry (1906: 22).
14 Ibid. (21).
15 Ibid. (15-16).
16 Tate (1999: 5).
17 Tate (1999: 5-6).
18 Berridge (2007: 13).
19 Hilton (2000: 75).
20 Walkley (1915).
21 Brandt (2007: 53).
22 Chesterton (1917: 374).
23 Sloterdijk (2009).
24 Chesterton (1917: 375).
25 Cited in Welshman (1996: 1380).
26 Brandt (2007: 51).
27 Ibid. (52).
28 Kiernan (1991: 148).
29 Briggs (1983: 260).
30 Owen (1967: 433).
31 Jerome (1984: 300-1).
32 Sassoon (1930: 27).
33 Kiernan (1991: 149).
34 "It's the Spirit, not the Letter, that giveth life" is the biblical allusion used (Kipling 1926: 62).
35 Pendarvis puts it baldly: "cigarettes were considered cheap and womanly until men started killing one another while smoking them, then everybody liked them" (Pendarvis 2016: 67).
36 Isherwood (1976: 143).
37 Gray (2008a: 58).
38 Svevo (2001: 8).
39 Davis (2006: 270).
40 I am grateful to Francis Thirlway for this insight.
41 Brandt (2007).
42 The recorded levels were 82 per cent for men, and 41 per cent for women (ASH, 2016a).

43 National Center for Chronic Disease Prevention and Health Promotion (US) Office on Smoking and Health (2014).
44 Tinkler (2006).
45 Heimann and Heller (2018: 70).
46 Bernays (1923: 171).
47 Brandt (2007: 88).
48 Tye (2002: 23).
49 Tye (2002); Brandt (2007: 84-5).
50 Stanford University (n.d.) contains all these examples.
51 Heimann and Heller (2018: 123).
52 Ibid.
53 Hess (1996) suggests that 80 per cent of the male population in the 1930s were smokers. Proctor (1996: 1450) states that "German per capita tobacco use between 1932 and 1939 rose from 570 to 900 cigarettes a year".
54 Proctor (1999: 283, n32). The physician's name was Schönherr.
55 Ibid. (219).
56 Quoted in Proctor (1996: 1451).
57 Lewy (2006: 1189). Proctor (1999) provides evidence of low levels of lung cancer amongst German women of the Nazi generation that are consequent on the low smoking rates amongst women during this period.
58 Larkin (2010: 24-5).
59 Proctor (1996:1451)
60 Proctor (1999: 209).
61 Quoted in Proctor (1997: 464-5).
62 See Chapter 4.
63 Schneider and Glantz (2008: 291); Bachinger et al. (2008).
64 Proctor (1999: 244).
65 Larkin (2010: 39).
66 Proctor (1999: 233).
67 Stratigakos (2015: 185).
68 David Schur was a Jewish cigarette manufacturer with excellent contacts in the Balkans. His company was taken over by Reemtsma in 1924, when he was invited to join the board. He escaped deportation arrest by the Gestapo in 1935 and ended up in the United States where he died in 1948.
69 Proctor (1999: 235-6).
70 Ibid. (235).
71 Davey Smith et al. (1995) provide a picture of a group of Edelweiss Pirates, all with cigarettes in their mouths.
72 Peukert (1987), cited in Davey Smith and Egger (1996: 110).
73 Proctor (1999: 219).
74 Rhodes (2002).
75 They were actually members of the 69th Division of the US First Army and the First Ukrainian Front.
76 One commentator on this photo remarked on cigarette parallels with Woody Allen's film Zelig.
77 Larkin (2010: 144).
78 Ibid. (143). Ironically these cigarettes were called 'Drug' in Russian, which translates as 'Pal'. Concern for the harmful qualities of 'inferior' cigarettes compared to 'normal' ones predates the rhetoric about counterfeit cigarettes in the later 20th century. In fact, their popularity was probably due to the fact they were cheaper than American brands.

79 De Grazia (2005) talks of the "American market empire" that came into being in the second half of the twentieth century.
80 Fay (2008: 24).
81 Larkin (2010: 153).
82 Indeed, so essential did Berg perceive the hybrid bond between habit and occupation, smoking and creativity, that he is reputed to have told a student that if he did not smoke, he could not call himself a composer.
83 To say "he died because of his habit" invokes the same complex web of causation the historian E.H. Carr (1961) ascribes to the smoker crossing the road to buy cigarettes who is killed on a blind corner by a drunk driver in a car with defective brakes.
84 Moldenhauer (1970: 880).
85 Cited in Larkin (2010). I have not been able to verify the source of this story.
86 Samuel (2002: 241-2 and 31), cited in Larkin (2010: 96).
87 Larkin (2010: 93).
88 Ibid. (137).
89 Ibid. (153). In a throwback to Virginian concerns of the 18th century, however, American tobacco traders expressed disappointment that the military government did not prioritize imports of quality tobacco over cheaper varieties. For the American authorities in Germany, though, the primary concern was to deal with Germany's post-war tobacco shortage and its related black market in the most effective way possible, within the limited budget at the authorities' disposal, leaving money to spare for vital food imports.
90 Larkin (2010: 169).
91 Ibid. (88).
92 Rates in 1990 were 50 per 100,000.
93 Adler (1912: 11). See also Timmermann (2014).
94 Sullum (1999: 43).
95 Proctor (1996: 1452).
96 In Berridge (2007: 23).
97 Ibid. (49).
98 Pal (1990: 151).
99 Carter (1985).

Chapter 8

Corporate voices: tobacco, 1950–2000

Introduction: "speaking as Philip Morris"

Tobacco was on the defensive. A Philip Morris internal memo written in 1989 articulated the need, given the issues it was facing,

> to talk in a variety of voices if what we want to say is to be heard, understood and acted upon. At times, we will speak as Philip Morris; sometimes we will need to speak as independent scientists, scientific groups and businessmen; and, finally, we will need to speak as the smoker.[1]

In this chapter I shall investigate this panoply of voices and what they say, under the guise of different forms of agnotology. Agnotology is a term coined by historian Robert Proctor and linguist Ian Boal as a counterweight to epistemology, and highlighting how what we don't know is just as much a construct of circumstance as what we do.[2] Not all agnotology is constructed in a deliberate way, of course. The ignorance about tobacco that existed in Europe when it first arrived was pure, what Proctor calls "native-state" agnotology. Then there is "agnotology as selective choice" – where "a focus upon object A involves a neglect of object B", as Proctor puts it.[3] "Active agnotology" involves deliberate attempts to mislead or create ignorance and confusion. This is where the power of the tobacco corporation or 'tobacco interests' more generally comes into its own: the deliberate attempts, by various means, to obscure and contest the nature of tobacco and the health risks of its long-term use.[4]

Tobacco has revealed the extent of active corporate agnotology through resolution of a US legal case in 1998 against the harms caused by tobacco. The "Master Settlement", as it came to be known, was a multistate decision which occurred primarily because it was in the interests of both parties – government and the tobacco industry – to avoid a mass of legal wrangling over individual liability suits. One of its outcomes was to subpoena and release to public scrutiny millions of industry documents,[5] now overseen by the American Legacy Foundation, a non-profit organization with an online document library that has become an illuminating trove of historical documents concerning the tobacco industry. The US Master Settlement was not the first time tobacco industry documents had been subpoenaed, but its scale was unique. It captures an era of tobacco industry lies and deceit, exposing the active agnotology in the tactics tobacco corporations use to control the agenda and mislead the public in myriad ways.

Anthropologists Pete Benson and Stuart Kirsch use tobacco and mining as examples of what they call "harm industries", those "capitalist enterprises that are predicated on practices that are destructive or harmful to people and the environment: harm is part and parcel of their normal functioning".[6] The harms of which they speak are not necessarily discrete events such as the Union Carbide gas disaster in Bhopal, India that killed nearly 4,000 people in the settlements one night in 1984.[7] Hughes comments *"if tobacco was understood to be more immediately and visibly dangerous*, then perhaps the contemporary picture of tobacco use in the West would look very different".[8] Most corporate harm comes in less obvious forms, which have variously been termed "slow violence"[9] or "slow death".[10] The production, marketing and selling of tobacco products is primarily of this kind. One of the key terms in critiques of corporate capitalism is the "fiduciary imperative". According to Wiist, "the primary purpose of the corporation is to increase shareholder value. It has no other obligation to individuals, societies or the planet".[11] The fiduciary imperative, then, involves the prioritizing of profits for shareholders over any civic concerns such as health, the environment or human welfare.[12] Because of it, Wiist argues, "in the absence of strong public spheres and the imperatives of a strong democracy, the corporation, lacking self-restraint, does not respect those human values that are not commoditized but that are central to a democratic civic culture".[13]

Some scholars consider the incompatibility between the fiduciary imperative and the health and well-being of the public to be irreconcilable, and that this makes the corporation an inherently pathological social form. For Bakan, a psychiatrist, the corporation's behaviour in the present economy fits perfectly with the psychiatric definition of a psychopath.[14] For Emily Martin, an anthropologist, "the corporation's only legitimate mandate is to exploit others for profit; people are treated like tools that can be used, depleted and thrown away. Its mandate is to dehumanize".[15] Such claims might seem a little far-fetched until one looks on the websites of some of the major tobacco corporations. The limited and amoral aspirations of Imperial Tobacco, for example, are summed up by the strapline "we're an international tobacco company focused on creating value for our shareholders".[16] Philip Morris International are equally open – but also opaque – about their goals, "to generate superior returns for shareholders, provide high quality and innovative products to adult smokers, and reduce the harm caused by tobacco products. We work toward this last goal by supporting comprehensive regulation based on harm reduction and developing products with the potential to reduce the risk of disease".[17]

The question then becomes – is tobacco unique in the degree of human mayhem it has created, or are all corporations and their products equally harmful, equally pathological? Some are happy to take the latter position; despite its title, *Killer Commodities*, Singer and Baer's edited volume devotes a surprisingly small portion of its content to tobacco, although they are the first to acknowledge that tobacco is "a product that kills its user on a scale unmatched by other commodities".[18] Yet a cursory analysis of how the tobacco industry compares with other corporate entities, such as those in the field of fast food, sugared drinks, alcohol or even pharmaceuticals, indicates there are many similarities between them.[19] They copy and even share tactics about how to deal with scientific and other challenges to their presence.[20] Only the nature (ontology) of their product(s) differentiates them significantly. Certain commodities, if not the means of obtaining and distributing them, fulfil a human need or requirement; but it is hard to justify the value of tobacco in these terms, particularly as an addictive product known to prematurely kill half its long-term users.[21]

The rest of this chapter will present a series of vignettes and examples of the many voices of the tobacco corporation, all of them geared to making an unnecessary product more appealing and better able to sell. Advertising has been a key way for tobacco corporations to make their unnecessary product more appealing. Revisiting Germany following the devastation of the Second World War offers the opportunity to see tobacco advertising promising a "taste of the big wide world" in both a literal (advertised) and political sense, through the strong links established between industry and government. Smokers' voices are represented through the ways cigarettes have transculturated and enmeshed themselves within particular ritual contexts, how tobacco causes people to act in ways that are not necessarily in their best interests, and the problems they have in attempting to quit.

"Scientific groups and businessmen" are represented by tobacco industry responses to its increasingly untenable position. The CEOs of the major tobacco companies met in New York City in 1953 and issued a "Frank Statement to Cigarette Smokers" about their commitment to the health of their consumers and their belief that their products were safe, while at the same time developing new technologies that appeared to address the growing body of health concerns. The meeting also spurred the formation of a jointly funded Tobacco Industry Research Committee (TIRC), an organization that would appear to be doing something while using science to confuse, in whatever way possible, the growing evidence of a connection between tobacco and ill-health.[22] The rest of the chapter will present examples of agnotology in practice, as revealed by the Master Settlement documents – the shifting nature and involution of tobacco advertising, tobacco's infiltration of academic life, its corporate presentation of apparent social responsibility, its shape-shifting into other goods ('brand stretching') and through the creation of faux grassroots 'astroturf' organizations. These are all examples of tobacco seeking to further enmesh itself into the fabric of everyday life during the second half of the 20th century, in the process deliberately fomenting ignorance and confusion. As important as such externally facing agnotology, however, are the ways in which tobacco maintains its workforce through what might be called internal agnotology. The different kinds of lies and deceit contained in the many voices of a corporation like Philip Morris culminates in a satirical cartoon character called Mr. Butts, a walking, talking cigarette. The chapter ends by considering the ways in which the many voices might be silenced, through a process I call "turning the policy network inside-out", as has happened to a certain extent in the UK.

"The taste of the big, wide world"

Launched across Germany in 1959, Peter Stuyvesant promoted itself as an international brand from the start. The internationalism and modernity is exemplified in an early advertisement for its filter cigarettes (Fig. 8.1). In this triumphant advertisement, people are on the move, and an Iberia Airlines plane has pulled in at the end of an international flight. The plane door opens onto a bright and breezy sunlit world and a collection of beautiful passengers walk down the aircraft steps. A man waves a newspaper (or is it a catheter bag?) to someone awaiting his arrival. At the bottom of the steps, past the sentry-like flight attendant, and overlaying a balloon-like barrage of colours, is the explanatory catchphrase "the taste of the big, wide world". This advertisement validates Schivelbusch's assertion that "as tobacco advertising evolved...it became increasingly detached from the thing or product it represented...With cigarette advertising, the item itself had become largely irrelevant".[23] Irrelevant, or simply more deeply 'hidden in plain sight', the better to make a powerful pitch for the glamour and modernity surrounding its product? All tobacco advertising has elements of fantasy and deception, and the public can be willing participants in this process, if they want to believe that they themselves could step out of a jet plane thanks to a cigarette. Simone Dennis points out the ubiquity of invitations to enticing destinations.[24] The English equivalent of this advert has the strapline "The International Passport to Smoking Pleasure".

The advertisement in question can be seen as more than a play on the magical glamour of modern life, such as we saw in immediate post-war German advertising (Chapter 7). It also makes a clever political statement offering cigarettes as a ticket for the rehabilitation of the (West) German people into the unbounded pleasures of cosmopolitan modernity. The Federal Republic joined NATO in 1955 and was a founding member of the European Economic Community in 1958. The much trumpeted 'economic miracle' was starting to kick in. This advertisement taps into this zeitgeist; it is little wonder that sales of Peter Stuyvesant increased by nearly 40 per cent in the first three years after the brand came to market, taking third place in the German rankings for total market share.[25] Both the nascent enthusiasm for

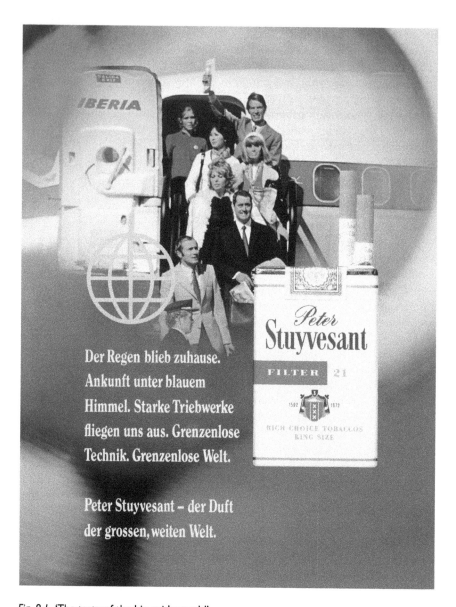

Fig. 8.1 'The taste of the big, wide world'
Source: Museum der Arbeit (Hamburg), Reemtsma-Archive

filter cigarettes, driven by a growing awareness of health concerns, and the success of Reemtsma in getting its brand into vending machines across West Germany,[26] were important factors in this growth, as well as the heavy advertising. Advertisers' magic meets health concerns and material circumstances in explaining the success or otherwise of tobacco products worldwide. However, political and economic factors can be seen operating at a higher level of government altogether. Germany offers a case study of some of the close relationships that can develop between government and industry, relationships that sustain bonds between users and product that can be equally difficult to break.

Germany – political economy of a smokers' heaven

It is not simply advertising that explains the surge in smoking rates in both West and East Germany from the 1950s onwards. Smoking became entwined with a desire amongst the populace on both sides of the Iron Curtain to distance themselves from all things Nazi, including the public health policies of the Third Reich. Additionally, the West German government desperately needed the tax revenues tobacco could be relied upon to provide.[27] People's abject experiences in the immediate post-war era made individual choice not only a right, but intrinsically pleasurable. The Marshall Plan led to increased shipments of tobacco from the USA to West Germany. There, the tobacco industry was also strongly influential in policy-making circles and, as was the case elsewhere, it used a number of strategies that sought not to deny the dangers but to minimize their significance.[28]

The West German government was not operating in a knowledge or policy vacuum over tobacco. The 1960s were the time that the first major US and UK reports about the health risks of smoking were released.[29] They prompted the West German Ministry of Health to explore the possibility of restricting, or even completely banning, tobacco advertising. The Economics Ministry, however, opposed all such measures. For that Ministry, marketing had become about more than just selling products – it symbolized being part of a liberal, democratic society, one that had successfully overcome the hardships of both its Nazi and immediate post-war past. Moreover, it had to demonstrate its superiority over the planned economy juddering along on the other side of the Berlin wall. East German circumstances were very different. Here, the Socialist Unity government of the German Democratic Republic felt it could not impose restrictions on smoking due to more general shortages in consumer goods people were experiencing.[30] It is interesting that smoking rates in the Eastern bloc countries increased at the same rate or faster than Western Europe, despite a lack of glamorous multimillion dollar advertising campaigns of the 'Taste of the Big Wide World' variety. Looking at the situation in another Eastern bloc country, Bulgaria, one historian writes that "the production of a desirable and inherently addictive product on both sides of the Iron Curtain clearly played a role" and, tellingly, "smoking also seemed to have a momentum all its own...a luxury and a freedom that was offered on a grand scale in a period when both were in short supply".[31]

In response to the growing health concerns, the West German *Verband der Cigarettenindustrie* ('Cigarette Industry Association', VdC) proposed its own voluntary advertising code which the Health Ministry, recoiling from the Economics Ministry's antipathy to a statutory code, welcomed. The code stipulated that no health-related claims or comparisons should be made about cigarettes, nor should special characteristics such as filter, mouthpiece, or casing be presented in such a way that implied added health benefits or enhanced pleasure. There were to be no prominent figures, celebrities or athletes in advertisements; nor were advertisements to depict athletic events or activities. Television and cinema advertising were prohibited before 7.00 p.m. and 6.00 p.m., respectively. Advertisements in publications oriented towards young people were prohibited, as were advertisements featuring models younger than 30 years (later reduced to under 25). Novelty schemes and gimmicks such as coupons, balloons and flags were outlawed, as was advertising on public transport within West Germany and at vending machines.

The industry slowly and strategically increased its self-regulation in response, in order to avoid any risk of the state taking a more active role in controlling tobacco marketing. Thus, TV commercials were withdrawn altogether in January 1973, much to the chagrin of advertising agencies who argued that cigarette advertising bore no relationship to cigarette consumption! The Federal government decided that, rather than countering other forms of advertising head-on, health education messages showing children and young people the errors of adult behaviour were the best way forwards. Young people were encouraged to follow *"Der neue Trend* ('The New Trend')—no smoking please".[32] This was a classic example of a neoliberal, pro-choice, and hence completely ineffectual anti-tobacco agenda; from having had the "world's strongest antismoking movement in the 1930s and early 1940s",[33] on both sides of what became the Iron Curtain, Germany became a post-war "smokers' heaven".

The Nazi past has created shadows beyond the immediate post-war responses to tobacco control, however. In a first example of agnotology, the industry was able to distort the complex history outlined in Chapter 7 by labelling all tobacco control policies as Nazi and labelling tobacco control advocates as "health fascists".[34] From the 1960s onwards, tobacco representatives on both sides of the Atlantic started making spurious connections between German fascists imprisoning and killing people with whom they disagreed and tobacco control advocates "persecuting smokers".[35] Demonstrating against No Smoking Day in the UK in 1992, members of FOREST, the tobacco advocacy group, dressed in Nazi uniforms and thanked the Secretary of State for health for "continuing the good work of his predecessors in Nazi Germany". City maps produced in advertisements by Philip Morris in a pan-European campaign in

1995 replaced the Jewish ghettos created by the Third Reich with "smoking zones", under headlines such as "Do we want another ghetto?"[36] It is easy to exploit a view that tobacco users are a 'got at' minority, using the immoral symbols of fascism to impute completely unfounded political doctrines on their supposed tormentors. It is a trope which we will see continuing in future chapters.

Smokers' voices – cravings and enmeshments

Tobacco's ritual practices

Cigarettes transculturated effectively across geographical domains, enmeshing themselves in the fabric and everyday practices of human life. In China, at least for the half of the male population in their thrall, cigarettes became a fundamental component of masculine identity and the building of social relationships (*guanxi*).[37] Kohrman identifies a word *fayan*, "to distribute smoke", which had "become a basic and highly ritualized feature of male performativity and *guanxi*-making".[38]

> In most settings, whenever men encounter each another and wish to engage in dialogue, it is expected that one or more will pull out a pack of cigarettes and offer a smoke to all men immediately present, with special attention given to participants' social status and the understood quality/ cultural coding of the cigarette pack being offered.[39]

Amongst Zimbabwean gangs in the oldest township in Harare cigarettes activated rituals of gang membership through a metaphorical 'cut' of one cigarette between four or five members.

> To actually cut the cigarette up – as one might a pie, for instance – would be to rob it of its very essence, its smokability...Before commencing, the group works out together how much each person's cut is – that is to say, what length of the cigarette may be smoked. Then the ritual begins, the cigarette is lit by the first person, who proceeds to smoke, precisely, their portion—no more, no less. If you refuse to cut appropriately, you might expect to find yourself in big trouble.[40]

However "the object is too powerful a presence to be just the sign of something else",[41] such as *guanxi* or a gang membership ritual. The biochemical reality of tobacco addiction and the individual tobacco craving that ensues are fundamental reasons for tobacco's perpetuation worldwide. "For many non-smokers, it is all too easy to underestimate the biochemical grip that cigarettes can have over people" writes Kohrman.[42] Tobacco craving is thus the prequel to a behaviour which takes place in a wider network of interpersonal, relational, and cultural significance, although the consequences of its 'grip' can occasionally be immediate and profound. An anthropologist who worked in Micronesia during a time when a lack of supply ships caused a tobacco shortage reports that people became so desperate in their desire for tobacco that four men set off in an outrigger canoe to obtain cigarettes from an atoll nine and a half hours' sailing time away. The canoe "had a fist size hole in the hull, which they stuffed with rags, but they still had to bail almost continuously for the whole trip". A similar trip in 1950 led to a canoe being lost at sea with the death of five men.[43]

Popular gifts and holiday life[43a]

While they were nothing new, cigarette coupons gave an added vitality to life with tobacco in the post-war era. Embassy Regal was a popular English brand in the latter quarter of the 20th century. Relaunched in 1962, part of its popularity stemmed from it offering coupons that could be used to obtain a range of different goods. Users of a Belfast internet forum report the compelling power of the coupons:

> Got my first microwave with Embassy Regal cigarette coupons, I had the world and their wives saving them up for me, it would have been cheaper to buy one. Wasn't I stupid.
>
> My father smoked for most of his life (finally gave them up in his fifties. Quit cold turkey!!) and [I] can remember him saving the coupons for a new electric kettle.

Cynicism also reigned, however.

> My uncle smoked 60 Kensitas per day...he eventually got a pine box.
>
> My late mother used to tell me, if I saved enough Embassy coupons, that I could get an iron lung with them.[44]

Another remembered the cards of a different cigarette company, and the poor quality of the goods they supplied:

> I had enough to receive a sleeping bag, kagoul, rucksack and lilo for a trip to Greece island hopping...and a snorkel kit...about 5 years of 20 a day...kagoul got me soaked in a wet Dublin en route to Greece, sleeping bag let in the sea breeze as I slept on the beach in Mykonos...lilo burst as I lay down to sleep on the deck of a Greek ferry...f***in snorkel...cheap and nasty and I got a burst ear drum when diving due to it...[I] no longer smoke.

As well as the coupons and their ability to translate into a 'free' gift, cigarettes particularly became inveigled into working-class family life and holidays. Pontins was a British holiday camp company founded in 1946. It divided guests into competitive 'houses' named after tobacco brands. Another internet forum member posted the following:

> When I went to Pontins in the 70s as a child...I was allocated a dining spot and house, you could either be in Embassy Regal house or Benson and Hedges house, this is no joke. You sat in the area designated with the ciggy signs at each end of the mass dining hall. As kids we would hang around the arcade and question other kids as to their cigarette house preference, quotes of "you Benson and Hedges b*stards" would go around and a few fights and attacks would take place all in the name of our respective cigarette house. This hate was propagated by blue coats [holiday camp entertainment teams]. At the swimming pool events we would be asked our cigarette house by the blue coats, only to be booed or clapped by Benson and Hedges people. I clearly remember kids chanting down the mic[rophone] "Embassy Embassy Embassy" and goading on other people from opposite houses...Kinda mad when I think about this...The loyalty to houses though was incredible. I remember the middle of the dining hall being empty, like a no man's land as each house sat at opposite ends of the dining hall...I remember being in some sort of children's club and being asked what house I was in, when I said "Embassy" down the mic all the other kids cheered and clapped.

This post prompted another forum user to remember "going to Pontins at Prestatyn in the 70s. The chalets were on two levels, the ground floor being Embassy and the top floor being Castella. Happy days".[45]

The Embassy Regal brand also created a cartoon character, a bald smoker called Reg, in a series of humorous advertisements that ran until the Advertising Standards Authority asked the company to stop. A study published in 1993 had found that 90 per cent of teenagers surveyed in the North of England had seen the ads compared with fewer than 50 per cent of adults.[46] The Embassy Regal catalogue coupons, cartoon advertisements and holiday camp experiences demonstrate how closely, until very recently, particular cigarette brands were bound up with working-class family life and 20th century memories.

One 28-year-old former smoker in Northumberland, UK, who started smoking at the age of nine, reflected on the power and significance of branding in her youth in an interview on a public health website[47] as follows:

> At school what you smoked said a lot about you – for instance the tough kids smoked JPS black, the 'hippies' Marlboros. We went for Lambert and Butler as we liked the shiny logos...Besides price, it was all down to what was on the packet and what you see on the shelves. The more eye catching the packs are, the more attractive they are.

Here we see the power of branding, of how easy it is for people, particularly when they have little else, to identify with and to a certain extent become tobacco, and for tobacco to be and become people.

Distentangling smoking identities

As people become long-term smokers, so the sense of tobacco constituting their whole being (Chapter 1) becomes stronger. Lesley Stern writes eloquently about her sense of embodied tobacco:

> It's a delicate balance. The way this body hangs together strung out on some hypothetical framework, sometimes called a skeleton. It feels to me, though, this matter I inhabit, it feels boneless. Not a Cartesian body, to be drawn and quartered, balanced by weights and measures. I imagine skeins of nicotine, sinuous threads of smoke woven through this matter, holding it all together. Organs infiltrated and protected. See the lungs as crocheted intricately, matter folded, padded with layerings of tar, every tissue exists as an elaborate crenellation, resilient, pliant. Like wrought-iron lacework, this twirling smoky edifice is strong, able to bear any amount of stress.[48]

In such a universe, with such an edifice (the body), it is hard to expunge something which is essentially part of yourself; your personhood in general will be compromised. "It's a very substantial part of my identity" says UK smoker Angela (26), who admits "being a nonsmoker...doesn't feel like me".[49]

The French philosopher Jean-Paul Sartre was similarly strongly entwined with his smoking identity. He took the view that

> to smoke is an appropriative, destructive action. Tobacco is a symbol of "appropriated" being, since it is destroyed in the rhythm of my breathing, in a mode of "'continuous destruction'", since it passes into me and its change in myself is manifested symbolically by the transformation of the consumed solid into smoke.[50]

Taking a philosopher's view on smoking, for him, "the act of destructively appropriating the tobacco was the symbolic equivalent of destructively appropriating the entire world".[51] Yet despite being an inveterate chain smoker, he tried several times to quit his habit. His approach was to try making tobacco as insignificant an object in his life as possible. In his book *Being and Nothingness*, he talks of reducing tobacco "to being nothing but itself – an herb which burns".[52] He talked about aiming to "decrystallize" the meaning inherent in smoking. However the auguries were not good. At another level Sartre was well aware of the hybrid bonds between himself and his smoking habit. His concern was that in giving up smoking I was going to strip the theater of its interest, the evening meal of its savor, the morning work of its fresh animation. Whatever unexpected happening was going to meet my eye, it seemed to me that it was fundamentally impoverished from the moment that I could not welcome it while smoking. To-be-capable-of-being-met-by-me-smoking: such was the concrete quality which had been spread over everything. It seemed to me that I was going to snatch it away from everything and that in the midst of this universal impoverishment, life was scarcely worth the effort.[53]

His way of disempowering tobacco – by regarding it as nothing but a "herb which burns", seems to have been singularly unsuccessful, long term.[54] Given the embedded nature of smoking in his life, and his rather abstract approach to the issue, any attempts to dislodge the 'me-smoking' and turning it into just 'me' seemed almost doomed to failure.

Richard Klein did manage to give up during the writing of his book *Cigarettes are Sublime*. But he shared Sartre's appreciation that

> the act of giving up cigarettes should perhaps be approached not only as an affirmation of life but, because living is not merely existing, as an occasion for mourning. Stopping smoking, one must lament the loss to one's life of something immensely, intensely beautiful, must grieve for the passing of a star".[55]

For others, though, giving up smoking, while tough, is not all doom and gloom. After all, writes anthropologist Lynn Meskell, "absence and loss do not have to be tied to mourning and nostalgia, rather, they can proffer a future-driven strategy to reimagine oneself, one's community and its practices".[56]

Sartre might have been more successful had he used a book such as Allen Carr's *The Easy Way to Stop Smoking*, which several smokers have told me helped them quit. One said she had been impressed by the book's undemanding, non-judgemental approach – on the front cover, the reader is positively encouraged not to stop smoking until they have finished reading the book. She found a chapter entitled 'The Advantages of Being a Smoker', which was immediately followed by a blank page, particularly effective. One of the ways in which Carr effects a transformation in people's relationship with tobacco is to downplay and decentre the significance of the craving sensation by personifying it as "the little monster". "It's not well written but that doesn't matter", said Colin, another non-smoker at the time of his interview. Almost as a result of the boredom it instilled in him, on reaching the end of *The Easy Way to Stop Smoking*, he threw the remainder of his tobacco pouch and all his other smoking-related paraphernalia away, vowing never to smoke again.

Token accommodation

The industry was far from oblivious to the image problems it was facing and the increasingly strong urges (if unsatisfied, in the main) that tobacco users had to give up. The industry adopted a tokenistic approach, experimenting through the TIRC and other bodies with a number of shape-shifting entities, including the development of filter cigarettes (such as Peter Stuyvesant, above). The first American filter cigarette was produced in 1936, but they remained essentially a novelty item until the 1950s. Cellulose acetate was finally settled upon as the main component of cigarette filters, although early varieties used asbestos.[57] Documents reveal that the major companies were initially optimistic that sophisticated engineering to filtrate some of the most dangerous components of mainstream cigarette smoke was a possibility, and collaborated with big textile and chemical companies such as Kodak to effect this.[58] At the same time, however, another corporate scientist was working on creating filter materials that would darken in colour when smoked, while acknowledging "the use of such a color change material would probably have little or no effect on the actual efficiency of the filter tip material".[59] The fundamental problem – "that which is harmful in mainstream smoke and that which provides the smoker with 'satisfaction' are essentially one and the same"[60] – only became apparent in the 1960s, when the "filter problem" shifted to one of sustaining the myth of cigarette filter efficacy rather than creating something that might actually work. "The illusion of filtration is as important as the fact of filtration", as one industry memo put it.[61]

Corporations made other spurious attempts to acknowledge and deal with the escalating knowledge of the dangers of cigarettes by changing the form and dimensions of their products. Philip Morris introduced Virginia Slims, cigarettes developed specifically for women with the advertising strapline "You've come a long way, baby", in 1968.[62] The diet theme was a metaphorical association created by advertisers rather than a substantive reality, however. There was no evidence that a 'slim' cigarette would contribute to weight-loss any more than a 'normal' cigarette.[63] Ditto with 'lights', a more widely targeted cigarette option based on claims they contained less tar and sometimes less nicotine, that came onto the market in the 1970s. Evidence quickly accumulated that any reduction in the tar and/or nicotine content of these cigarettes was compensated for by the smoker either taking deeper 'drags' or smoking more. Another message that played out well to female audiences in particular was that of 'time out' and escape. An advertisement for Eve Lights Slim 100s argued, from a woman's bath-tub: "It's not just a cigarette. It's a few minutes on your own".[64]

Turning on and sustaining the tap

R.J. Reynolds could be speaking for all tobacco companies in a 1984 memo that reminds readers that no more than 5 per cent of smokers started after the age of 24, and how the brand loyalty of 18 year-olds far outweighs any tendency to switch with age.[65] This highlights one of the key demographic priorities for the continued fiduciary success of tobacco corporations, namely the need for a reliable stream of young people to start smoking, either to replace those who die from their 'habit' or those who quit. According to the rationale for a 1975 advertising campaign:

> For the young smoker, the cigarette is not yet an integral part of life, of day-to-day life, in spite of the fact that they try to project the image of a regular, run-of-the-mill smoker. For them, a cigarette, and the whole smoking process, is part of the illicit pleasure category...[a] declaration of independence and striving for self identity.

The anonymous author of this report argues that advertising should present the cigarette as one of the few initiations into the adult world. It should take the cigarette seriously as one of the products and activities in the illicit pleasure category, and should endeavour to create scenes and situations taken from the day-to-day life of the young smoker, "but in an elegant manner". These circumstances should touch on basic symbols of growing-up and maturity.[66]

The many faces of advertising

The growing epidemiological evidence of tobacco's harm was sufficient for a few countries to introduce bans on tobacco advertising of the 'Taste of the big wide world' type in national radio, TV, billboards, and print media during the 1970s. However, these kinds of direct advertising are only a subset of the plethora of ways in which tobacco advertising, promotion and sponsorship (TAPS) can occur.[67] The term "involution" has been used to describe how, as the range and scale of agricultural production in Bali (Indonesia) became geographically constrained, production efforts intensified around a more limited range of agricultural options.[68] A similar process can be seen with tobacco since, where its direct advertising has been restricted, tobacco corporations have increased their spending on other forms of indirect or opaque advertising, the tactics of the 'silent salesman'. Cigarette packaging is a case in point, with an increasing sophistication of shapes and colours in cigarette packets making them as alluring as possible to an increasingly segmented consumer market – cigarettes specifically for women, for example, or cigarettes targeted at young people (despite their purchase being illegal). Why in the UK, for example, did a package selling 14 Benson and Hedges cigarettes portray the number '14' in something reminiscent of Lego bricks? Did it, perhaps, suggest the age of consumer at which it was aimed? Lambert and Butler started using a hologram on their packets, with beams of light emanating from the logo that were almost religious in their iconography.

Then came the collective appearance of cigarette sales venues. Point-of-sale advertising is all the ways tobacco products can be promoted at the place where they are sold, and displays such as 'tobacco walls' with eye-catching illuminations became increasingly common in shops and super-markets. Advertising can also take place through product placement, such as cigarettes and their brands appearing in films, TV and other media. This became an increasingly lucrative source of funding for film makers, with millions of dollars changing hands in order for a specific product to be featured. Cigarette smoking on celluloid was nothing new, of course. Sometimes it acted as a signifier, as well as something signified – signifying, for example, the sexually available, vampish woman.[69] At other times it could be an expression of individual control and power. The ability of Sharon Stone in the film *Basic Instinct* to carry on smoking in the presence of police authority while under suspicion for murder, for example, "stands out as a 1990s testimonial for smoking in the face of oppressive regulations".[70] However, it is the consumer who, if s/he can be encouraged to smoke in places where others can see them, is perhaps the greatest sales pitch of all, as the examples in Chapter 7 of women marching through New York with their 'torches of freedom' and the GIs acting as 'American billboards' in post-war Germany attest.

Tobacco goes academic

Financial connections between academia and the tobacco industry have been large, deep and complex. Duke University in Durham, North Carolina, is founded on the wealth of its James Duke namesake (Chapter 6).[71] Harvard University has long been indebted to the tobacco industry for funding, its medical school having received some hefty endowments, while in Mexico, the Instituto Carlos Slim de la Salud, endowed by large amounts of tobacco money,[72] is an example of a research centre that remains "resoundingly silent on issues of tobacco and health".[73]

The influence of tobacco in research and teaching establishments does not derive only from endowments, however. In the late 1990s, Philip Morris attempted to legislate 'sound science' in an effort to question the link between second-hand smoke and lung cancer. "The campaign involved enacting data access and data quality laws to obtain previously confidential research data in order to reanalyse it based on industry-generated data quality standards".[74] Since then, tobacco-corporation interests have targeted individual scholars where their work has offered a particular challenge to the tobacco industry. For academics in the UK, compulsory release of the data they have collected is in prospect, under the Freedom of Information Act.[75] Good researchers will have entered into ethical agreements with informants at the time of their involvement in the research concerning the further use or dissemination of the information they provide.

The rise of Islamic fundamentalism has posed a threat to tobacco interests in some parts of the world. Tobacco corporations have sought to influence Muslim thinking by recruiting allies. A 1996 BAT memo suggested that the company identify "a scholar/scholars, preferably at the Al Azhar University in Cairo, who we could then brief and enlist".[76] This person would then be teamed up with a Muslim writer or journalist. "This is an issue to be handled extremely gingerly", the memo went on. "We have to avoid all possibilities of a backlash".[77] Meanwhile, Philip Morris was seeking allies at the Islamic studies department of McGill University in Montreal, one of several efforts by lobbyists to create a panel of scholars tolerant of tobacco. Industry-funded lawyers searched Koranic verses for loopholes. A presentation from the firm Shook, Hardy and Bacon found no prohibition against smoking and argued that "making rules beyond what Allah has allowed is a sin in itself". Consultants in Islamic countries have worked hard to prevent health warnings making mention of the Koran. A BAT consultant wrote that he had prevented publication of several booklets on the subject. "Once the religious aspect is conveyed to the public it will be very difficult to reverse the situation", he warned.[78]

Some academic disciplines were particularly well-disposed to tobacco corporation interference[79] or to adopting theoretical positions that cast tobacco in a more favourable light. Anthropology is an example of the latter. One disciplinary trend has been to downplay or challenge concepts like 'dependency' and 'addiction', seeing them as social constructs, while at the same time playing up the power of human agency and consigning a substance like tobacco very firmly to the passive, inert, non-human category. Such a trend can be seen in anthropological studies of other corporate fields.[80] Anthropologists, and social scientists more generally, are quick to criticize more 'hard science' approaches for their intrinsic biases, while many 'social studies of science' emphasize the way in which scientific results are dependent on the social, political and economic circumstances that dictate what kinds of studies are undertaken, how they are carried out, and what the research in question actually reveals. While at some level bias cannot be avoided, how much more is it likely to bias research that has been funded by groups or organizations with vested interests in the outcomes? Seltzer's Harvard Anthropology research received more than 50 payments totalling $1.7m from the US Council for Tobacco Research, a solely tobacco-industry-funded institute, over the period from 1959 to 1990. His research mainly involved looking for examples of propensity to smoke correlated with body types, and contesting the science of smoking and heart disease.[81]

Tobacco corporations can also make trouble by attempting to undermine or cut short academic research that is unfavourable to their cause. A public health specialist active in the field of tobacco control relates how in the 1970s the chairman of a major tobacco company offered him funding to work on any campaign issue other than tobacco.[82]

Corporate social responsibility (CSR)

Numerous efforts have been made to polish the reputation of the industry through philanthropic acts and good deeds. There are plenty of examples of tobacco industry magnates making philanthropic donations, frequently of very large sums. If tobacco executives have trouble living with themselves,[83] making amends through giving money away might act as a form of conscience-salve. One example is Albert Lasker, "a titan in the history of tobacco sales and promotion. He and his wife Mary directed their considerable largesse to cancer research and the prolongation of life, a telling irony in the history of this product".[84] The Lasker Foundation "envisions a healthier world through medical research".[85] The President, Claire Pomeroy, does an excellent job of promoting the value of certain medical advances (such as the MMR vaccine), developed by "Lasker Laureate" Maurice Hilleman in 1983. In a *Fox News* opinion piece she went on to write, "the story of once conquering measles in the U.S. is one of triumph of biomedical research and public health policies. The tragic story of its resurgence is a reflection of the dangerous attractiveness of pseudoscience and of parents who refuse vaccination for their children".[86] Sad then, to reflect on the pseudoscience on which the money that led to the formation of the Foundation is based, for Lasker was responsible for the advertising account for Lucky Strike cigarettes during the time of the "Reach for a Lucky instead of a sweet" slogan (Chapter 7). Links may not always be apparent, but tobacco permeates the organization. One of the Lasker Awards society Members is Robin Chandler Duke, fourth wife of Angier Biddle Duke, grandson of Buck Duke.

Corporate social responsibility is inherently confusing to members of the public concerned about the moral worth of the tobacco corporations. When the die was cast and evidence about the health risks of smoking was nigh on irrefutable, in 1991, R.J. Reynolds started a campaign "Kids Shouldn't Smoke". Yet beneath the veneer of responsibility, even nobility, that such an initiative promotes, evidence of success in direct efforts to discourage 'kids' from smoking seems quite minimal. Evidence from Malaysia demonstrates how companies engaged in youth smoking prevention programmes in that country, while duplicitously increasing their efforts to promote smoking amongst that same audience.[87]

Brand stretching and other forms of promotion – the case of Dunhill

Dunhill is well-known for its 'brand stretching' into luxury goods. In the 1990s, Dunhill beamed matches from the English Football Association Cup to clubs and bars in Malaysia. The posters advertising this series were thrilling – professional footballers in full colour with lightning flashes coming out of their torsos.[88] At the same time, the Malaysian Tobacco Manufacturer's Association produced a health promotion poster suggesting that a young footballer could be "On top of the world without smoking". The confusing juxtaposition of a tobacco-sponsored football series and a tobacco-sponsored campaign arguing against smoking aside, if you were a young person (and maybe you are) which of the posters is more appealing?

Dunhill's name has featured in other promotional/CSR work – in fact the boundary between the two is almost inevitably blurred, since CSR also almost invariably acts as a form of corporate promotion. The Dunhill Medical Trust is a UK charitable trust with funds established "for medical research and the furtherance of medical knowledge", and is closely linked to the Dunhill family. Mary Dunhill, who was Chairman of the Dunhill group of companies for 14 years from 1961-1976, wrote in her memoirs in 1979 that she was still "intimately involved" in the administration of the fund, which had been set up by her uncle Bertie. "Now amounting to some £5 million, [it] continues to support research projects in a number of hospitals".[89] Its contemporary focus, with some degree of irony perhaps, is "mechanisms of ageing and treating age-related diseases and frailty", and supporting "community-based organisations which are working to enhance the lives of those who need extra support in later life".[90] Somewhat like the Instituto Carlos Slim de la Salud (above) there is no mention of smoking, or of any of the smoking-related diseases, in the list of grants the Dunhill Medical Trust has awarded.

Astroturfing

Astroturfing is the term given to the creation of an apparently grassroots movement or organization with a strategy and agenda that is controlled by a hidden company or organization. One such UK-based tobacco example is FOREST (Freedom Organization for the Right to Enjoy Smoking Tobacco), an industry-funded smokers' rights group founded in 1979 with 96 per cent of its money coming from the tobacco industry.[91] A memo released by the public relations committee of the industry's joint Tobacco Advisory Council in 1981 stated how its members "acknowledged the need for FOREST to have a considerable degree of independence of action but that this would ultimately be controlled by the industry's funding".[92] In all areas, the funding dependence of FOREST on the industry is reflected in the strong alignment of the organization, which has a strongly neoliberal political agenda. This is a set of political beliefs in which human well-being is considered best advanced by intensifying and expanding the use of markets; government intervention in any sphere (including health policy) is seen as unwelcome and ill-judged, and professional interest groups such as doctors are accused of manipulating state mechanisms for their own benefit.[93] A more international variant, ostensibly representing the interests of tobacco producers rather than consumers, came into being as the International Tobacco Growers' Association.

Internal agnotology – maintaining the ethical animation of employees

In 1978, R.J. Reynolds inaugurated a campaign centred on the tobacco fields of North Carolina called "Pride in Tobacco". Its aim was to counter anti-tobacco sentiments through the development of a more positive image for the crop, particularly amongst those in tobacco-producing states "whose way of life depends on this important commodity".[94] Using bumper stickers, placards, billboards, press conferences and rallies in major tobacco towns, the company aimed to create "wider and more favourable coverage than the tobacco industry has enjoyed in many years". By these means, the company intended to become "the primary friend of the grower".[95] Their goal was to develop "'complete industry unity' in the face of the 'health scare'",[96] and "to unite these interests into a cohesive force that will help ensure all viewpoints receive a fair hearing when the industry and its people are threatened by anti-tobacco activists".[97] Their public argument was as follows:

> The issues that surround smoking are so complex, and so emotional, it's hard to debate them objectively. Over the years, you've heard so many negative reports about smoking and health...that you may assume the case against smoking is closed...[We] think reasonable people who analyse it may come to see this issue not as a closed case, but as an open controversy. We know some of you may be suspicious of what we'll say, simply because we're a cigarette company...But we have confidence in the ability of people to reason after they have been presented with all points of view.[98]

The call for multiperspectivalism in a dualistic arena apparently consisting of "the industry and its people" and "anti-tobacco activists" is intriguing. Despite its language as one of breadth and inclusivity, the reality is the 'points of view' to be expressed are deliberately limited to those that contribute to the ongoing development and expansion of the tobacco corporation. And these may be at odds with the interests of the people it claims to represent and whom are expected to subscribe to this modern version of 'tobacco ideology'. At the same time as their "Pride in Tobacco" charm offensive was taking off, R.J. Reynolds was making moves towards buying cheaper leaf tobacco from overseas. Causing the market price of leaf tobacco to fall was part of a global trend towards increased tobacco production in low-income rather than high-income countries, thus boosting company profits (the fiduciary imperative again).[99] By 2004, more than half the tobacco used in the manufacture of American cigarettes came from outside the US.

Mr. Butts – challenging agnotology through satire

In 1989 (April 19th 1989, to be exact), cartoon rookie advertising executive Mike Doonesbury was reputedly asked by the R.J. Reynolds company to work on promoting its products to teenagers. From out of his dreams about this request comes Mr. Butts, a walking, talking cigarette, "always smiling, always lying".[100] Mr. Butts gets around a lot. He takes part in a congressional hearing concerning the ban on cigarette advertising (June 27th 1990) in which he claims "the ban is unconstitutional...People have a right to know which image their cigarette brand projects...The ban will bring chaos! Cowboys will start smoking Virginia Slims! Blacks will smoke white brands!" He then travels to the Middle East during the time of the Iraq war on a recruitment drive.

A marine company commander's memoirs from the war in Iraq recount how "during Desert Shield, as a show of support for the troops, several tobacco firms had shipped complimentary cigarettes to Saudi Arabia. Doonesbury's creator, Garry Trudeau, had mocked it in his comic strip as he portrayed Mr. Butts...handing out smokes to the soldiers in the desert". One soldier declined Mr. Butts' offer for fear of dying of lung cancer. "Lung cancer?!" Mr. Butts exclaims. "Hey, I hate to tell you this, but you're a soldier. You might not be alive twenty *minutes* from now! Why worry about twenty years from now? Besides, you can always quit".[101] The parallels with the attitudes towards smoking in the military expressed during the First World War (Chapter 7) are obvious.

Then on January 1st 1996, Mr. Butts appeared on the cover of *The Nation* magazine, delivering a Federal Express box with a cheery "Hello? Anyone Home?" This reflected an eerie story in which "Mr. Butts crossed over from the comics to real life".[102] In 1994, Stanton Glantz, a university tobacco researcher, received a Fedex box with the return address "Mr. Butts". "The box...contained 4,000 pages of documents that one of world's largest cigarette makers – Brown & Williamson (B&W) – later claimed were stolen from its files. B&W, the nation's third-largest tobacco company, makes Kool, Pall Mall, and Lucky Strike, among other brands".[103] These documents proved that the tobacco corporations had known for 30 years that nicotine was addictive and that smoking causes cancer, information that was deliberately withheld from the public in a conspiracy of silence.[104] Mr. Butts' delivery was the start of the process that led to the Master Settlement five years later.

Silencing the voices – turning the tobacco policy network inside-out

Germany was not alone in having an overly cosy government/industry network. Up until the 1980s the UK too had a situation in which saw the tobacco industry closely integrated with the government at the core of a UK 'policy community' (Fig. 8.2). Around the edge of this network is a 'producer network' of those immediately dependent on the industry, including retailers and distributors, sports and arts (then very often dependent on tobacco for sponsorship), the unions, and the media.

On the periphery are what are called 'issue networks', groups and organizations such as the Department of Health and Social Security (DHSS), Action on Smoking and Health (ASH) and the British Medical Association (BMA) for whom tobacco is an 'issue'. Other government departments took active, passive or (in some cases) antagonistic positions on these issues. The examples given in Fig. 8.2 are transport, employers and local authorities. This was hardly the kind of policy-making environment that could hope to have much impact in terms of separating tobacco control from the antithetical interests of those for whom the fiduciary imperative was paramount.

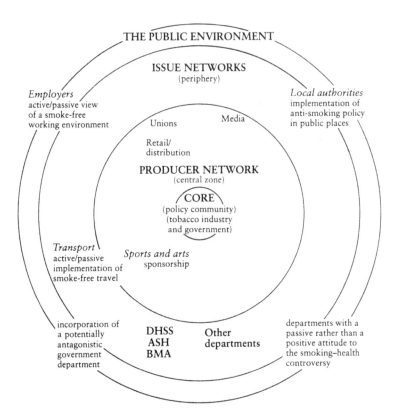

Fig. 8.2 The UK tobacco policy network in the 1980s

Source: Read, 1992: 129; © OUP

The tide was turning politically, however. The cosy relationship between industry and government that Fig. 8.2 portrays was epitomized by Margaret Thatcher's Conservative government appointing a Secretary of State for Health who went on to become a non-executive director of British American Tobacco between 1998 and 2007. Things were becoming fraught, however. A Labour party election victory in 1997 opened a short window of opportunity, as the new government sought to establish its distinctiveness from what had gone before. A government White Paper finally started to move forwards on an agenda to tackle health inequalities, something set out but largely ignored by the previous government in its 1992 report *The Health of the Nation*,[105] inequalities which smoking was widely regarded as playing a key role in maintaining. The Report of the Scientific Committee on Tobacco and Health published in 1998 highlighted the dangers of passive as well as active smoking, and was backed up by a government White Paper, *Smoking Kills*.[106]

Scientific evidence normally only has an oblique and selective influence on policy making, but further research had showed that cigarette smoke was not only harmful to individual smokers but to anyone in the vicinity who might find themselves passive or second-hand smokers.[107] The smoke that many had taken for granted or regarded as normal, swirling around pubs, clubs and workplaces worldwide, started to take on a more sinister edge. From an individual danger, science had rendered smoking a potential problem to the entire gamut of a smoker's associates: in anthropological terms, smoking had shifted from being an individual to a *dividual* issue.[108] This was something of a game changer in public health terms because it recast smoking as something relational rather than with purely individual consequences. This had implications for people who smoked (Chapter 9) as well as for those working in the nascent field of tobacco control (Chapters 10 and 11).

Conclusion

Tobacco in the second half of the 20th century was indeed able to speak through a myriad of corporate and other voices. It was during this time, though, that the long-term dangers of tobacco use (particularly, but not exclusively, cigarettes) became increasingly clear and, grudgingly in many cases, acknowledged. It was also the period in which the incorrigible behaviour of the tobacco corporations was exposed. The Master Settlement documents, which revealed the attempt to create a plenitude of Philip Morris voices amongst many other examples of industry skulduggery, offer a treasure trove of information about corporate maleficence in the recent past. The main achievement of the Settlement, though, was to generate a growing cadre of researchers and activists galvanized by the revelation that here was a conspiracy theory about the tobacco industry colluding to deny the link between smoking and lung cancer that, unlike most conspiracy theories, had turned out to be true. As the Millennium approached, tobacco control was forming as a non-tobacco entity, energized as never before by the many disclosures being made about its common source, tobacco. Benson and Kirsch propose "resignation" as the political emotion that is the primary public response to problems of corporate capitalism.[109] Yet there were other responses to the longer-term understanding and fresh revelations about the corporate world of tobacco. The following chapters (Part 2) will explore some of these, via contemporary perspectives of tobacco users and people who have become part of a growing movement for tobacco control (one local and one global). The final chapter discusses how the future may be envisioned as a world without tobacco and the further shape-shifting that has taken place as, paradoxically or understandably, tobacco in both individual and corporate hybrids has sought to embed itself in tobacco control.

Notes

1 Quoted in Ulucanlar et al. (2016: 6/21).
2 The subtitle of the book in which the longest exegesis of agnotology appears is "The making and unmaking of ignorance" (Proctor and Schiebinger, 2008).
3 Proctor (2008b: 7) quoting Burke (1935: 70). Meadows et al. (1972) make the point that our attention tends to be limited to more immediate temporal and spatial concerns rather than more distant ones.
4 Proctor and Schiebinger (2008).
5 Formerly known as the Legacy Library, these are now in a publicly accessible archive, Truth Tobacco Industry Documents, UCSF Library (n.d.).
6 Benson and Kirsch (2010: 461).
7 See Rajan (1999).
8 Hughes (2003: 135), his emphasis.
9 Nixon (2011).
10 Berlant (2007).
11 Wiist (2010: 6).
12 Indeed, corporations would argue they have a legal duty in this regard.
13 Wiist (2010: 5).
14 The subtitle to Bakan (2004)'s book, for example, is "The pathological pursuit of profit and power".
15 Martin (2006: 284).
16 Imperial Tobacco (2011).
17 Philip Morris International (Pakistan) Limited (2014). This derives from an earlier mission statement produced in 2011. For more on PMI's further corporate shape-shifting intentions, at least in higher income countries, see Chapter 12.
18 Singer and Baer (2009: 3).
19 Brownell and Warner (2009). See also Hastings (2012a, b).
20 See, for example, Cowlishaw and Thomas (2018).
21 Kohrman and Benson (2011). We shall return to this argument in Chapter 12.
22 Benson and Kirsh (2010) call this 'strategic engagement' with critique, a third stage after denial and token accommodation.
23 Schivelbusch (1992: 186).
24 Dennis and Alexiou (2018) gives examples such as 'Marlboro Country' and the 'Road to Flavor'.
25 Larkin (2010: 200).

26 Vending machines accounted for nearly half of all cigarette sales in Germany in the 1970s and were poorly regulated by the Federal government (Larkin 2010: 178-9). They were a notoriously good way for younger generations to access cigarettes free of adult surveillance (Hanewinkel and Isensee 2006).

27 Elliot (2012).

28 Simpson (2002).

29 These were published by the Royal College of Physicians (1962) and the US Department of Health, Education, and Welfare (1964) respectively.

30 Hong (2002). 'Ossis' ('Easties') had to content themselves with relatively little choice and brands such as the f6 cigarette (Landsman 2005: 219). F6 has now become an object of nostalgia for some Berlin bohemians.

31 Neuburger (2013: 198).

32 Elliot (2015).

33 Proctor 1996: 1450.

34 Schneider and Glantz (2008).

35 Harris (1991).

36 Schneider and Glantz (2008: 294).

37 Gender is the most significant variable in whether a person in China smokes or not, with smoking amongst young women being coded as "transgressive and...sexually suspect" (Kohrman 2008: 19) and making the ratio men to women smokers approximately 45:1 in the country.

38 Kohrman (2008: 19).

39 Ibid. (19-20).

40 Sterns (1999: 67).

41 Pels (1998) in Reed (2007: 33).

42 Kohrman (2008: 16).

43 Marshall (2013: 99; 232 n. 19). Compare this with Hume's suggestion that tobacco, like love, 'makes men sail from shore to shore' (Chapter 2).

43a The argument in this section is from Thirlway (2015: 153–154).

44 Belfast Forum (2010)

45 hotukdeals (2009-12)

46 ASH – Action on Smoking and Health (2017: 31).

47 The website is run by FreshNE (Chapter 10).

48 Sterns (1999: 76).

49 Hughes (2003: 171).

50 Sartre (1958: 596).

51 Ibid. (597).

52 Ibid.

53 Ibid. (596).

54 Klein comments drily that, "like many stories of success, the happy ending leaves unspoken tobacco's eventual revenge...[Sartre] continued to smoke for the next forty years" (1993: 36).

55 Ibid. (3).

56 Meskell (2010: 212).

57 Proctor (2011: 343-4).

58 Harris (2011).

59 Quoted in Brandt (2007: 245).

60 Harris (2011: i15).

61 Quoted in Brandt (2007: 245).

62 This strapline – both feminist and condescending – led to subsequent problems for the brand when younger women in the 1990s, so crucial to the brand's

future, started to find it out-of-date compared to their older sisters. Philip Morris could afford to alienate neither group (Toll and Ling 2005).

63 Proctor (2011: 410).

64 Greaves (1996: 25).

65 Burrows (1984).

66 Ted Bates Marketing agency, Viceroys cigarette campaign, New York (1975) – Glantz (1996) traces this back to a US Federal Trade Commission report in 1981.

67 The others include packaging and point of sale advertising, other forms of merchandising, brand stretching, product placement, loyalty schemes and coupons, free samples and other forms of marketing and communications, corporate social responsibility programmes and sponsorship, and (latterly) internet advertising.

68 Geertz (1963).

69 Isenberg (2004: 248).

70 Greaves (1996: 29).

71 Benson writes poignantly and poetically of the disconnect between "the dormitories and athletic fields" of Duke University campus and the "neighborhoods that were built up and then gutted by the tobacco industry" just a few exits further up the highway (Benson 2012: 6).

72 See Braine (2007).

73 Burch et al. (2010).

74 Baba et al. (2005).

75 See, for example, S. Connor (2011).

76 Petticrew et al. (2015: 1089).

77 Ibid.

78 Petticrew et al. (2015).

79 Proctor (2011: 460-3) lists no less than 48 US historians who have testified as expert witnesses for the defence in American tobacco litigation.

80 One example, funded by the drinks industry, is a study that argued dysfunctional relationships fostered "alcohol-related" domestic violence, rather than the other way round (Fox 2008).

81 Kohrman and Benson (2011: 337).

82 Daube (2012: 877).

83 Rosenblatt (1994).

84 Brandt (2007: 515, fn 16).

85 Albert And Mary Lasker Foundation (2018).

86 Pomeroy (2015).

87 Assunta and Chapman (2004).

88 See Assunta (2002).

89 Dunhill (1979: 122).

90 Dunhill Medical Trust (2018).

91 S. Clark, D. Swan and C. Ogden, of FOREST made these points during the Select Committee on Health session, 'The Tobacco Industry and the Health Risks of Smoking', held at the House of Commons in London in 2000. (Clark et al. 2000).

92 UCSF Library (1981).

93 Harvey (2005); Treanor (2005).

94 Benson (2010: 504).

95 R.J. Reynolds internal documents quoted in Benson (2012: 108).

96 Quoted in Benson (2012: 109).

97 R.J. Reynolds internal memo quoted in Benson (2012: 109).

98 R.J. Reynolds public newsletter (1984) quoted in Benson (2012: 110).
99 Between 1977 and 1997 the share of tobacco production in high-income countries declined from 30 to 15 per cent, while rising from 40 to 60 per cent in the Middle East and Asia, and from 4 to 6 per cent in Africa. In certain countries, tobacco became a dangerously high proportion of export revenue – more than 60 per cent in Malawi, and 23 per cent in Zimbabwe (1994 figures – World Bank 1999: 58).
100 Wiener (2010).
101 Folsom (2006: 249).
102 Wiener (2010).
103 Ibid.
104 Haapanen (2003).
105 Secretary of State for Health (1992).
106 Department of Health (1998).
107 The key piece of research was Hirayama (1981). For an exegesis on the wider meanings of smoke-free legislation, see Dennis (2016).
108 For elaborations on Strathern's original concept and its significance, see Rohatynskyj (2015).
109 Benson and Kirsch (2010); see also Fisher (2009).

Part II

Times

Chapter 9

Host and parasite

Introduction – "I am your friend"

This is the first of four chapters that will look at the changing nature of tobacco-human hybridity in the 21st century using a variety of examples from my own and others' ethnographic research, written and visual sources. The argument throughout is that the current century marks a sea change in the relationship that has been the central focus of this book. It is as if knowledge and experience of tobacco's potential for harm, particularly through the ways in which the 20th century world was swamped by industrially produced cigarettes and the subsequent revelations of the tobacco corporations' agency and subterfuge in this process, is finally being acted upon. The outcome is the emergence of a new assemblage – tobacco control – as the third pole in a triumvirate of tobacco-human relationships (the others being persons and corporations) identified so far.

The changing nature of the relationship is epitomized by tobacco's vocal role in a 2003 book published by Richard Craze, a dedicated smoker who intended to quit and decided to write a diary about the experience. Nearly four centuries had elapsed since tobacco itself, rather than its paraphernalia, had spoken in any kind of work published in English, despite it having had plenty of opportunities to do so. Craze's tobacco speaks with a very different vocal quality to the "Emperor Tobacco" that came on stage talking an alien language in the 17th century (Chapter 2). Craze's tobacco speaks only too comprehensibly in Craze's head, undermining in any way it can the likelihood of his success at quitting.

For Craze, the unexpected trigger to attempting to give up cigarettes is watching TV nature programmes about parasitic lifecycles, of which that of the *Hymenopimecis* wasp larva is one of the most bizarre. The larva feeds off a spider, injecting it with a hallucinogenic anticoagulant which causes it to spin a strange web that then becomes the larva's cocoon. Craze is both fascinated and appalled by the parallels he sees between the larva and tobacco in terms of mind control. "Tobacco is just another parasite with a bizarre breeding cycle. I am just the host for it. The more I smoke, the more it gets planted.

A successful crop trading its strange pleasure for increased growth",[1] he writes. Craze tries using his revulsion at the idea of tobacco's parasitism as the lever he needs to overcome his dependence on it. Tobacco's voice becomes cajoling, almost hurt, at this point:

> I'm not a parasite [it says], I don't reproduce in your lungs. I don't live in you as a plant of infection. I am a gift from the gods to give you pleasure, ease your pain, help you relax, protect you from colds and chills, make you fear less and enjoy more. I am your friend.[2]

Tobacco also suggests ways in which Craze might save his self-esteem by actively choosing to have a cigarette rather than feeling a failure should he crack, or conversely by becoming a secret smoker so he can continue his habit without others knowing. Over three months of abstinence, Craze reflects on his smoking history, his health, a family history of premature smoking-related deaths (something which seems to silence tobacco's voice), the tobacco industry, and the conflicts that became part of the tobacco experience in the 20th century. He points out the fundamental paradox of 21st century smoking, that it is "cool, grown up, relaxing, enjoyable and smart. But it is also life threatening, dirty, smelly, addictive, uncool, expensive and unfair on others".[3]

Tobacco thus has multiple and ambivalent symbolic and practical meanings for individuals in the 21st century. To a decreasing minority in the 'western' world (but to increasing numbers overall if we take low- and middle-income countries into account), tobacco delineates and traverses boundaries between our bodies and the external world. It facilitates interaction between people in some cases but, in others, blocks it. It is a "resource for negotiating identities, and…a signal for communicating emotive states".[4] Smoking represents a significant relationship between 'thing' (the pipe, cigar or, for the majority in the Anglo-American world in the 20th century, cigarettes) and context (such as a physical place, or smoking signifying 'time out' or leisure time). In the mould of tobacco constituting persons, smoking can mediate what is sometimes a strong sense of identity for people who smoke – of both themselves, and others, of what they are and what they are not. However, it has also come to inspire a sense of enslavement, disgust, guilt and, increasingly, stigma. No wonder, in many ways, that a fairly steady 70 per cent of tobacco smokers surveyed, wherever in the world they might be, express a desire to give up or regret that they ever started.[5] Yet giving up can be very hard to do, as Craze's experience makes plain.

Another of the remarkable things about Craze's book is that he identifies corporations, as well as people, as the hapless hosts enabling tobacco's spread. For him, "the tobacco corporation bosses are as much its victims as us, the poor smokers at the end of the chain".[6] Craze's argument makes sense from an ontological point of view – we could add governments to his list of tobacco's hosts/victims. However, the power and influence of these different actants vary markedly (something which a Latourian flattening is not terribly good at handling). User experiences risk becoming increasingly marginalized and, in some circumstances, stigmatized in the dominant corporate and health discourses about tobacco. The 21st century is also marked by the perspectives of increasing numbers of people who have first- and second-hand experience of premature deaths and incapacitating illnesses caused by tobacco.

This chapter firstly returns to the contemporary experience of tobacco's hybridity, and the shifts that can be observed in terms of who is smoking, where and why. It then goes on to look at the worlds of tobacco manufacture, with further examples of corporate agnotology that continue to mystify and obscure, and a changing technoscientific assemblage of which these processes are a part, particularly the rise of the internet. Counterpointing these are examples of non-corporate tobacco manufacture. It ends with a consideration of the e-cigarette as the latest example of tobacco's shape-shifting. Might the e-cigarette turn out to be for the 21st century what the cigarette was for the 20th?

Being and becoming a tobacco user in the 21st century

There is an increasingly tense paradox in the lives of 21st century tobacco users – their entwinement with a *pharmakon*-like substance that both "works to promote…well-being while threatening their physical health".[7] Both tropes – well-being and danger/ill-health – are found in contemporary accounts of tobacco users. Simon Gray focuses on the former. He expresses no regrets about smoking, only about the way his habit became routine, involving "hundreds or thousands of cigarettes that I never experienced, inhaled and exhaled without noticing".[8] Gray saw smoking as "an integral part of his identity",[9] not only as a person but as a writer. Like the writers and composers portrayed in previous chapters, he saw tobacco as both embodied and embedded in the creative process. He writes of sitting with a Cross ballpoint pen in his right hand, in his left a cigarette "held between the two middle fingers in the classic smoker's grip".[10] Yet Gray did try, unsuccessfully, to quit during his life, only ever managing to cut down. His diary volume, titled *The Last Cigarette*,[11] is misleading; he had further cigarettes, dying of lung and prostate cancer in 2008, aged 71.

The pleasures tobacco can provide and that Gray writes about so wistfully are frequently overlooked.[12] Richard Klein talks of "the release and consolation that cigarettes provide, with the mechanism they offer for regulating anxiety and for mediating social interaction".[13] Such pleasures, however, are not always unadulterated. As a 35-year-old mother in Hughes' account puts it

> [I]f you've not had one for a while, a short while, it's very enjoyable to have a cigarette. If you've gone an extremely long time without a cigarette, then you're going to feel giddy for a couple of minutes and that's when it highlights to me just how much of drug it is, cos you, sort

of 'whoooo', and I wouldn't say that's particularly nice either, it's a very off-putting experience when you're feeling wobbly.[14]

Sometimes their pleasure can be what Immanuel Kant calls "negative pleasure". According to Klein, such "a darkly beautiful, inevitably painful pleasure...resides precisely in the 'bad' taste the smoker quickly learns to love".[15] At the root of the relationship with tobacco lies a craving which at base fulfils the criteria of what Lacan calls "pure desire" – no utilitarian calculus, or universal goodness, its fulfilment both uncountable (an "incommensurable measure")[16] and unaccountable. An action motivated by pure desire is, in Lacan's terms, "literally motivated by no good".[17] Men in Bomana gaol, Papua New Guinea, "claim to be constantly 'hungry for cigarettes'", living for the next smoke, "thinking and dreaming on how to get it".[18] It is a hunger that cannot be forced into categories and their variation counted. As Klein puts it, "cigarettes...resist all arguments directed against them from the perspective of health and utility".[19] Klein captures the paradox well in his consideration that

> cigarettes are bad for you. But if they were not also good for you, so many good people would not have spent some part of their lives smoking them constantly, often compulsively. One thinks of the many great men and women who have died prematurely from having smoked too much: it does them an injustice to suppose that their greatness did not depend in some degree on the wisdom and pleasure and spiritual benefit they took in a habit they could not abandon.[20]

Matthew Kohrman is struck by how many thoracic surgeons in China, whom one might expect to be acutely aware of the dangers of cigarettes through their direct experience treating people with tobacco-related diseases, still smoke regardless. One such surgeon he interviewed in 2004 had this to say:

> To tell you the truth, with such a pressure-filled job, smoking is extremely helpful, at times soothing, at times energizing, at times helping me focus my attention when preparing for a complex surgery or facing a stack of paperwork at 10:30 at night. Once addicted, nicotine is a pretty useful thing.[21]

As well as its enmeshment in the principle of *guanxi* (Chapter 8), the constancy of tobacco over a period that has encompassed civil war, occupation, liberation, totalitarianism, cultural revolution and ongoing neoliberal economic transformation is striking. Meanwhile, the Chinese government at regional and national levels has become dependent on the income from tobacco production and distribution. There is a strong sense, as in other countries with nationalized tobacco corporations, of 'smoking for the nation'.

Tobacco constitutes relations – and divisions

Another relational aspect of smoking is the anthropomorphic conversion of cigarettes into friends and companions of the "I am your friend" variety that tobacco expresses to Craze (above). In a statement resonating with the Lucky Strike advertisements of the 1930s (Chapter 7), Pippa, a 35-year-old smoking mother, speaks of tobacco as a friend and mate, "something that will always be there for me".[22] The companionship offered by cigarettes is ambivalent, but frequently more reliable and trustworthy than that shown by other (human) friends. Here is a woman describing her cigarette in Rio de Janeiro, for example:

> [It is] the best and worst friend you can have...he is the best because he is with you when you are sad, when you're happy, when you have insomnia...It is worse because it kills you, but it causes great pleasure.[23]

Similar language is found in other studies: "everytime you get stressed...I'll have a cigarette. It's always a way out, so I see that as like a partner".[24] "I love stroking this lovely tube of delight", said the playwright Dennis Potter about the cigarette he was holding during the final interview he gave before his death from pancreatic cancer in 2007.[25] Spanish filmmaker Luis Buñuel expresses similar sensuous pleasure in tobacco-related things, almost as if speaking of a lover: "I love to touch the pack in my pocket, open it, savor the feel of the cigarette between my fingers, the paper on my lips, the taste of tobacco on the tongue".[26]

The reliable companion, the friend, the lover that brings pleasure as well as, eventually, death, are particularly pronounced tropes for many people living in adverse circumstances, such as the women smokers caring for children in low-income households in Hilary Graham's pioneering work. For one woman in her study, smoking was "an excuse to stop for five minutes...a moment of self caring which, unlike a cup of tea of coffee, needed no preparation".[27] As Klein describes it,

> The moment of taking a cigarette allows one to open a parenthesis in the time of ordinary experience, a space and a time of heightened attention that give rise to a feeling of transcendence, evoked through the ritual of fire, smoke, cinder connecting hand, lungs, breath, and mouth. It procures a little rush of infinity that alters perspectives, however slightly, and permits, albeit briefly, an ecstatic standing outside of oneself.[28]

Opportunities to experience the infinite and "an ecstatic standing outside oneself" are generally limited for people living in disadvantaged circumstances. Yet they come with an increased likelihood of dissonant pressures from people who do not smoke, such as non-smoker Rebecca in the North East of England who said she didn't like visiting her grandparents any more because they smoked while her children were present. It was not the grandparents them-selves who were the problem, but the cigarette smoke they produced, that came as an inherent package on visiting. In a world where 'smoke free' is becoming a watchword for health and environmental purity, arguments about the dangers of second-hand smoke are becoming increasingly well-rehearsed, and increasing numbers of people talk spontaneously about tobacco causing some kind of interpersonal dissent in their family.

Tensions may occur within couples as well as families. In discussing her family's smoking history with me, Gina reported her nephew Jack's continued smoking was causing discord between him and his wife, who was only too keen for him to stop. Smoking for him was a secret activity, not least because of his job as a junior sports coach. Tobacco is becoming increasingly hidden, increasingly stigmatized – its use, as described in the next section, increasingly associated with specific, generally disadvantaged, population groups.

Smoking islands?

Another reason for people carrying on smoking is not necessarily pharmaco-logical or relational but because their experience of smoking is simply normal, or a mark of either aspiration or rebellion. In some parts of the world, smoking is so common that not smoking may be remarked upon as different, rather than the act of smoking.[29] Some researchers have suggested that, as people who smoke become increasingly marginalized and stigmatized, with poor and minority populations becoming further segregated in a world of increasing economic disparities, so "smoking islands" can be formed where smoking as a behaviour is reinforced rather than discouraged.[30]

Frances Thirlway conducted research for her PhD dissertation in a former coalmining community in County Durham, North East England, where she expected to find the 'smoking island' model worked well. However, she found the crucial thing in her community was history rather than geography – smoking was indeed common, but smokers felt most linked to other smokers through time and kinship links (e.g. smoking parents and grand-parents), rather than through geography.[31] She suggested that family histories of smoking made it difficult for villagers to distance themselves from tobacco, should they have wanted to do so, or to feel sufficiently alienated from it to be able to give it up. In a situation of adverse circumstances, where ill-health was likewise normal and unremarkable, some of the usual motivations for giving up smoking were lacking too.

The 'smoking islands' model works better in Kwanwook Kim's study of female call-centre workers in South Korea.[32] Women's smoking is still heavily stigmatized in South Korea and women's smoking rates, like those of their female counterparts in China, have historically been very low. Hence Kim, a physician and medical anthropologist, was surprised to be asked by a multinational corporation to deliver a stop-smoking programme for its mainly female call-centre workforce. The company had received complaints from residents in a luxury apartment building nearby because they could watch female workers smoking on an 11th floor balcony at company headquarters. Kim was surprised to find that, rather than the usual discouragement of women smoking, the call-centre workers were actively encouraged to smoke if they felt like it: one woman called it a "smokers' heaven". He found smoking rates five times higher (35.2 per cent) amongst these employees than they were for women in the rest of South Korea (7.4 per cent). Cigarettes had become a 21st century "drug food",[33] seen as a way to help women get through the day in a stressful working environment. The 11th floor balcony was the company's comfortable, easily accessible outdoor smoking area where women who smoked could take a break at pretty much any time during the day.

Call centres the world over are places demanding a considerable amount of "emotional labour".[34] Korean call-centre workers generally have few qualifications and receive relatively low pay for their low-status job. Ninety per cent are women. Numerous physical and electronic surveillance systems were in place in Kim's study. Workers leaving their desks had to set a 'time out' icon (in the form of a coffee cup) on their computer screen, which triggered a timer on the manager's monitor accurate to a second. Incentive payments were based on the number and quality of calls answered (all of which were recorded). Every employee had a mirror at their workstation and were expected to keep smiling throughout every call they answered to ensure they always spoke to the caller with a 'smiling voice'. Workers were therefore under a lot of pressure to recover their exhausted emotions as quickly as possible, and women became accustomed to taking only short, but relatively regular, breaks in the smoking area, and appreciated the social contact and break time cigarettes afforded them. "We usually talk together in the smoking area because we can't talk while working" said one employee. The call-centre manager did not smoke himself, but often advised women in distress to "go outside for a minute" to have a smoke. He also pointed out the cognitive effects of tobacco – its ability to help workers stand outside themselves and think reflexively about their recent experiences. The fact that cigarettes were a third cheaper than a cup of coffee, the other regularly used 'break' marker, probably helped cement the presence of tobacco in this environment.

At a more micro level, island-like associations have been observed between numbers smoking in a household and the likelihood of a child starting to smoke. Sharing a house with parents or siblings who smoke is one of the most reliable predictors of whether you yourself will become a smoker.[35] In fact, longitudinal evidence from the British Household Survey indicates that in the UK it is the mother who has a stronger influence on whether or not her children smoke, an effect which is stronger for girls than boys.[36] Those in the UK living with parents or siblings who smoke are around 90 per cent more likely to become smokers themselves than children raised in non-smoking households. Peer pressure is also a strong influence, as studies that have taken place in the USA testify.[37]

"One of the few day-to-day pleasures"

The physiological entwinement of tobacco with individual smokers in an addictive dependency is matched by the hybrid relationship it has forged with personhood and identity. Consider Guy Grieve's account of having a coffee break during his annual fishing boat refit:

> With work like this, one survives on small comforts, and around mid-morning I would climb the ladder onto the boat and head for the snug shelter of the wheelhouse. Inside, the diesel stove would be purring, creating a warm fug. Kettle would clank onto the hob, and here I would embark on my chief indulgence: rolling a cigarette. As tendrils of steam rose from the kettle my frozen fingers would roll rich, sweet-smelling Virginia tobacco into a delicate made-to-measure smoke. Sugar would be stirred into my mug of coffee, and I'd step out onto the deck, still in the shelter of the wheelhouse door, and light up. Toasted tobacco smoke, coffee and a view out across the sea. Pure bliss.[38]

What we see in Grieve's account are the constrained horizons of his workplace ("one survives on small comforts") and what a powerful, blissful combination tobacco, coffee and sea view are. One can find resonance between Grieve's account and the following statement by a doctor in Kunming, China:

> I started smoking because it was important, so important for being a man. It was important for developing my life...I started to smoke when I finished high school and began working. Then, once I started, I just kept smoking, because it was important for keeping my life on track, getting along with people, managing problems. And I kept smoking because it was one of the few day-to-day pleasures I had.[39]

Giving up (is very hard to do)

As tobacco use becomes increasingly problematic, giving up becomes increasingly common. People report different triggers to quitting (rather like the notion of triggers in Zola's work on "triggers to consult").[40] The final trigger can be very different for different people, and is not always what one might think. A health scare of some sort is very often an epiphanic moment. One inhabitant in Thirlway's work recalled:

I was coughing until I threw up, so I packed up...I was in the Club one night sitting coughing away, I said here, there's your tabs, I'm smoking no more, it's making me ill. People say to me they can't stop, I say if you took ill you would. That was it.

Another man had an epiphanic moment as an ambulance driver while transporting a patient with advanced lung cancer, who begged him "don't end up like me!". He was so shocked by the patient's suffering and emaciated appearance that he and his wife stopped smoking immediately. A father had given up smoking cold turkey from smoking "120 cigarettes a day seven days a week". His wife had an angina attack, and so the man took early retirement to look after her. When the doctor said he should give up on her account, he picked up his packet of 20 and threw it in the fire saying: "That's it!".[41]

Sometimes it can be a non-human species rather than other people who exert more of a quitting trigger. At a health promotion meeting I attended, a smoking cessation expert recalled how one burly, tattooed man living in Newcastle-upon-Tyne had made several quit attempts without long-term success. His final trigger to giving up was the message that his second-hand smoke might be endangering the life of his dog (a brown pit-bull terrier). Sometimes, more abstract arguments can be effective. A fellow humanist confronted sociologist Laurie Taylor with the question: "How can one call oneself a rationalist and still be a smoker? I mean, how can you talk about the value of planning other people's lives when you can't take control of your own?"[42] Laurie Taylor quit smoking.

Those less successful at giving up frequently say that social utility is the most complex issue for them to deal with – how to manage in situations where they would normally be invited to smoke, particularly where tobacco facilitates social interaction. The situation is a common one – but how to handle it varies across cultures and settings. How can one establish a positive non-smoking identity? Here are Kohrman's thoracic surgeons talking about the problems of giving up in Kunming, China. One reports:

I have tried to quit numerous times. I know that cigarettes are dangerous and that they could be ruinous for my family if I fall seriously ill. But what am I to do? Smoking is such a big part of being a doctor here. The director of our hospital smokes. The party-secretary smokes. The chair of my department smokes. And whenever I walk into the duty office, most of my colleagues are smoking.[43]

Another explains:

My quit attempts have often begun during Spring Festival holiday or when I've been on business trips away from the hospital or out of the country for a conference. These quits have all been painful, and I've tried to cope with that discomfort as best as I can, drawing on all my willpower. That's all one can do, depend on one's willpower. Those Chinese herbs sold to help you quit are worthless. I've heard of other techniques and medicines, but nothing like that is available here. So, I quit, and then…aiya!…I get back here [to the hospital] and everyone is politely proffering cigarettes (*fayan*) – colleagues, supervisors, patients' relatives. How can anyone sustain a quit under such circumstances?…I'm just not strong enough…It leaves me disgusted with myself.[44]

Here is tobacco enmeshed in deeply felt emotional exchanges such as *fayan* and *guanxi* and the tendency of the individual user (in this case, a surgeon) for self-blame in explaining and responding to his lack of success. Smokers can be preoccupied with themselves and the sense of an individual self (networked with tobacco) against non-self (without it). Yet there are other determinants of smoking behaviour apart from individual actors' relationship with the substance itself, and with their peers. The efforts of individual tobacco users trying to quit are also being made in the context of tobacco corporations, whose goal is that as many people as possible should start and continue to use their products. We need different perspectives on the tobacco corporations too.

Tobacco's corporate worlds

The first edition of the *Tobacco Atlas*, published by the World Health Organization in 2002, contains a striking map of the world carved up by both multinational and state tobacco corporations, neo-colonial style.[45] After an extensive period of merger and acquisition activity in the 1990s and 2000s, the map shows just four major transnational tobacco corporations – Philip Morris International (PMI), British American Tobacco (BAT, represented in the US market by a 42 per cent stake in Reynolds American, Inc.), Japan Tobacco International (JTI), and Imperial Tobacco. In a fast-moving constellation of products, brand names do not equate with corporations in any simple fashion because rights to a brand can be sold or assigned. Camel, Salem and Winston cigarettes, for example, are all resolutely Reynolds' brands within the USA, but are sold by JTI elsewhere in the world. Benson and Hedges is a particularly mobile brand, sold by BAT in Australia, New Zealand and Asia apart from Taiwan and the Philippines, by PMI in the USA, and by Gallaher (a subsidiary of JTI since 2006) pretty much everywhere else.

'Big Tobacco', as it is sometimes known, consists of more than private equity corporations. State-owned tobacco corporations (SOTCs) are the principal tobacco suppliers in 16 countries worldwide, with the China National Tobacco Corporation controlling a staggering 37.1 per cent of the world tobacco market, almost as large a share as the 'big four' private corporations combined.[46] India also has its own major player, ITC Limited, formerly the India Tobacco Corporation,[47] postcolonial scion of the Imperial

Tobacco Corporation. The different segments of its operations include hotels, paperboards and packaging, agribusiness and information technology industries, but nearly two thirds of its revenues still come from tobacco, under the guise of what it euphemistically terms "fast-moving consumer goods". It has 81 per cent of the Indian cigarette market.

Other tobacco corporations have diversified their interests beyond purely tobacco products. BAT (for example) is now a stakeholder in 40 other companies including Marks and Spencer, Coca-Cola, Diageo and Rolls-Royce. What we might call 'corporation stretching' is matched by an equivalent, 'brand stretching', diversification of the products that are sold under the label of particular brands. Dunhill, for example, once a small family business trading tobacco out of Duke Street, London has become the Dunhill Group, its name associated with a diverse range of luxury goods of all kinds.[48]

One constant in this changing array of alliances, brands and products is the agnotology the tobacco corporations continue to perpetuate, but in changing and increasingly sophisticated technological and informational contexts. One of the most astonishing elements of 21st century tobacco promotion (at least to someone living in a country where overt advertising is a temporally distant memory) is PMI's "Be Marlboro" campaign, launched in 64 countries worldwide in 2011. I shall look at this first, before going on to present other ways in which, despite the new technologies, it is still a case of '*plus ça change*' ('the more things change, the more they stay the same').

"Be Marlboro"

An example of contemporary cigarette hybridity promotion is PMI's "Be Marlboro" campaign. Launched in Germany in 2011, it is particularly targeted at young people. The explanation given by the company for starting the campaign was that "as a brand, Marlboro was not resonating with adult smokers. Smokers missed the cowboy…Live the Marlboro Values – to be true, bold, and forever forward". The accompanying slogan runs "Don't be a maybe. Be Marlboro".[49]

Millions of dollars have been spent by PMI promoting this message in 64 countries. Favoured images show glamorous, attractive young people falling in love and partying. Adverts link the Marlboro brand with adventure (sports such as skiing and surfing), risk-taking (a young person with torn jeans jumping into a 'mosh pit' at a pop concert), defying authority (jumping over a fence into a place unspecified) and sex. All the classic advertising tactics, outlawed for tobacco in some parts of the world, feature in the campaign, including billboard advertising (in Germany, Indonesia and the Philippines), point-of-sale advertising in Brazil and Indonesia, concert sponsorship, brand ambassadors, commercials and promotional videos, social media marketing, and 'brand stretching'.

On Tunisian beaches an attractive team of brand promoters were seen interacting directly with young people, using electronic tablets to collect consumer information from them. Respondents were asked to declare whether they were a "yes", a "no", or a "maybe". If they said "yes", they were allowed to compete for "Don't be a Maybe" branded tee-shirts and hats. Meanwhile in Switzerland, a Marlboro Beat lounge featured at three international music festivals. On Atlantic coast beaches in Latin America, DJ David Guetta performed at a 2012 Marlboro-sponsored summer tour. Online promotional videos included one of young men at a hip-hop-themed party in Saudi Arabia. Interactive promotional booths at shopping malls in Ukraine featured large cigarette displays and promotional videos. After buying cigarettes, customers could register to play interactive games on iPads and win various prizes. PMI's own ethical code states "we do not and will not market our products to minors, including the use of images and content with particular appeal to minors". Germany banned the promotional images in October 2013, ruling they were designed to encourage children as young as age 14 to smoke. PMI appealed the ruling, without success.

Affordances of the internet – from astroturf to sock puppets

'Astroturf' is the term applied to faux grassroots interest groups that are actually sponsored by corporations or other political interests. The growth of the internet during the 21st century has made it possible for such groups to become increasingly sophisticated. One of their tactics is 'conflict expansion', where single issues such as smoke-free public places (Chapter 10) bifurcate into broader, non-health arguments such as "the freedom to smoke in private establishments has become a signature issue for proper liberals".[50] Alternatively, a problem with multiple causes may end up reduced to just one issue, such as attributing the 18 per cent fall in the number of pubs in the UK since the introduction of smoke-free legislation between 2006 and 2013 solely to that factor, ignoring less convenient explanations such as the growth of cheap supermarket alcohol sales and the economic downturn of 2008. The advent of the internet has also permitted the formation of denialists, a more dispersed, looser band of individuals and technologies than astroturf organizations. Denialists tend to operate as individuals, but they are fractal persons, able to use the affordances of the internet to shift into and between multiple identities in order to give the appearance of a large denialist 'community'; the idea of multiple individuals puppeteered by a 'master' controller gives denialists their nickname 'sock puppets'. Sometimes a post from one person can appear copied and pasted on websites around the world, many thousands of times. The hidden hand of industry (if such a thing exists) is less apparent amongst them than it is amongst the front groups discussed in Chapter 8.[51]

Tobacco corporations and the state

In 2010, BAT followed in the footsteps of PMI and JTI by signing an agreement titled The Final Non-Confidential BAT Main Agreement with the European Union (EU).[52] The UK's Economic Secretary to the Treasury signed the agreement in Brussels. It was intended to combat tobacco smuggling and was designed to develop better relationships between BAT and EU Member States. According to the press release, the EU States would "hold the tobacco manufacturers accountable for their actions and encourage responsible trade by requiring BAT to make substantial annual payments to the EU and participating Member States over a period of years and to put in place measures to control the supply and distribution of their products". BAT was also required to make supplemental payments to Member States if its product was found smuggled in significant volumes. In return, however, the manufacturers were "released from any civil claims arising out of past conduct relating to illicit trade".[53] The latter statement was later retracted for a period, but many news media outlets had picked up on the original release, and so it was subsequently reinstated in the government's account of the Agreement. Releasing tobacco from risk of prosecution in this way is rather astonishing. One legal analyst suggested the statement might have been included by mistake, or referred to a separate agreement not included in the publicly available BAT Agreement. The fact that it was called "Non-Confidential" and "Main'" agreement probably signifies that there were other, confidential subsidiary agreements being made less transparently. Could the payment being made by BAT to the EU (reportedly US$10 million a year over 20 years) have originally been meant to support such an arrangement?

Tobacco goes academic, again

In 2000, Nottingham University in the UK received £3.8 million from BAT.[54] Durham University, UK, received a £125,000 donation from the same company to support its Afghan women's scholarship fund – a much smaller amount than Nottingham, but equally controversial and divisive.[55] Despite BAT's evident enthusiasm to support academic endeavours, rival firms were attempting to stymie them. The UK's Freedom of Information Act (FOIA), a law originally designed to help individuals garner information from government or corporations deemed in the public interest, can be used by corporations *qua* individuals seeking access to research data. In 2011, PMI used the FOIA to attempt to force a tobacco-control researcher working in the UK to release data from research undertaken with teenage smokers to explore their reasons for smoking. Understanding such motivations would undoubtedly have helped PMI to market their products more effectively and hence get more teenagers to smoke. Moreover, the researcher had gathered her data with the prior agreement of the young people concerned that what she recorded would remain confidential and anonymised, and only used for her own research – not someone else's.[56]

Maintaining the 'ethical animation' of employees in China

The China Tobacco Museum, built in the Mayan style, opened its doors to the public in Shanghai, China in 2004. It was built, somewhat symbolically perhaps, on the site of a former BAT factory.[57] It was the first of three in China and probably the largest museum of its kind in the world. While it can easily be interpreted as an attempt by the Chinese authorities to promote a positive image of tobacco to the public at large, if this is its aim, it has been singularly unsuccessful.[58] In fact, the museum was created primarily for the education and inspiration of tobacco industry employees across China, in order to reinforce a positive, valorising perspective on the product they manufacture for the largest (state) tobacco corporation in the world. Nearly half the cost of building the museum (equivalent to US$ 23 million) was contributed by branches of the State Tobacco Monopoly Association – that of Yunnan (China's largest tobacco-producing province) giving the most.

In a world increasingly hostile to the charms of the cigarette, the museum provides employees with the ethical nurturance to bolster their comparatively large salaries.[59] It does so through emphasizing the "gorgeous and colourful tobacco culture"[60] that has developed as tobacco has become Chinese, and by lauding individual workers whose patriotism and bravery, by pushing forwards the production of tobacco in China, have animated the party-state, economy and culture. It emphasizes the "great men and celebrities" who have smoked, such as Chairman Mao and Deng Xiaoping. Health concerns are dealt with under a modernization rubric that claims cigarettes have been made progressively cleaner and more scientific over time, while agronomists have involved themselves in the production of tobacco of improved quality. The Chinese tobacco industry, the exhibition claims, has been at the forefront of tackling the dangers of cigarette smoking with the advent of 'light' and 'low tar' cigarettes (see Chapter 8). Under a banner heading "why people smoke cigarettes", a 1948 American Medical Association article is quoted to justify the assertion that "tobacco can relax mental tensions. Therefore there is no need to object to cigarette smoking". Concerns about dangers such as addiction and passive smoking receive no substantive coverage. The museum aims at "cultivating industrial employees' self-perception that they are noble individuals".[61]

Chapter 8 discussed 'Pride in Tobacco' as a means for increasing support for tobacco amongst farming communities in the US. Here we see internal agnotology at work in the ethical animation of tobacco employees through the messages presented at a tobacco museum in China.

Resistance, and counter-resistance

While scientific knowledge has been important in generating increased confidence about working to dissolve the multiple bonds between tobacco and its human hosts, the direct and indirect experience of increasing numbers of people with someone near to them succumbing to an early, and frequently painful, death from tobacco, particularly since the introduction of cigarettes from the 1890s onwards, has also been important. At the birthday party of a practitioner active in the field of tobacco control, the speech-making suddenly raised the memory of her father, who had died of smoking-induced emphysema some 15 years earlier. His absence became a grave and spectral presence at the party, the raw emotion of loss which surged into the narration of thanks for the evening opening up a deep and previously hidden dimension about what drives people to enter into this kind of work. However, personal bereavement amongst kin-relations (often euphemistically and sometimes dishonestly called 'loved ones' in public health rhetoric) is but one of the experiential drivers motivating people's passion against tobacco. A GP friend remembers her early years in Australia as "a young GP doing some locum work in the western suburbs of Sydney". She continues:

> I was asked to visit a family where the man had lung cancer. There were two young boys playing happily in the garden at the front of the house. The man was only in his thirties but had been a heavy smoker. He was dying but clearly his wife hadn't been told how close to death he was. I examined him and had to break the bad news to her. Her reaction, as well as shock, was to ask me if I could help explain what was happening to the boys. At that point I could gladly have strangled the CEO of Benson and Hedges with my bare hands.

Her counter-tobacco narrative, which resonates with Rosenblatt's work on tobacco executives (Chapter 8), is based on first-hand experience of the effects of tobacco on both the individual and that person's social relationships. Her perspective owes little to a sense of needing to rectify the behaviour of individual tobacco users and treating the diseases it causes (too late by far in the story she tells). For her, tobacco corporations (in the persona of the CEO of Benson and Hedges) must shoulder the bulk of the blame. Another Australian doctor, Bronwyn King, argues this most strongly:

> In my early time as a doctor, I did a placement on the lung cancer ward of the Peter MacCallum Cancer Centre in Melbourne. Despite being able to offer the very best medicine available, the majority of my patients died, many of them in their 50's and 60's [sic], some as young as 40. It was shocking to bear witness to the true impact of tobacco. Whilst the treatment and care of patients is paramount, we must deal with the source of the problem – tobacco and the companies that manufacturer it.[62]

As the tide turns against tobacco, both experientially as well as cognitively, some counter-resistance to the myriad arguments against the substance can be discerned. In an article much used by medical students to better understand some of the cognitive 'buffers' generated by tobacco users "in the face of overwhelming pressure from the general public, their loved ones, the local and national press, and the medical establishment" to abstain, DeSantis identifies five arguments regularly used by male cigar smokers at an independently owned cigar shop in a southern US city that enabled them "to light up without being paralyzed by fear or ridden with guilt".[63] The arguments, he concludes, only work because they are used in a disconnected manner from one another and are essentially incoherent. One commentator uses the term "cognitive embodiment" to describe how people with methamphetamine develop cognitive processes that differ from those of people who do not use the drug.[64] The same could be said of tobacco's "kinship with its human host", to revert to Craze's terminology again.

It is not just the use of tobacco and its consequences that promotes statements and acts of resistance amongst those involved with these issues. There is also resistance of various sorts amongst producers, where technological shape-shifting can be discerned. Two kinds of product characterize the alternatives to industrial-scale tobacco production in the 21st century that I present here – one is home-grown, the other is the e-cigarette phenomenon.

Local production – Nepal and Durham, UK

Although I didn't pay attention to it during the time, I was aware that production as well as consumption of tobacco might be carrying on 'under the radar' of contemporary tobacco control initiatives, having spent 21 months doing fieldwork in East Nepal in the 1980s. Many people in the dispersed settlement where I worked smoked a distinctive smelling home-grown tobacco, which they rolled in maize leaves. However, more-recent research has introduced me to Fred and Ed, who live in a village just outside Durham City, UK, where I work. They are local tobacco growers, cultivating the plants along with more conventional crops such as onions, leeks and potatoes, in three allotments on an area of waste ground that the local council asked them to take over. They grow their tobacco from seed – they purchased seed the first year, but five years later they haven't had to spend any more money on the cultivation side of their hobby. Since tobacco seeds are tiny, with one of the highest seed to biomass ratios of any plant on the planet – they use a pepper pot to scatter them, cover the seeds with a centimetre of soil, water them in and wait for up to eight weeks for germination to take place. They usually permit around 100 plants to grow to maturity.

In a manner akin to how tobacco leaves were hung from the rafters of the house where I lived in Nepal, they spear the spines of their harvested tobacco leaves with a pointed cane before hanging them in their greenhouse to 'air dry' (Fig. 9.1).

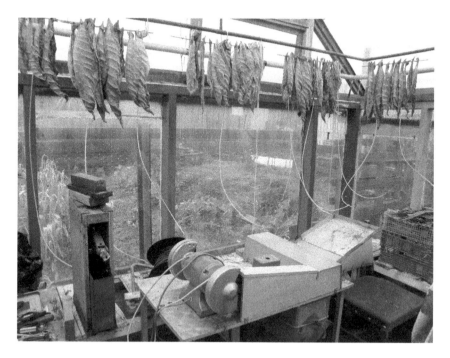

Fig. 9.1 The shredding machine, with tobacco leaves drying above
Source: Photo by the author

The shredding machine, of which they are justifiably proud, sits beneath the hanging leaves, powered by a generator that they keep under a cover shaped like a dog kennel so as not to draw attention to itself.[65] The shredder cuts their tobacco up into strands just like ordinary rolling tobacco – to my eyes, their product is indistinguishable from a commercial variety. They take out the thick central spines of the leaves before shredding them.[66] Retirees from the engineering sector (Fred retired early due to rheumatoid arthritis), they have tried all sorts of implements in their quest for shredding perfection. They started with a guillotine that needed arm-wrenching effort, so next they tried a second-hand bacon slicer, but this lasted all of three minutes shredding tobacco leaves before it was "knacked".[67] Their latest shredder is a combination of old lawnmower blades and a car windscreen wiper motor protected by a steel covering, for safety. A transformer, purchased for £6, slows down the machine without changing its shredding power. They have also made a press, worked by an old car jack. This compacts the shredded tobacco (moistened with alcohol) into a solid brick from which one can tear off what one needs – the old-fashioned 'twist'.

They blend their own tobacco with varying amounts of commercial rolling tobacco – not only because of the shredding problem, but because what they produce isn't as strong as what they buy. In other words, they use their home-grown as 'filler'. They like the idea that what they grow comes straight from the garden, without additives – after all, says Fred, what you buy contains saltpetre, the ingredient of gunpowder, as well as arsenic. He recently saw a television programme that had reported some Trading Standards' raids on illicit tobacco sellers in Manchester.[68] They found all sorts of additives in the smuggled cigarettes they seized, which hailed from countries such as Russia and Bulgaria. By contrast, he said, they don't even need to use fertilizer on their plants.[69] When I visited, their current crop was standing in the allotments at over six feet tall and had produced leaves nearly two feet long. They showed me nine freezer bags full of their harvest, shredded, waiting to be consumed. A friend came in to get some of the less-well-shredded tobacco for his pipe, and took some of the more finely shredded away with him for a friend who smokes roll-ups. The resourcefulness, creativity and dedication Fred and Ed showed towards their hobby was truly remarkable.

Having visited Fred and Ed, I looked further into the legalities and otherwise of what they were doing. One book I read turned out to be wrong, or at least very out-of-date, in stating that growing tobacco at home purely for one's own use was legal.[70] I enquired of a friend in the Trading Standards field about the situation and he forwarded me a letter that had been sent by Her Majesty's Revenue and Customs to a seed importer in 2001 responding to a query he had raised about home-grown tobacco. Apparently the UK government, with its EU partners in 1992, agreed "that there should be no exemption from duty for tobacco products intended for the tobacco grower's personal consumption". The letter went on to assure the correspondent that this was not:

> an attempt to generate revenue from a previously untaxed product. Tobacco use is detrimental to health with significant wider social costs. Growing tobacco at home for personal consumption has, potentially, particularly adverse health consequences as its manufacture is totally unregulated and is not subject to the same limits on tar and nicotine levels as commercially produced tobacco. It is appropriate, therefore, to deter such tobacco consumption in the same way as the Government seeks to deter consumption of commercially produced tobacco.

As if for reassurance, the letter ended

> there is not a great deal of home-grown tobacco smoked in the UK and we will certainly not be targeting potential domestic tobacco producers. Nor do we wish to devote a disproportionate amount of resource to the

control of hobby growers and manufacturers...Duty only becomes due once the tobacco can be smoked, i.e. when the cured tobacco leaves have been shredded.

Robert Proctor's analysis of the "cigarette catastrophe and the case for abolition"[71] concludes, contrary to expectation, that "people should be free to grow, cure and smoke whatever kinds of substances they like, for personal or non-commercial use".[72] A Customs and Excise Notice[73] I found, however, indicated that Fred and Ed would be liable to duty of £180.46 per kg,[74] which seemed quite punitive for a processing system they have spent years developing. It was also somewhat at odds with efforts to decriminalize other forms of home-grown substances that were going on in the Durham region during that time.[75]

E-cigarettes – "disruptive innovation"

Can a leopard change its spots? Can a tobacco product shape-shift into a nicotine product and what are the catches to doing this?[76] Truth be told, e-cigarettes caught public health practitioners by surprise. From a patent issued in China in 2003, the development and sales of e-cigarettes globally have expanded dramatically, from $20m to $1bn in the four years 2009 to 2013 in the US,[77] with use rates in the UK following a similar trajectory. Various kinds of e-cigarettes are available. They include one-use, disposable e-cigarettes, but a survey of 667 current e-cigarette users in the UK in 2016 reported that only 3 per cent regularly used this kind.[78] There are two main types of rechargeable e-cigarettes, which are much more popular. They have various titles, but I shall refer to them by their colloquial names in the UK, that is 'cigalikes' and 'tanks'.

'Cigalikes' very clearly model the form of a traditional cigarette. They have replaceable, pre-filled cartridges in the 'filter' part and sometimes even a light at the end that glows when the user draws on the device. The 'tank' variety has a tank or reservoir that has to be filled with 'e-liquid'. In the 2016 survey, ex-smokers appeared to prefer 'tanks' (81 per cent compared to 63 per cent of current smokers) while current smokers preferred 'cigalikes' (29 per cent compared to 16 per cent of ex-smokers).[79] According to Action on Smoking and Health UK (ASH), in 2014 there were 446 different brands of e-cigarette and 7,700 different flavour variations. Meanwhile, developers in China have moved on from devices mimicking or substituting for cigarettes to devices mimicking pipe and cigars – 'e-pipes' and 'e-cigars' (Fig. 9.2).

E-cigarettes may prove to be the "disruptive innovation'" of the 21st century that machine-produced cigarettes were in the 20th.[80] The name 'e-cigarette' is potentially misleading. Only a subset of the wide array of technologies that have come onto the market in the last ten years or so actually resemble cigarettes, and hence in public health the whole conglomerate is often referred

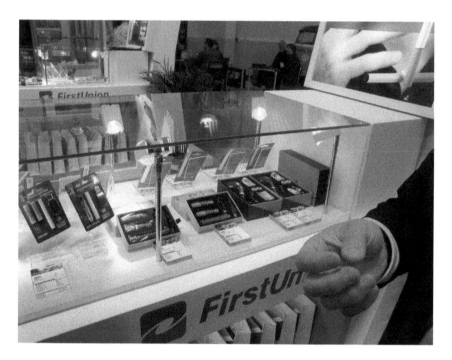

Fig. 9.2 'This is not a pipe (or a cigar, or a cigarette)' – e-cigarettes, e-cigars and e-pipes on display at Eurotab 2014, Krakow, Poland

Source: Photo by the author

to as "electronic nicotine delivery systems" or 'ENDS'. All ENDS contain a liquid made up of a mixture of propylene glycol, vegetable glycerin and a liquid containing nicotine in varying strengths and flavours. A battery-powered element heats the liquid to produce a vapour which the user then inhales: this gives the products a variety of English colloquial names such as vaporizers or 'vapes' (with their users, correspondingly, known as 'vapers'). In the UK, 'vape shops' have expanded and become more sophisticated. The industry producing them is changing in ways that may not be best for public health (see Chapter 12).

What might explain the popularity of e-cigarettes compared to other forms of non-combustible nicotine ingestion devices such as nicotine patches, gums, and other existing nicotine-containing products? One obvious thing is how well they mimic the form and associated actions of cigarettes. The President of the UK Faculty of Public Health talks of e-cigarettes satisfying "the primitive roots of oral gratification".[81] There is much more to a nicotine vaporizer than oral gratification, however.

Unlike other nicotine delivery alternatives – or replacement therapies – it can produce a similar experience to that of a traditional cigarette, in that it provides a nicotine 'hit', at the same time as providing something to hold and also allowing the user to draw 'smoke', or vapour into the body and watch it leave the body as it is exhaled.[82]

The opportunities to individualize one's vape – in ways which are unavailable to cigarette consumers – is another popular feature.

A vape user at a mid-West college in the USA who had smoked for nearly 35 years writes of the bodily changes she has noticed since switching to vapes nine months before. She writes that after only two weeks she found her breathing had got better and she had more energy when she woke up in the morning. Now moreover,

> I feel so much better. I have noticed my skin looking healthier, my teeth are whiter, and my breathing is so much better with no more cough. The one thing that I have really noticed is my asthma. When I smoked regular cigarettes, my asthma would flare up more often. Now that I have switched to e-cigs, I rarely even noticed my asthma...I truly believe e-cigs are safe and a great tool to quit smoking.

She is also pleased at the social consequences of her switch:

> According to the research I have done, there are no harmful chemicals in the vapor. I used to feel guilty about smoking around my friends because of the smoke. Now that I have switched to e-cigs, I don't have that problem.[83]

Others speak highly about the money they save vaping, compared to the cost of cigarettes. Many users on internet forums comment on these savings, although their enthusiasm is tempered by the frequently quite hefty 'up front' costs of buying the initial paraphernalia necessary. Some (who can afford it) even develop a collection. While the variety of different types and flavours available can lead to heavier spending than users might initially envisage or hope for, in the longer term, someone spending (say) £16 per day on two packets of cigarettes can reduce their outgoings by up to two thirds. Vapers often also start to consume less of their product, particularly when they are using it as a means of quitting nicotine altogether, which many try to do. Fifty-six per cent of e-cigarette users/former smokers in a survey conducted by ASH in 2014 said the principal reason for moving onto e-cigarettes was to help them stop smoking entirely. Subjectively, e-cigarettes might have a role to play in absolute smoking cessation. But objectively they are also better for health in a relative way, something of a conundrum for future public health efforts in this area (Chapter 11).

"Find out how Megan can smoke…"

An online e-cigarette forum member reports that most of his friends who once smoked have moved on to e-cigarettes. "Their health has improved and they enjoy vaping, with different flavours and nicotine levels that they can control more effectively. The level of enjoyment has increased tenfold because of the control and choice e-cigarettes offer as well as the health benefits". The user adopts a telling metaphor to refute public health concerns that e-cigarettes might be a gateway to young people smoking by saying one might as well propose mobile phones as a gateway to children using an antiquated popular computer, the Commodore 64. Why would they want to go backwards from e-cigarettes to tobacco?

Worries persist, however, that e-cigarettes lead to a 'renormalization' of smoking or at the very least make it harder to enforce smoke-free legislation.[84] These points are all contested by those who favour harm reduction – and, presumably, by vapers themselves, who see their actions as normalizing vaping, a different action to smoking. At the same time nicotine, long held to be the harmless (albeit addictive) component in cigarette smoke is under the microscope once more with fears that it might impede apoptosis (the process of programmed cell death) and hence increase the risk of cancer, but enhance angiogenesis – the growth of new blood vessels which is a factor in the development of cancerous tumours.[85]

In January 2014, an advertisement began appearing unsolicited on people's computer screens worldwide. Megan, "attractive, slim, elegant, professional, confident and happy",[86] sits on a jet aeroplane with a 'No smoking' sign in the background, holding what is apparently a smoking cigarette. The slogan invites viewers to "find out how Megan can smoke anywhere". Fifty years after Virginia Slims suggested "you've come a long way baby" (Chapter 8), and 12 years after such advertising was eliminated from UK print media, the 'baby' is back – except this time, she is 'smoking' a 'cigalike'. The renormalization agenda, then, is alive and well and animates this advertisement (Fig. 9.3).

Adverts like this raise concerns that the tobacco industry is muscling in on what is clearly a potentially lucrative market, buying up companies and encouraging the sales of 'cigalikes' rather than 'tanks' because of a perception that the former is more likely to attract people back, or lead new users on, to the 'real thing'.

On September 12th 2014, the UK Medicines and Healthcare Products Regulatory Agency gave the first medicines licence to a nicotine inhaler. The product, Voke, is not a 'vape' since it depends on a heat-free, breath-operated miniature valve technology to deliver nicotine to the lungs. Action on Smoking and Health, the tobacco control lobbying group, welcomed the news, hoping that it would pave the way for e-cigarettes to be given licences as medically approved stop-smoking aids and give companies the confidence

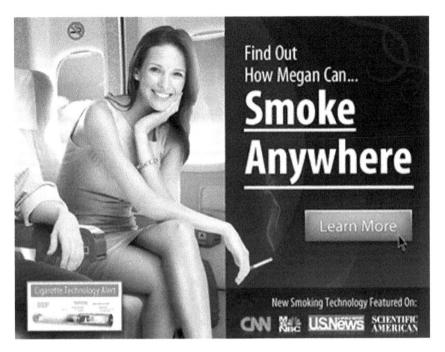

Fig. 9.3 'Find out how Megan can smoke anywhere'
Source: From the collection of Stanford Research Into the Impact of Tobacco Advertising
(www.tobacco.stanford.edu)

to follow the process through. The developer, a company called Kind Consumer, has a worldwide exclusive distribution agreement with Nicoventures, a wholly owned subsidiary of BAT. This brings what for many campaigners may be the ultimate paradox, an item produced by a tobacco giant for doctors to prescribe to patients on the National Health Service, as a means for them to stop smoking.

So are e-cigarettes another kind of tobacco product, or something different? The answer to this ontological conundrum has implications for how they are handled, and who handles them. For some, they are a potential life saver for millions of people currently addicted to tobacco smoking; for others, they are devices with dangers as yet unknown which pose a number of serious risks, not least that they may be a 'Trojan horse' for the tobacco industry to get back into diminishing markets by the back door, and create new ones, by renormalizing behaviours that are like smoking. Amongst some in tobacco control there is extreme concern about what will happen as the tobacco industry starts to muscle into what is currently a patchwork of small, independent companies, and some argue against the over-regulation of the e-cigarette market in consequence. That is before one even gets to safety and health-risk arguments, which are liable to overlay or be influenced by these other issues.[87]

E-cigarettes in the 21st century, like cigarettes in the 20th century and indeed tobacco itself ever since it moved beyond its New World origins, have thus been an extraordinary 'disruptive innovation'. They have been beamed and branded around the world far more rapidly than tobacco in the 16th century. There are further comparisons with tobacco to be made – the way e-cigarettes have spread in 'under the radar', so to speak, and created an amazing and rapidly evolving market – both of producers and consumers. For some, vaping is a time-limited alternative – for example, something to use in restricted spaces where smoking is forbidden, a practice referred to by those in public health, somewhat disparagingly, as 'dual use'. For others like those in the quotes above, 'vaping' is a permanent alternative to smoking, and may be a prelude to quitting altogether.

Conclusion

Craze's book ends 100 days after his quit attempt with no triumphal sense of addiction conquered and cravings overcome. "Will I go back to it?" asks Craze. "I don't know, I really don't know".[88] Tobacco's voice reveals its most menacing aspect at this point:

> You will smoke again. There is no doubt about that. I am your Dark Lord and you will obey. It is only a question of time. I will catch you off guard one lonely cold winter's evening and you will come back to me. You will return to the fold and I will be triumphant.[89]

The "question of time" was to become irrelevant however. An obituary in the London *Times* reveals that Craze died of a heart attack, three years after publication of *The Voice of Tobacco*, aged 56.[90]

Tobacco's voice in Craze's account reflects the growing unease of people about the long-term bond with tobacco. It sets the scene for what it is like being a tobacco user in the 21st century, in China and the UK, and the increasing divisions and inequalities associated with its use. Giving up emerges as a challenging analytical theme, although success in disrupting the tobacco-human amalgam is difficult. Meanwhile, the tobacco corporations maintain their relentless search for market expansion and domination worldwide. Resistance is multifaceted, however. As well as the scientific evidence against tobacco, people have more personal experiences of the substance's harms, but embodied cognition, home-grown produce, and the strong biochemical grip tobacco exerts all serve to counter the strengthening resistance to tobacco's individual and corporate worlds. The arrival of e-cigarettes provides another example of tobacco's shape-shifting abilities and raises both ontological and epistemological issues which will be the subject of further exploration in the following chapters.

Notes

1 Craze (2003: 6).
2 Ibid. (36).
3 Ibid.
4 Nichter (2015: 2).
5 See for example CDC (2017).
6 Ibid. Cf. Goodman (1993)'s multiple 'cultures of dependence' (Chapter 3).
7 Graham (1987).
8 Gray (2008a: 58).
9 Pattison and Heath (2010).
10 Gray (2008a: 54).
11 Gray (2008b).
12 Bunton and Coveney (2011).
13 Klein (1993: 17).
14 Hughes (2003: 166).
15 Klein (1993: 2).
16 Lacan (1996: 388).
17 Ibid. (296).
18 Reed (2007: 36).
19 Klein (1993: 2).
20 Klein (1993: 2).
21 Kohrman (2008: 30).
22 Hughes (2003: 170, 171).
23 Trotta Borges and Simoes-Barboas (2008).
24 Hargreaves et al. (2010: 464).
25 Bragg (2007).
26 Buñuel (1984), cited in Walton (2000: 181) as Buñuel 1982.
27 Graham (1987). Note the potent resonance between this and advertising for a woman's 'me-time' in the bath (Chapter 8).
28 Klein (1993: 16).
29 This is no longer the case in some jurisdictions – in the US, for example, more people are now ex-smokers than current smokers (CDC 2017).
30 Thompson et al. (2007).
31 Thirlway (2015).
32 Kim (2017, 2018).
33 Jankowiak and Bradburd (1996).
34 Hochschild (2003).
35 Leonardi-Bee et al. (2011).
36 Loureiro et al. (2010).
37 Alis and Dwyer (2009).
38 Grieve (2017: 72).
39 Kohrman (2007: 98).
40 Zola (1973).
41 Thirlway (2015).
42 Feldman (2007).
43 Kohrman (2008: 29-30).

44 Ibid. (30).
45 See Mackay and Eriksen (2002: 50).
46 SOTCs may have future advantages when it comes to tobacco control – see Hogg et al. (2016).
47 The corporation insists on being known by its acronym rather than its previous, full name. This reflects its diversification away from purely tobacco products while hiding its continued association with them.
48 Dunhill (1979).
49 Tobacco Free Kids (2014).
50 Salter (2010). Salter is a member of the Adam Smith Institute, which follows the economic principles established by Adam Smith during the Enlightenment.
51 Neither have documents been released at the volume and scale of the Master Settlement millions in this century, so later *relazione* (Strathern 2014) of the major tobacco corporations have become ill-apparent again.
52 Joossens et al. (2016).
53 HM Revenue and Customs (2010).
54 Cohen (2001).
55 Mathews (2012).
56 S. Connor (2011).
57 This had closed down in 1949, the year of the Chinese Communist Revolution.
58 Varma et al. (2005) and Wang et al. (2016) seem to assume the museum is aimed at the general public. According to the latter (118), however, during the ten days of World Expo in 2010, 2,500 people, most of them middle school students, visited the museum. This is hardly a phenomenal number for so large an enterprise at so critical a time. Kohrman (2017: 2) likewise comments that during most of his visits to the museum in 2011 it was "a near ghost town", only open to unscheduled visitors two days a week.
59 Kohrman (2017: 12) states in a footnote that a Yunnan cigarette factory worker is likely to earn a salary about three times that of a steel worker or civil servant.
60 Varma et al. (2005: 5).
61 Kohrman (2017: 11).
62 King (2016).
63 DeSantis (2003: 460). Heikkinen et al. (2010) identify a different set of five protective/defensive arguments used by cigarette smokers in Finland to justify their habit.
64 Bennet (2009: 2).
65 They previously kept the generator in the shed but it proved too difficult for Fred to carry it outside on his own "when he got bad".
66 This, Ed points out, is unlike some commercially produced products such as 'Drum' which "you can see use all parts of the leaf".
67 'Knacked' is a variant of 'knackered' in the north-east of England.
68 Trading Standards is the department in every UK local authority charged with consumer protection and investigation and prosecuting traders who operate outside the law.
69 In this, Fred is demonstrating a common belief worldwide that less chemical treatment of home-grown tobacco means lower health risks. See, for example, Aitken et al. (2008).
70 Gately (2001: 363). This is not the only error in Gately's book: he claims the city of Glasgow, Scotland, is "affectionately known by its inhabitants as 'Auld Reekie'" and suggests that it is located on the banks of the River Spey (105), neither of which are correct.
71 Proctor (2011).

72 Ibid. (10).
73 HM Revenue and Customs (2017).
74 HM Revenue and Customs (2018).
75 Gayle (2015).
76 For more on this topic, see Bell and Keane (2012).
77 Stimson et al. (2014).
78 ASH (2016b: 10).
79 Ibid.
80 Stimson et al. (2014) coined the term "disruptive innovation" with regard to e-cigarettes.
81 Ashton (2014: 8).
82 Lewis (2014).
83 Edem (2014).
84 On normalization see Chapter 10.
85 Chapman (2014).
86 Hunt and Sweeting (2014).
87 We shall see the international debates on this topic in Chapter 11.
88 Craze (2003: 106).
89 Ibid. (105).
90 Anon. (2006).

Chapter 10

Becoming Fresh: a regional platform against tobacco

Introduction – becoming tobacco control

We saw in the previous chapter how 20th century revelations about the multiple harms wrought by tobacco generated not only indignation but some practical responses in the 21st. New social forms were charged by governments and society to deal with what had come to be called the 'tobacco epidemic' at local, regional, national and international levels. This chapter will present the work of Fresh, Smoke Free North East (hereafter "Fresh"), the UK's first regionally based tobacco-control programme. I and colleagues have worked with Fresh, its personnel and campaigns in a variety of different contexts ever since its formal establishment in 2005. Two concepts – denormalization and 'wicked issues' – have been lynchpins of Fresh's activities and are the focus of this chapter. Denormalization, as the word implies, aims to make tobacco less normal in society; it is something that has been at the heart of Fresh's activities from the beginning. Also important has been Fresh's readiness to approach aspects of tobacco's presence as 'wicked issues', problems that "defy easy or single bullet solutions—if, indeed, there are any solutions at all or ones of a lasting nature. Wicked issues have complex causes and require complex solutions".[1] However, an office such as Fresh does not operate in a vacuum. The wider political economy also has implications for tobacco control and its future expansive presence in the tobacco landscape. With financial and structural changes in the way public health is organized, Fresh's progress in both denormalization and tackling some of the wicked issues with which tobacco is entangled are under threat.

Tobacco control – introducing denormalization

In 2002 the Deputy Medical Director of the Northumberland, Tyne and Wear Strategic Health Authority (SHA)[2] stood up at a conference and presented a graph showing how, if National Health Service (NHS) Stop Smoking services remained the only means of reducing smoking prevalence in his region, it was going to take more than 20 years for the smoking prevalence targets set by the government to be met.[3] He argued that the health risks of tobacco, while compelling, had led to tobacco control becoming siloed as a purely 'health services' problem. He argued that a stronger legislative approach at the national level was needed to reduce tobacco use, and a broader-based, region-wide tobacco control programme was required in order to counteract tobacco's influence in a more comprehensive, cross-sectional way. A major bid to the European Union Public Health programme was supported by partners such as the Regional Development Agency, the Government Office for the North East, the Association of North East Councils and the North East Regional Assembly. Although the bid was unsuccessful, the consensus for action that had built up in the process of its development permitted a determined rationale to implement something, albeit with a smaller budget.[4]

His thinking resonated with a number of emerging tobacco control initiatives elsewhere in North America and Europe, for example California,[5] Massachusetts,[6] Canada,[7] Ireland and Scotland. California had taken a pioneering role. A 1988 state ballot initiative had led to the creation of a Tobacco Control Office with an annual budget of $90m. The results of investing this money mainly in cessation services proved disappointing,[8] leading to a more broad-based approach using principles that came to be known as 'denormalization', i.e. changing the norms and values that made tobacco desirable, acceptable and accessible. Despite the efforts of industry lobbyists (amusingly called 'tobacco-people') to counteract it, tobacco control in California achieved some noteworthy results: smoking rates in the state between 1988 and 1995 declined at a rate almost double that of the rest of the United States, for example.

The California office was not the only exemplar Fresh had to follow when it came onto the scene in 2005, but it was a key one. Other examples it followed closely were the Republic of Ireland's introduction of legislation on smoke-free public places in 2004 (and Scotland two years later).[9] The FCTC's inauguration (Chapter 11) and the UK Department of Health's World Bank-derived six-strand tobacco programme were both influential in the formation of Fresh's strategy too. Tobacco control, even at this sub-national level, was becoming international: following a job share, Fresh's first sole Director was a tobacco-control expert who had previously worked in Australia, where tobacco control had been equally dynamic in its approach.[10]

The Canadian government, through Health Canada, already had prevention, cessation and protection as the three 'pillars' of its National Tobacco Strategy when it added 'denormalization' as a fourth in 1999.[11] It identified two strands to the concept, both of which challenged the taken-for-granted nature of tobacco in Canadian society.[12] While in some places denormalization aims "to reposition tobacco products and the tobacco industry",[13] elsewhere the concept is a more person-focused one. Thus "denormalization, in the context of social behaviour, aims to change attitudes toward what is generally regarded as normal or acceptable behaviour...When attitudes change, behaviour will also change because humans generally want to act in ways that are acceptable to others".[14] And "there is clear scope to consider further behavioural denormalization, particularly where it focuses on the consequences for others, rather than just the person smoking".[15]

Taking the latter approach to denormalization risks developing policies and strategies that buy into the tendency to focus on inequalities at the behavioural rather than structural level, what has come to be known in public health circles as 'lifestyle drift'.[16] This has been described as

> the tendency for policy to start off recognizing the need for action on upstream social determinants of health inequalities only to drift downstream to focus largely on individual lifestyle factors. Coupled with this is a move away from action to address the social gradient towards activities targeted at the most disadvantaged.[17]

People who have been absorbed (or absorbed themselves) into tobacco control are frequently acutely aware of this issue but feel powerless to do anything about it. 'Focusing upstream' swims against the current, a trend that makes health and disease a matter of individual responsibility rather than the result of wider social, cultural, political or economic determinants. Critics decry denormalization, despite its dual 'person+corporation' approach, for focusing too much on the 'person' side. Yet the claim that "stigma has not been a historic concern regarding tobacco use",[18] is belied by the history of tobacco use in England which demonstrates plenty of people for whom tobacco use was never a 'normal' activity. Stigmatization was undoubtedly present well before the concept or (in some cases) policies of denormalization came into play. In other cases, as we shall go on to see, tobacco users can be seen actively subverting their feelings of stigmatization as they fit increasingly straightjacketed tobacco-personae into ever more de-tobacconized worlds.

Fresh has had to contend with all these issues during the course of its work. But let us first look at how Fresh has worked in practice, the interactions and exchanges between this sub-national (UK regional) initiative and national and international policies and concerns, some of the unique programmes and campaigns it has run, and some of the shape-shifting and other transformations of tobacco that its staff and supporters have had to follow, a theme that will continue in the remaining two chapters.

Fresh in practice

The image conjured up by the term 'tobacco control office' might be a very grand one, at least in a place like California where tobacco control covers a state that, if independent, would be the seventh largest economy in the world. Fresh, by contrast, was initially an office comprising six members of staff. These six people, however, had strong relations with others involved with tobacco control across North East England and beyond. When Fresh was launched in May 2005 the region had a headline smoking rate of 29 per cent, one of the highest in the country. The only government money funding tobacco control was the NHS Stop Smoking Services and a £94,000 grant for a Regional Tobacco Control Manager. To create Fresh, this latter sum was crucially supplemented by contributions from the 16 Primary Care Trusts in the region, based on a rate of £0.32 per capita. The budget for 2005-06, by this means, was £837,275, of which approximately half was allocated for staff and half for programme costs. Accommodation for the office was provided by a district council in a central location in the region.

The title 'Fresh' and its associated branding were important – offering the positive aspiration of freedom from smoke, rather than focusing on the negative penalties of smoking. The location of the office, separate from NHS premises, was also an important symbol, demonstrating tobacco control was more than just a 'health' issue, a point further reflected in the diversity of groups and organizations involved in the different strands of its operations, and a Fresh strapline that tobacco control was "everybody's business". Key to this was the support of 12 local alliances across the North East region; no other part of the UK was able to maintain such a level of devolved commitment to tobacco control. The governance arrangements also reflected the importance of non-health partners, with a Strategic Advisory Panel made up of representatives from 18 NHS and non-NHS organizations in equal measure.

Three other committees performed more specialist roles within Fresh. A management committee, chaired by a member of the Local Authority Chief Executives' Group, was responsible for the day-to-day running of the Office. An Intelligence Sub-Group had representatives from four of the five regional universities and key NHS partners (such as the NE Public Health Observatory, until its closure due to government cuts – or, as its spectral website encourages us to think, its 'absorption' by a national body, Public Health England). The Intelligence Sub-Group was concerned with research and evaluation – both of the Office itself and the effectiveness of some of its individual initiatives. The Communications Sub-Group looked at the all-important ways in which media messaging was organized and delivered. Latterly a strategy group, titled "Making Smoking History in the North East" was formed.

Denormalization underpinned Fresh's whole approach, with its expressed goal "to change the social norms around smoking to make it less desirable, less acceptable and less accessible". In aiming "to motivate and support smokers to stop", provision of Stop Smoking services and media campaigns to encourage quitting were both important. But Fresh also aimed "to turn off the tap of new smokers, and to protect individuals and communities from tobacco related harm". Its focus in doing this was on "changing community norms rather than just changing individual behaviour",[19] and to be 'anti-smoking' (a behaviour) not 'anti-smoker' (an individual). We shall return to the implications of this distinction for tobacco control practice towards the end of this chapter. First it is important to understand how Fresh's creation and campaigning took place in a context of and engagement with national and international tobacco control initiatives and concerns, before going on to look at its attempts to tackle the 'wicked issues' in tobacco control, and what some of these are.

Exchanges and interactions with national and international concerns

Second-hand smoke

In June 2005, only a few weeks after the inauguration of Fresh, the government published a Health Bill that proposed measures to control smoking in enclosed public places. This had a galvanizing effect on Fresh and its supporters, and enabled them to take advantage of its status as a quasi-independent rather than a civil service or health organization to engage in debate and lobbying about the proposals. The bill offered several options. The UK government, and many regional MPs, initially favoured a "ban with exceptions". This proposed exempting private members' clubs and pubs that did not serve food (so-called "wet pubs") from the need to comply with the smoke-free legislation. However, doing so would have excluded more than half of all pubs in some parts of England; in the case of one NE local authority, the sixth most deprived in the country, 81 per cent of pubs would have been classified as 'wet'. Thus the prospect of a ban with exceptions threatened to widen rather than narrow health inequalities.

Fresh started intensive advocacy work amongst North East primary care organizations, local authorities and other key regional agencies, encouraging them to declare their support for a comprehensive ban, and offering media training to support this. Many members of the Advisory Board were involved in this work, some of them travelling to London to present the scientific evidence in favour of smoke-free legislation to Parliament and other bodies. Fresh distributed 145,000 postcards, calling for a comprehensive ban, that members of the public were encouraged to complete and send in. At the end of the government consultation on the proposed legislation, it was revealed that approximately 18 per cent of the 60,000 responses received by the government had come from the North East, a region with only 5 per cent of the country's total population.[20] Fresh did extensive survey work monitoring public opinion about the proposals; during the consultation period support for a ban grew to 70 per cent of the NE adult population. A clinching argument was that people with jobs forcing them to remain in smoky environments often had no choice but to do so, thus making second-hand smoke an occupational health issue. The comprehensive ban option was eventually voted for in Parliament and came into effect in England on July 1st 2007.

As well as the expected changes – making public places generally more pleasant and healthier to be in, and the incentive it gave some people to give up smoking altogether – the smoke-free public places legislation had more immediate impacts on people's health than anyone had expected. In Scotland, where legislation was initiated a year earlier than England, researchers observed a surprising 2.4 per cent reduction in hospital admissions for heart attacks in the 12 months immediately after the ban compared to the five years before it came into force.[21] Converting this into real figures, 1,200 fewer people went through an emergency admission to hospital in Scotland with a heart attack in 2007-08 compared to 2006-07. The observed reductions in England, while still present, were smaller than in Scotland. This may have been because of a greater reduction in exposure to second-hand smoke in England in the run-up to enacting the legislation, since many public and work places went smoke-free in advance of the all-out ban.

The lobbying work in support of the Health Bill provided an instant, emotionally charged 'issue' that drew Fresh and its partner organizations closer together. In interviews afterwards, several Board members described the experience of working with Fresh on the Health Bill as the most exciting thing they had done in their professional careers.[22] They had become 'tobacco control persons', a counterweight to the different kinds of 'tobacco-persons' and 'tobacco corporations' who had ruled the roost until then. However a downside of the successful passage of the legislation was a misperception amongst some policy makers on the periphery of its work that tobacco control was now achieved whereas, for those at its heart, tobacco control in a real sense had hardly started.

Fresh needed to identify new issues that mobilized similar energies to those unleashed in lobbying for the comprehensive version of the Health Bill. The Health Bill was not the only form of national level policy making with which Fresh engaged: the organization also played a mediating role between national and local tobacco-control activities concerned with the sale of tobacco products from vending machines (2011),[23] point-of-sale displays and associated advertising in large (2012) and small (2015) shops, and standardized ('plain') packaging (2017).[24] Meanwhile those working in tobacco control were being forced to address new (or not so new) forms of opposition to their actions developing with and through new forms of social media. As we saw in Chapter 8, tobacco corporations are subtle and not-so-subtle agents of denial, able to marshal arguments apparently from grassroots people and organizations that seek, wherever possible, to portray anti-smoking agendas as conspiracies against beleaguered smokers based on philosophical principles of individual freedom and personal choice. Fresh had to counteract the development of such perceptions and the associated arguments that spun out from them.

Tackling some 'wicked issues'

"Get some answers" – illicit tobacco

There were several meetings and conferences where I found myself talking with public health professionals and other researchers about smuggled and counterfeit tobacco being an 'elephant in the room' – a big, complex problem 'hidden in plain sight' but largely unacknowledged because it was seen as extremely difficult to tackle. An article published at the turn of the millennium had suggested that, in the eyes of many people in poorer communities in the UK, people who smuggled cigarettes were modern-day Robin Hoods, robbing the taxman to give to the poor.[25] People young and old in low-income communities in North East England seemed only too happy to acknowledge and talk about the presence of what they called the "snidey ones". All were illicit, some were smuggled, others counterfeit, others 'white goods' – like the brand Jin Ling – made purely to target the illicit market. All were sold 'duty free' and were available for about half the price of cigarettes from a normal shop. As one 13-year-old girl said in a discussion with an ethnographer, "I'm glad we can buy them cheap – I wouldn't be able to smoke otherwise". The availability of illicit tobacco was and continues to be a serious hindrance to reducing tobacco use by fiscal means since illicit offers alternative, cheaper sources of supply.

The black market in tobacco sales took diverse forms. A common way of obtaining cigarettes and hand rolling tobacco was to visit a house, known in the North East as a 'tab' house, where cigarettes and other merchandise were sold without tax. Sometimes car boot sales were the venue. Sometimes people would come into pubs and clubs with a carrier bag full of cigarettes and rolling tobacco. In some cases, people would trade in the work place. While this was clearly frowned upon, little would usually happen. As one man put it, "quiet words would be had...you know. But by the nature of it, this sort of stuff...it's not the arms trade". Magistrates, too, tended to take a lenient approach in how they sentenced tobacco smuggling. Early campaigns in other parts of the country had proved largely ineffectual or misleading. One particularly graphic poster had featured a woman with a rat's bottom sticking out of her mouth, under the caption "some people put anything in their mouths", and continuing with the message "dodgy cigs may contain rodent droppings, bugs and dirt". Smokers themselves would sometimes comment on the quality of illicit cigarettes. "They taste horrible... I mean, I've smoked ones before where it burns the back of your throat off, they're like really bad so what's in them? I dread to think", said one male smoker in a community setting. Customs and Excise, being less concerned about health than fiscal benefit, were quite fond of including such arguments in their campaigns against illicit tobacco. However they were anathema to those working in tobacco control since they implied non-illicit tobacco was some-how 'safer' or 'cleaner' than illicit,[26] when there was neither evidence that this was so nor any transparency from the industry about the contents of legal tobacco products. The choice between illicit and legal tobacco was sometimes likened to that between whether one should jump out of the fifteenth or fourteenth floor of a burning building.

Fresh thus initiated the North of England Illicit Tobacco Programme, a world first set up in collaboration with colleagues in the North West and Yorkshire and Humber regions that, with the North East, comprised a population of 14.3 million people. The programme aimed at a comprehensive approach focusing on reducing demand as well as supply. Like the smoke-free campaign, the programme involved a range of stakeholders beyond the 'usual suspects', such as the police, judicial services, customs and trading standards officials. One common perspective – or maybe it was something people wanted to believe – was that most of the cigarettes and hand rolling tobacco sold on the black market was surplus from people's 'duty free' allowance brought back from trips abroad. There were indeed some interesting trips undertaken: one apocryphal story was of a pensioners' special coach party which left from outside a regional newspaper office early every Saturday morning, taking its charges down to Dover and across on a ferry to France. Here they stocked up on their individual 'duty free' allowances of tobacco products, paid for by the trip organizer. When they returned to the North East very late in the day, the same organizer relieved them of their purchases, but since for the old people it was a free day out, everyone was happy.

Most of the tobacco products sold as contraband came from very different sources to this, however. Various kinds of petty criminals and gangs were involved, frequently in a range of illegal activities of which selling smuggled tobacco was only one.[27] The tobacco corporations were complicit in this trade, and remain so.[28] There were apocryphal stories of factories in some parts of Europe producing cigarettes in two shifts – the day shift for the legal market, and the night shift for illegal distribution. Lorries would divert on their way to the channel ports (a process known as 'swerving') so that the product they contained could be shipped from cheaper jurisdictions. If a smuggler chartered ten lorries to transport his merchandise, it only needed one of these to get through for the marketer to make a profit. The market has always been very quick to adapt to changing circumstances and opportunities.[29] During the mid-2000s the proportions of cigarettes and hand rolling tobacco sold illegally reached nearly 20 and 60 per cent respectively. As well as counterfeit and 'cheap whites' produced abroad, authorities discovered illegal factories producing counterfeit tobacco in towns such as Grimsby, Glasgow, Aberdeen and Chesterfield.[30]

The different stakeholders all had their own philosophies and ways of working that were sometimes at odds with those of tobacco control. For example, as mentioned above, the primary concern of those working in Customs and Excise was with eliminating lost tax revenues, not the health problems illicit tobacco caused. They also tended to have a more restrictive approach to intelligence sharing, honed through years of running clandestine operations, not to mention a scandal with a lost computer data stick in 2005 which had allegedly risked divulging private information about thousands of legitimate tax payers across the country. The first task was to establish a protocol to which everyone could sign up. This greatly facilitated the flow of intelligence about the supply of illegal tobacco. The programme went on to develop two social marketing campaigns: "Get Some Answers" and "Keep It Out"; these were based on two messages that research had shown resonated with the widest public constituency: that illegal tobacco brought criminal elements into the heart of people's communities, and the risks posed to vulnerable children from their sale. During the second decade of the 21st century, due both to the campaign and increased pressure on suppliers, amounts of illicit tobacco consumed in the North of England, based on comparing revenue receipts against smoking prevalence rates, dropped by around 50 per cent.

Protecting the pre- (and post-) natal child

Midwives were a group of UK health professionals who had tended to be very poor at raising the issue of smoking in the course of their daily work. Smoking during pregnancy is associated with a higher risk of miscarriage, premature delivery and stillbirth, and lower birth weight – a baby born to a mother who smokes is, at time of delivery, on average 200g lighter than one born to a mother who does not smoke.[31] Scientific knowledge about the later effects of foetal exposure to damaging toxins in the womb (and what some of these toxins are) has become more sophisticated as longitudinal, population-based studies reveal their secrets. For example, lung function (LF) is a crucial issue in human physiology. Peak LF is normally achieved in the second decade of an individual's life, after which it plateaus until their 40s. However, people who don't reach their full potential LF find it declines earlier and more rapidly than those who do. The complex of developmental factors that can impede LF include premature deliveries, low birth weight and childhood asthma.[32] These are themselves frequently (but not always) the result of smoking during pregnancy and the exposure of the foetus, infant or young child to toxins found in cigarette smoke. Chronic Obstructive Pulmonary Disease (COPD), an umbrella term for emphysema and chronic bronchitis, is a largely smoking-related disease caused by the restriction of airflow due to inflammation and excessive mucus in the bronchial airways, or by damage to alveoli (air sacs) in the lungs. It can either result from an overly rapid decline from a normal LF level in early adulthood (frequently as a result of smoking), or because of a normal decline from a lower initial starting point.[33] Thus smoking in pregnancy increases the risk of a child going on to experience COPD in later life, whether or not that child goes on to smoke themselves and, whatever the cause, there are clear hazards in life if one does not reach optimal LF.

North East England had much higher rates of smoking in pregnancy than the rest of the country – 22.2 per cent of women in 2009/10 compared to 14 per cent elsewhere. Fresh commissioned a training package from a consortium of public health practitioners, Improving Performance in Practice, called 'Baby-Clear'. The package introduced more stringent checks on women's smoking status when pregnant, with automatic referral to NHS Stop Smoking Services for women who smoked and more robust 'risk perception' advice given by the midwife at the time of the first scan. Since there is a frequent mismatch between what a woman might say to a midwife about her smoking status and the reality, a carbon monoxide (CO) monitor was issued to every midwife for routine use in the ongoing tests and measurements administered to every woman during pregnancy, giving a more objective picture of whether the woman was smoking or heavily exposed to second-hand smoke.

Ahead of launching the initiative, Fresh sought the views of 1300 midwives in the region. Some expressed concern that raising the smoking issue might fracture what they saw as the all-important relationship between midwife and pregnant woman; some claimed they had no time to do so, and others felt that nothing they said would be likely to make a difference anyway. They were also uncertain about the symbolism adhering to using the CO monitors – would they imply the midwife did not trust the woman to tell the truth about her smoking status?[34] However, in practice, midwives found using the monitors helped them to separate their 'empathy inhibition' – i.e. a feeling of passing moral judgement – from a technical clinical action designed to help get the best outcome for the women concerned. Pregnant women also found the routine use of the CO monitors reassuring – an expected part of antenatal care, something which they saw as part of a coherent system of messaging across the entire NHS. Over a seven-year period from the commencement of the intervention, smoking rates in the North East at the time women delivered their babies dropped to 15.6 per cent, nearly one third in real terms when changing demographics during this period are taken into account.[35]

Epistemic injustices

Inequality is an archetypal 'wicked issue' and there is far more evidence about the extent of inequalities in tobacco use than there are effective policy responses.[36] Smoking in the UK began to decline amongst the upper classes from 1948 onwards, well before the well-publicized links between smoking and lung cancer were established. Women's smoking rates in the UK only began to decline following a peak in the 1970s, and did so at a slower rate than men's.[37] Now the rates are almost similar. But with the concentration of tobacco into areas that score low on what is known as the IMD ('Index of Multiple Deprivation') or, in occupational terms, amongst those employed in 'routine and manual' jobs (if they are employed at all), new ways of dealing with this as a problem were required. The forms of 'cognitive embodiment' (Chapter 9) that set people with a smoking addiction apart from those without one, produce epistemic injustices that contribute to perpetuating their dependency.[38] Fresh has taken on some of these knotty aspects of tobacco's hybridity and tried to pick them apart.

"Don't Be the One"

Street surveys of 500 regular smokers in four different places in North East England revealed a number of perceptual biases about the risks of smoking. One was the assumption that smoking was something which would only catch up with them in old age, rather than, quite possibly, their 30s, 40s or 50s. Moreover nearly half those quizzed said they thought the risk of dying prematurely from smoking was somewhere between one in 10 and one in 20. More than half, when presented with the real statistic (one in two), found it alarming, and queried whether 40 or 50-year-olds can die due to diseases related to smoking. Comparisons such as "you could be hit by a bus" (likely chance in the UK: 1:500,000), or "it's a lottery" (chance of winning the National Lottery in the UK: 1:14m) were more usually, and comfortably, made. There is a deep irony here, which works in favour of tobacco. Basically, the cognitive embodiment of tobacco-using people means some appear either not to know, or prefer not to recognize, the increasingly heavy price exacted by long-term engagement with their product. Straightforward ignorance (Proctor's "native-state agnotology" – Chapter 8) is unlikely, although occasionally Fresh staff came across younger people who expressed surprise on being told about links between, say, smoking and heart disease. 'Selective agnotology', where people recognize the dangers posed by tobacco and do nothing or come up with counter arguments against it, like DeSantis' cigar smokers (Chapter 9) is more likely. Others may decide more proactively to take the gamble that they won't be one of the losers in this two-barrel game of Russian roulette, assuming they know that these are the odds they are playing to in the first place.

Fresh addressed the perceptual bias through its "Don't be the One" campaign, humanizing the one-in-two statistic in the most person-centred way possible. In it Michelle Barthram, a 47 year-old Gateshead woman, told her story, something she had volunteered to do after learning that she had developed small cell lung cancer.

"Smoking has been…my downfall" she states at the start of a powerful video about her situation. "At 47 I definitely didn't expect a terminal lung cancer, and especially small cell, and it is totally related to smoking". She had smoked from the age of 13 and had continued it into her 40s, to her deep regret. She reflects on the physical limitations, recurrent illnesses and other consequences of long-term tobacco use. "I could walk miles; now I struggle; sometimes I have to use a chair. At the minute I'm suffering with a chest infection which probably I wouldn't have had. I don't think you realize just how quickly a disease can come". She then goes on to reflect on the effects of her premature demise not only on her but her family: a keen 'individual'/ 'dividual' approach shines through the story she tells.

> It is in the back of my mind that obviously there are things I am not going to see...potentially there might not be grandchildren, I don't know...Under 50 I think it's just pathetic that I'm in this position, but like I say I did it, I can't change it. The best thing I did was stop. I would never ever touch a cigarette, and like I said before I would urge anybody out there, "Don't do it".

She continues in a more hopeful mode. She would like to see cigarettes in a museum, she says, as "something that [used to be] done that was bad". She was hopeful too of her lung cancer treatment. "You don't know, do you, what's around the corner?" The truth of this statement lay both in Michelle coming to terms with her small cell lung cancer diagnosis and how quickly a serious disease like that can come on, and in her hope that "they're coming up with new drugs all the time, and we'll give anything a go". She concludes "all you can do is live with it, get up every day, give it your best shot and that's it, just carry on".[39]

Unfortunately Michelle died two months after the film was made. She left behind a husband, two children and a dog. The campaign represents an increased focus on the stories of people whose voices against tobacco tend to go unheard. We are less likely to hear the stories of those who die ten years prematurely, most likely following a difficult illness. Barthram makes the point that the premature death and illness from using tobacco are both avoidable and unnecessary. "Don't be the one [of two]", the voiceover says.

"Every Breath"

With COPD it is not so much a question of whether you will acquire it as a long-term smoker, but when.[40] Yet 67 per cent of regular smokers in North East England expressed ignorance about COPD and its debilitating effects. Partly because of this agnotological lacuna, the North East has the worst rates of COPD in England, and the majority of people nationwide who have the disease remain undiagnosed. Despite COPD being destined to become the world's third biggest killer by 2030, funding for research into this, like other respiratory conditions, is pitifully small compared to cardiovascular diseases or cancer.[41] Fresh's "Every Breath" campaign represented the office joining forces with the British Lung Foundation charity to showcase this relatively unknown, underfunded and chronically debilitating disease. In many disadvantaged communities where smoking is the norm, smokers, and maybe the public more generally, seemed to feel that shortness of breath was a normal part of ageing rather than being an early sign of irreparable lung damage.[42] The rock musician Sting, who hails from North East England, gave permission for the lyrics from his song *Every Breath You Take* to be used in the campaign, which featured local actors.

The song continues "every step you take, I'll be watching you". A critical public health expert might query who is watching who here? The caption is ambiguous. It is the pervasive sense of surveillance which is paramount, the statements at the top of the poster linked to the lower caption "every cigarette is doing you damage". This is innovative, if sinister, advertising.

Tobacco use and the NHS

We saw in the case of the BabyClear programme how the public perceives the NHS as an organization (some would say behemoth) that, despite some resistance from smokers,[43] should be at the forefront not only of treating but preventing the health problems associated with tobacco use. Yet many staff in the NHS lack the knowledge, skills and confidence to raise the smoking issue with patients effectively. Fresh is currently hosted by an NHS Foundation Trust, but at an early stage of my involvement I heard a shocking story of a man who had been admitted to a leading hospital in the region following a heart attack. His wife had a 40-a-day 'habit'. Yet despite the proven risks of second-hand smoke, particularly for someone in a vulnerable position like him, after a week in hospital he was discharged without anyone having raised the smoking issue with him (or her) at all. There is evidence that, given the cognitive embodiment (or perhaps we should call it disembodiment) tobacco causes, people regard not being given a message that smoking is a health hazard during a medical encounter as tacit agreement from the medical profession that smoking is alright, or something about which the clinician in front of them is willing to cast a blind eye. Despite an NHS campaign to make every encounter a health-promoting encounter, in some areas of the NHS staff were falling short of fulfilling this obligation.

Thus in some ways tobacco in the NHS generally had become an elephant in the room as big as illegal tobacco for those working in tobacco control (see above). A dismal sight on visiting many NHS hospitals (non-NHS hospitals might have different approaches) was to see the number of patients, often connected to drip stands, sitting around the entrance having left the premises to smoke. Times were changing, though: new technologies such as nicotine patches meant nicotine levels could be managed when patients were in hospital such that there was no physiological need for them to smoke (whatever psychological elements regarding their hybrid relationship might remain). Mental health services were particularly problematic. Despite smoking rates amongst those with a mental health condition being akin to what the UK as a whole was experiencing 30 years ago, according to Health Survey England data the same proportion of people with mental disorders who smoked wanted to quit as did smokers in the general population (i.e. roughly two thirds). New evidence was starting to link tobacco and mental illness in a causative way rather than seeing tobacco as a passive response or human attempt at self-medication.[44] Whether or not tobacco caused mental health problems, there was undoubtedly evidence that smoking cessation improved people's mental health.[45]

There were other increasingly sophisticated ways of understanding tobacco's harms. For example, more than one in three childhood asthma deaths in the UK were in families where one or both parents smoked and, perhaps even more alarmingly, one in ten less than ten year-old asthma deaths was to a child who smoked.[46] It made sense for the NHS to become the place where more tobacco prevention as well as treatment work took place – after all, statistically speaking, tobacco users were more frequent visitors to NHS premises than the general population. The aim of a project started by the London Clinical Senate in 2014 was simple – for every clinician in London to know the smoking status of every patient they care for and have the competence and the commitment to encourage and support that patient to stop, either through direct action or referral. There were simple logarithms to follow with each patient. The "3 As" (ask, advise, act) was the 'very brief advice' mnemonic applied to every patient, which had come to overrule the older "Stages of Change" model in which whether or not a tobacco user should be advised to quit was dependent on first appraising their readiness to do so.[47] The underlying logic of the London campaign was to talk of "tobacco dependency" as "a long term and relapsing condition that usually starts in childhood. Treating it is the highest value intervention for today's NHS and public health system, saving and increasing healthy lives at an affordable cost". Fresh has taken up this medicalized approach through supporting and servicing a Smoke Free NHS Regional Taskforce. Jointly chaired by a Director of Public Health and an oncologist, it aims to get ahead of the national curve by implementing a variety of evidence-based measures a year ahead of the national target set within the Tobacco Control Plan for England. It aims to treat tobacco use as a dependency issue within the NHS, to encourage better record keeping and to promote policies such as completely smoke-free grounds in hospitals.

Resisting the denormalization of tobacco

People are complex and their ideas about what makes them who they are and able to live well may not necessarily be related to what makes their bodies healthy. Sometimes these opinions may counteract the logic whereby tobacco control has become something of a tornado on the tobacco landscape. We should always be aware of the cognitive embodiment of the long-term tobacco user, and how this might lead to reasoning at odds with dominant public health narratives based on individual responsibility for health. Simone

Dennis has worked extensively with people who smoke, exploring their responses to pictures of blackened lungs on a mortuary table which formed a central feature of an Australian anti-smoking campaign. She found people resistant to such a single-image reduction of their bodily potential and feeling – and possibly fearing – a fissure or disconnect between their future aspirational, non-smoking self (with an 'ex-smoking' past) and their current smoking, embodied self.[48]

Some of her interlocutors have gone to great lengths to avoid the machinations of plain packaging: some choose a packet with a particular image from the sales cabinet where they buy their cigarettes; others have started to decant their cigarettes into some kind of alternative container. Sometimes this can have the same kind of 'travel' motifs as did former cigarette advertising (Chapter 8). The tobacco-control messages in the Australian campaign and in the graphic warning labels that have become an increasingly prominent feature of tobacco packets since their introduction in 2012 aim, Dennis argues, to shift the viewer's perspective inside, rather than outside, their body.[49] They have had the effect, as Hill and Carroll argue, of connecting "the thought, act, or sight of *inhaling* a cigarette" with "the sticky walls of arteries, genetic damage to lung tissue, of the 'rotting' that characterizes chronic lung disease".[50]

Not everyone will be consuming tobacco in such a state of assumed dream-like ignorance (or native-state agnotology), however.[51] Others may smoke deliberately and intrinsically *because* it is a risky activity. Crucially, though, "it is a risk for later in life, and not for the here and now. It can be seen as a way of *expressing* that 'I am not investing in my future, I'm *living for now*'".[52] This overt courting of risk and potential damage to themselves and others can easily be linked to spirits of contrariness or rebelliousness. Sometimes this can even shift into rejoicing at the failure of tobacco control at effecting a rescue from one's potentially fatal behaviour. We can glimpse this in Dennis' interviews with smokers on their response to anti-smoking advertising: "The ads have the reverse effect on me; it reminds me that it's probably time for one".[53] A study conducted in New Zealand identified a similar response from a lapsed former smoker having a surreptitious smoke on a night out: "There must be an element of wanting to belong to that crowd...those health-conscious nut cases are behind me... It's like regaining youth and Bourbon drinking".[54]

Freedom to take risks; a legal product; regaining youth. These are tropes of resistance that tobacco industry representatives seize on and milk mercilessly whenever they get the chance to promote tobacco messages of their own. Initiatives to discourage youth smoking are also taken up, with ineffectual results, as we saw in Chapter 8. However, in other parts of the world we can see tobacco-control initiatives that appear to be effective in their context; we shall look at one of these, 'Respira Uruguay', in the next chapter.

The wider picture: survival in a neoliberal economy

Fresh was not operating in a bubble or vacuum. In 2012 its director and her North West regional colleague in charge of Tobacco Free Futures, Manchester, contributed to an anthology marking the 50th anniversary of the release of the *Smoking and Health* report. In it they criticized the coalition government of the time's decision to scrap all semblance of a middle, regional governance tier in public health, leaving just two tiers – national and local – that were deemed sufficient to cover all public health work.[55] The authors were justifiably sceptical about the "duplication of effort, fragmentation of resources, under-prioritisation of tobacco issues or, ultimately, low population reach" that local approaches risked perpetuating.[56] They pointed out the importance of a regional tier using the North of England Illicit Tobacco Programme as an example. Since their words were penned, however, Tobacco Free Futures turned into a social enterprise initiative and has subsequently been forced to cease trading, while the devolution of public health responsibilities to local authorities has presented challenges for Fresh as pressure on public sector funding gets tighter as a result of the government's austerity measures.

Unlike other regions that lacked a Fresh equivalent, most local authorities in the North East have thus far maintained a commitment to working collaboratively and recognizing the added benefits that Fresh offers. The success of Fresh stimulated the creation of Balance, an equivalent programme for alcohol. One way of coping with the financial pressures has been for Fresh and Balance to come together as a single team of nine staff, based within a big NHS Foundation Trust while maintaining their quasi-independence. However the political landscape continues to present challenges due to the loss of some key regional support agencies and the impact that the government's devolution policies are having. While the programme continues to deliver an extensive range of initiatives it takes time to secure the necessary funding from each local authority as well as to diversify the income streams. And, ironically (given the Smoke Free NHS Regional Taskforce mentioned above) the transfer of public health responsibilities to local authorities has given some recidivist sections in the NHS permission to say tobacco control is not their job.

There have also been changes to the organization of smoking cessation services too. While not the sum total of Fresh's identity by any means, stop-smoking services and campaigns to get people to quit remain a central plank of Fresh's work. Durham County Council decided to commission its smoking cessation services from a private company, Solutions4Health, a transglobal organization with offices in New York, London and Dubai. Performance has improved since this move, but there are potential problems. A big company has the resources to 'pump-prime' a bid, for example, undercutting anything that smaller or not-for-profit companies might be able to afford. There are also risks from using long and complex transglobal financial supply chains. It would be deeply ironic, for example, to find a tobacco corporation had invested in a company designed to make money out of curing people of an addiction that same corporation had caused in the first place. There is evidence this has been happening in the case of e-cigarettes, as we saw in Chapter 9.

Fresh has also had to mediate some of the emergent technologies and markets that e-cigarettes represents. A head teacher had contacted the health promotion adviser in charge of a local alliance meeting I attended in April 2014, concerned because children had been bringing e-cigarettes into her primary school that they had bought at stalls in the town's twice-weekly market. "*They're quite safe, Miss*" had been the riposte when she confiscated them. Although what she had confiscated were nicotine-free, they looked like felt-tipped pens and were clearly designed to appeal to children. Very little information or instructions about safe use came with the product. A Trading Standards officer present at the meeting said that, while some retailers were scrupulous about maintaining an over-18s only policy, not all were and that this was a future regulatory issue that would need to be tackled. Would a voluntary code amongst retailers work, or were tougher, statutory regulations necessary? Fresh has kept abreast of developments in the e-cigarette market and ran a series of evidence sessions for practitioners on the subject, as well as maintaining an up-to-date position statement on the issue.[57]

These are some of the ways in which wider political and economic factors can be seen to have impacted on the work of Fresh. However we saw in Chapter 9 that there were some issues that did not fall seriously within the purview of Fresh but which were nonetheless present. One of these was the presence of local tobacco growers in the area. Over the first decade of its work tobacco control became a much less partisan political issue. In one debate in the House of Commons, the Minister and Shadow Public Health Minister united in praising Fresh and its success in supporting the largest decline in smoking rates of any region in England.[58]

"Take Seven Steps Out" – the micropolitics of denormalization

Canada's National Tobacco Strategy talks about how, "traditionally, anti-smoking social marketing efforts have been directed at making smoking a less socially acceptable behaviour *without blaming the victim*".[59] Researchers working in the field known as 'critical public health' tend to find even the implication that denormalization might apply to an individual alarming. They are concerned that, as tobacco control develops, the "without blaming the victim" clause may find itself quietly dropped.

This chapter has shown something of how denormalization has played out in Fresh's work, in the context of it having addressed some 'wicked issues' surrounding tobacco such as the smoke-free public places legislation, smoking in pregnancy, and its work in the illicit tobacco field. However, just as the "without blaming the victim" clause in the Canadian case might be inadvertently dropped in practice, so can the division between 'smoking' (the behaviour) and 'smoker' (the individual) become easily elided in everyday life.[60]

'Take Seven Steps Out' was an award-winning media campaign developed by Tobacco Free Futures in partnership with Fresh, following insight that suggested people were sometimes unaware of or ignored the harms caused by second-hand smoke in the home. The campaign acknowledged the importance of lay health practices, highlighting the inadequacies, however well intentioned, of a number of these aimed at protecting others from the effects of second-hand smoke. A report based on work in a suburb of Gateshead, however, showed that things had gone further than the maintenance of a smoke-free environment in the domestic realm. "Local women have been heard to shout at local smokers 'Take 7 steps out' when they feel that smokers are not respecting this message and are smoking too close to the entrance to the community centre", said one report.[61] Elsewhere, "local volunteers have endorsed the pledge scheme and have been heard to shout at peers who are not moving away from public buildings to smoke 'Oi you – take 7 steps'".[62]

Such examples of what sounds eerily like street vigilantism serve to reinforce calls for a debate on the question of "not could we but should we?"[63] One argument against denormalization could be that it is an abstract concept which has become divorced from the reality of its effects on people's lives, a potentially dangerous marriage between what is ideologically irresistible and financially expedient. In this it is reminiscent of another well-known movement in public health, deinstitutionalization.[64] In both cases, the overall goal was population health benefit, but the experience for some individuals was likely to be negative, quite possibly stigmatizing.

Allied to this is the trend for tobacco to become an increasingly class-based, health inequalities issue in recent years. With some notable exceptions, use rates have fallen most quickly amongst those at the higher end of the social spectrum, and more slowly amongst those in more disadvantaged circumstances. For these reasons, denormalization as a strategy may become increasingly problematic.

Another point those working in critical public health also make is the paradox that in other domains of (generally illicit) substance use, it is destigmatization, both of people and product, that is seen as crucial to reducing barriers and improving access to healthcare. In tobacco, the reverse is true, since denormalization of what is a generally licit substance leads to increased stigmatization of the individual smoker. There is also the issue of second-hand smoke and the harm it causes, a substantive public health issue that is not faced in the case of most other drug products, although public health is now adopting a more sophisticated, 'social harms' approach to tobacco,[65] as well as accepting the harms, at least temporarily, that may be produced by public health interventions themselves.[66] Some are alarmed by the intrinsic impact of certain new concepts in tobacco control such as 'third-hand' smoke, the term given to tobacco smoke residues left on surfaces and materials.[67] Denormalization is not without its critics, and the concerns about stigmatization of people who smoke, particularly in disadvantaged communities where the bulk of regular smokers now live, is a live issue.

Conclusion

Fresh presents an example of a uniquely configured tobacco control programme acting at the regional level as a bridge between local areas and national/international levels in a situation of increasing concern about the presence of tobacco. The three campaigns unique to North East England highlighted in this chapter – "Get Some Answers", "Don't Be the One" and "Every Breath" – were all designed to change tobacco users' and non-users' perspectives, where these were identified as somehow limiting the potential of tobacco control for success. They were based on challenging some of the embodied cognition of tobacco users as well as more-general impressions about tobacco amongst societies in general. Other programmes such as the North of England Illicit Tobacco Programme and BabyClear attempted to address 'wicked issues' in tobacco control, some of which also supported the denormalization agenda.

Fresh's activities have perforce primarily involved acting locally while thinking globally. We have seen what a lot of international exchange fed through Fresh's work from its inception to deliverables. It follows a 'denormalization' agenda to tobacco control, but with a greater focus on denormalization of tobacco use as a behaviour than on denormalization of the upstream tobacco industry that feeds it. The 'regional level' has a very different meaning for the World Health Organization (WHO), namely a platform and mediator between national entities and the global system. The WHO, the global United Nations representative for health, operates a much more nurturing environment for its seven international regions than we have seen in the case of the UK government for its nine English ones. Denying the importance of the regional meso-level, in both cases, risks the loss of micro-level alternative scenarios and ontologies. The fundamental question of this book, "what is tobacco?", is shifting to "what is tobacco control?". We have looked at Fresh's credentials in this field in this chapter. In the next we shall venture into the world of the Framework Convention on Tobacco Control (FCTC) and how it operates. But to answer the "what is tobacco control?" question, we need to consider a range of global imaginaries that are attempting to move the agenda on from 'control' to 'elimination', even as we seek to encompass it. Tobacco's deep past (without tobacco) and the deep future come together in considering the prospects for a world without tobacco in the final chapter.

Notes

1 Hunter (2009: 202).
2 Strategic Health Authorities were subsequently scrapped in a 2013 coalition government move to disband regional entities wherever possible.
3 Milne (2005). The targets in question aimed at reducing adult smoking rates from 26 per cent in 2002 to 21 per cent or less by 2010, and the rates for those in "routine and manual" socioeconomic groups from 31 per cent, significantly higher than the national average, down to 26 per cent in the same time period.
4 Russell et al. (2009).
5 Bal et al. (1990).
6 Robbins and Krakow (2000).
7 Cunningham (1996).
8 California Department of Health Services (1998: 6).
9 For more information, see Russell et al. (2009).
10 See Studlaw (2005).
11 Prevention, cessation and protection are the other three pillars.
12 The strategy seeks to render abnormal "the addictive and hazardous nature of tobacco products, the health, social and economic burden resulting from the use of tobacco, and practices undertaken by the industry to promote its products and create social goodwill towards the industry". In another definition, denormalization "can be described as all the programs and actions undertaken to reinforce the fact that tobacco use is not a mainstream or normal activity in our society", Lavack (1999: 82), cited by Bell et al. (2010).
13 Health Canada (1999: 3).
14 Ibid. (24).
15 Ibid.
16 Popay et al. (2010); see also Baum and Fisher (2014).
17 Popay et al. (2010).
18 Bell et al. (2010).
19 Fresh website, About Us (2012).
20 Heckler and Russell (2008b: 339).
21 Sims et al. (2010); Humair et al. (2014) observed similar reductions for acute respiratory and cardiovascular admissions in Geneva as restrictions on smoking in public places were implemented.
22 Heckler and Russell (2008b).
23 There had been a voluntary agreement that such machines should only be sited in places not regularly used by children. Informal investigations, however, had revealed young people had little difficulty in making purchases since the self-service machines were rarely supervised.
24 Standardized packaging takes away all scope for visual brand marketing. In fact, plain packaging is something of a misnomer (rather like 'smoking ban') since, despite the removal of all but the brand name in a standard font, and the enforced olive green colour of the packets, the graphic and verbal warnings overlaying the packets make them far from plain. Research in Australia, which introduced standardized packaging three years before England, revealed some smokers attempted to counteract the agency of the new packets by limiting their exposure to them, e.g. by selecting (or avoiding) particular graphic images, and by decanting their plain-packaged cigarettes into alternative containers, some of which perpetuate the sense of 'travel' that was such a common motif in earlier cigarette promotion (Dennis and Alexiou 2018). However such acts of resistance are interpreted as a sign of success by tobacco control researchers, since avoiding

the warnings has been found to predict subsequent quit attempts (Wakefield et al. (2015: ii 23).
25 Wiltshire (2001).
26 Scientific evidence is now starting to accumulate that suggests there might be significant differences in the composition of 'normal' and counterfeit cigarettes – see for example Stephens et al. (2005) and Stephens (2017).
27 One of the few published descriptions of this illegal activity is Hornsby and Hobbs (2007).
28 See for example, Joossens and Raw (1998); Lee et al. (2004); Novotny (2006).
29 Hornsby and Hobbs (2007).
30 Antonopoulos and Hall (2016).
31 Lower birth weight is associated with a range of increased health risks such as early breathing and feeding difficulties and problems in later life, such as heart disease and diabetes.
32 McGeachie et al. (2016).
33 Lange (2015).
34 Beenstock et al. (2012).
35 Bell et al. (2017).
36 Smith (2013: 68).
37 Russell (2015).
38 For more on epistemic injustice see Carel (2016), Chapter 8.
39 See Don't Be The 1 (2014).
40 Lundbäck et al. (2003) were amongst the first researchers to reveal COPD as a massively under-reported, under-diagnosed and under-acknowledged problem.
41 British Lung Foundation (2016).
42 This may instead have been a convenient fiction, of the same order as that tackled by the "Don't Be the One" campaign.
43 Pilnick and Coleman (2003).
44 See for example Fluharty et al. (2017).
45 Taylor et al. (2014).
46 Royal College of Physicians (2014).
47 The stages of change model (also known as the transtheoretical model) assumed advice to quit was reckoned only to succeed when the person targeted was at the appropriate stage of readiness to follow it (DiClemente et al. 1991). Not receiving advice every time was identified as confusing to people who smoked, potentially legitimating their practice. There was evidence that people who might not be ready to quit immediately according to the tenets of the stages of change model were likely to be influenced by the "Three As" messaging nonetheless.
48 Dennis (2011).
49 Dennis (2013).
50 Hill and Carroll (2003: ii 9) in Dennis (2016).
51 To coin Proctor (2008b)'s phrase again.
52 Hughes (2003: 135), his emphasis. This was also a minority expression amongst certain dispossessed young people, that "my life is hopeless/there is nothing to live for, hence why bother?"
53 Dennis (2006).
54 Thompson et al. (2009).
55 Rutter and Crossfield (2012). Even the title of their entry uses 'sub-national' for 'regional'.
56 Ibid. (48).
57 Fresh Smoke Free North East (2018a).

58 Fresh Smoke Free North East (2018b). Rates declined from 29 per cent in 2005 to 17.2 per cent in 2017.
59 Health Canada (1999: 24), my emphasis.
60 Cf. Macnaughton et al. (2012).
61 Malcolm and Goodman (2011: 12).
62 Ibid. (15).
63 Bayer (2008) does this.
64 See for example Dear and Wolch (1987); Mathieu (1993); Desjarlais (1997).
65 Hillyard and Tombs (2007).
66 Bonell et al. (2015).
67 E.g. Bell (2014); Dennis (2016).

Chapter 11

Becoming the FCTC: global solutions to a global problem

Introduction: eeriness and the FCTC

This chapter takes the story of tobacco control from a UK regional tobacco control platform (Chapter 10) on to a significant global stage. The World Health Organization (WHO)'s Framework Convention on Tobacco Control (FCTC) is the first global health treaty ever negotiated by the WHO. Since its inauguration in 2005, it has been one of the fastest growing treaties in the history of the United Nations (UN), with over 180 signatories representing more than 90 per cent of the world's population. Every two years the Convention Secretariat, based in Geneva, organizes a Conference of the Parties (COP). This is the governing body of the FCTC, consisting of representatives of all the governments ('Parties') which have signed up to its obligations. While the FCTC and the COPs are supposed to be antithetical to the production and use of tobacco, there is nonetheless an eeriness to the COPs, where by 'eeriness' I mean a "failure of absence"[1] (in this case, of tobacco) in what are supposed to be spaces for the control of, and freedom from, tobacco. This failure of absence is manifest in a number of ways – through the infiltration of tobacco interests into the debating chambers, through the troublesome relationship between health and trade, and the 'disruptive innovation' of e-cigarettes, here transmogrified into 'electronic nicotine delivery systems', or ENDS.

This chapter is based on attending four of the biennial COPs (COP4 to COP7 inclusive) from 2010 to 2016. Each COP took place in a different part of the world – Uruguay, Korea, Russia and India. Ethnographic methods for research in these kinds of settings have been widely championed,[2] but ethnography is still under-represented as a methodological approach in the field of global health diplomacy. The research for this chapter followed a modified form of Collaborative Event Ethnography (CEE),[3] which takes a team approach to fieldwork, covering as many micro-events as possible in the transnational "mega-event"[4] that is the COP. The description and micro-analysis of real-time negotiations that ethnography offers illuminates some of the processes and contexts within which a treaty such as the FCTC is negotiated and performed. Has the international community managed to counter the influence of the global tobacco industry, and how has the tobacco industry responded to this emergent, antithetical force appearing on the world stage? What are the points in the COP where particular 'failures of absence' can be discerned? What are the areas that are supported, and what left out, by the treaty's focus on the transnational tobacco industry? The chapter ends with a visit to Respira Uruguay, an exhibition targeting young people which was displayed at COP3, and considers the extent to which its success is contextual to its place and the creativity of its designers.

Bringing a tobacco control treaty to life

The fact that there is an international health treaty concerned with a single commodity is remarkable in itself. So normal was the presence of tobacco amongst health planners and policy makers when the WHO formed in 1948 that tobacco was not included in the list of major health problems within its remit to address at that time.[5] Delegates at the 23rd World Health Assembly (WHA) held in Geneva in 1970 expressed concern that, wherever records were being kept, the incidence of lung cancer appeared to be increasing. Other known effects of smoking included chronic bronchitis, emphysema and heart disease. A resolution from this meeting requested the Director-General to investigate to "what extent and by what educational methods young people might be persuaded not to begin smoking", and to encourage the UN's Food and Agriculture Organization to start looking into crop substitution programmes.[6] However, the first proposal made in the resolution simply asked all those attending the WHO to refrain from smoking in its meeting rooms.

The notion of developing a tobacco control treaty came much later,[7] and again was partly stimulated by the revelations contained in the Master Settlement documents. "It came as a shock to all of us to realize how early on the tobacco industry had been tracking us, looking at us, criticizing WHO internally, much earlier than we ever dreamt of", is how one leading tobacco control activist put it at a 'witness seminar' charting the history of the FCTC in 2010.[8] She also reported her sense of betrayal at realizing how many of her public health colleagues had been in the pockets of the tobacco industry.

Although its 1948 charter gave it the power to do so, the WHO had never sought to create a legally binding treaty.[9] In the early 1990s, a small group of influential policy makers, dismayed at tobacco's relentless progress around the world, began lobbying at the WHO's headquarters in Geneva for some kind of international agreement for better, more consistent and above all global tobacco control.[10] Deciding the best format for such an agreement was only one of the challenges they faced. The WHO had developed a nonbinding 'code of conduct' for the marketing of formula milk for babies worldwide, and many in the WHO thought a similar initiative for tobacco was the best way forwards. The more radical amongst them favoured a treaty, but opponents argued it was not the place of the WHO to develop such a document or, if a treaty was the preferred option, it should be under the auspices of the UN as a whole rather than the WHO. Progress in this direction was slow until the appointment of former Norwegian Prime Minister Gro Harlem Brundtland as WHO Director-General in 1998.[11] She took tobacco control very much to her heart, and to the heart of the WHO.[12]

In the epidemiological language used to justify the treaty, the WHO Expert Committee was explicit about what they saw as the distinctive features of the 'tobacco epidemic': "tobacco use is unlike other threats to global health. Infectious diseases do not employ multinational public relations firms. There are no front groups to promote the spread of cholera. Mosquitoes have no lobbyists",[13] they said. Other powerful messages emerged to support the push for international tobacco control. Tobacco had become "the world's greatest cause of preventable death".[14] Estimates are that tobacco will be responsible for almost 1 billion premature deaths in the 21st century, 70-80 per cent of these in what is known in development terms as the global South. As legislation squeezes tobacco use in the richer countries of the Global North and public tastes change, so the industry doubles its efforts to infiltrate and manipulate new markets in order to carry on fulfilling its "fiduciary imperative" (Chapter 8). The FCTC then was very much seen as a global solution to a global problem, and the tobacco industry did everything its power to undermine it.[15]

Industry representatives worked to inhibit progress on the FCTC in various ways, particularly through governments they saw as champions of tobacco. Germany, China, Japan and the United States became the 'Big Four' countries seeking to water down the wording of the text.[16] The strong reliance of Malawi on tobacco cultivation – accounting for 61 per cent of its export revenues and rising in 2006 – was another leverage point for tobacco industry activities against the FCTC.[17] Despite these hindrances, the WHA agreed the documentation prepared for the FCTC in 2003 and, once the necessary 40 signatures from different countries ('Parties') required for an international treaty to enter into force were secured, the FCTC came into being in 2005.

The FCTC in its final form was enshrined in 38 Articles which between them address most, but not all, the production and consumption measures necessary for there to be effective control of tobacco. Demand-focused elements such as price and tax increases, protection from second-hand smoke, advertising, packaging and labelling, health education, and provision and support for smoking cessation were complemented by the Articles dealing with supply issues such as sales by and to children, illicit tobacco, support for economically viable alternatives, and measures to deal with the environmental problems tobacco causes.[18] One of the central principles of the Convention is enshrined in Article 5.3, which states that: "In setting and implementing their public health policies with respect to tobacco control, Parties shall act to protect these policies from commercial and other vested interests of the tobacco industry in accordance with national law".[19]

In what follows I shall look at the ways in which tobacco attempted to infiltrate the FCTC through some of the gaps in its provisions as these became manifest in the discussions and decision making at the COPs, divided into three sections – trade, e-cigarettes and personnel. Trade was not included as a 'supply-side' issue in the Articles and as such came back to haunt the progress of the FCTC. E-cigarettes emerged as a disputed presence on the global stage, and tobacco, despite attempts to control its presence, has remained *in situ* through some of the personnel attending the COPs. But first I shall outline the organization and nature of global health policy making as a response to the tobacco epidemic – or, looked at in a different way, how tobacco has shaped the FCTC and its COPs.

Creating spaces for global tobacco control

Participants at a COP consist of "Representatives of Parties" and "Observers" (Fig. 11.1), the latter subdividing into representatives of states that have not signed the treaty but are permitted to send observers (non-Parties), Intergovernmental Organizations (IGOs), and representatives of Non-Governmental Organizations (NGOs, also termed "civil society"). Representatives of Parties have the right to speak first in plenaries, known as "having the floor", with those who speak on behalf of one of the WHO's six regions prioritized over those who speak on behalf of their own country. In order not to give spatial preference to one country over another, the seating plan for the Parties starts from a randomly chosen letter of the alphabet. However, it has become customary for countries' representatives to sit according to their regional groupings rather than alphabetically, for ease of consultation during the COP.

The main NGO group represented at the FCTC COP is the Framework Convention Alliance (FCA), a consortium of over 500 civil society organizations working in tobacco control around the world. Observers have a right to speak (a "voice") once all Parties who wish to speak have done so but, unlike Party representatives, observers have no voting rights. "Non-Party" representatives are permitted to speak ahead of the IGOs and NGOs. Such is the volume of business (and the number of Parties in attendance) at a COP, however, that it is unusual for an NGO to have the opportunity to take the floor. It is extremely unusual for a vote to be called at a COP, moreover, since the primary way of achieving agreement is through consensus: calling for a vote is seen as a mark of failure in global health diplomacy circles in that it implies irreconcilable disagreement and lack of flexibility in different Parties' positions.

The other two categories represented in Fig. 11.1 are "Members of the Public" (MoPs) and "Members of the Press". We encountered MoPs the very first morning my colleague, Megan Wainwright, and I attended a COP. As researchers we felt our status was most appropriately MoP, so joined a line in the conference hotel lobby to acquire the day passes MoPs were permitted. We quickly figured out that most of our fellow MoPs were part of the

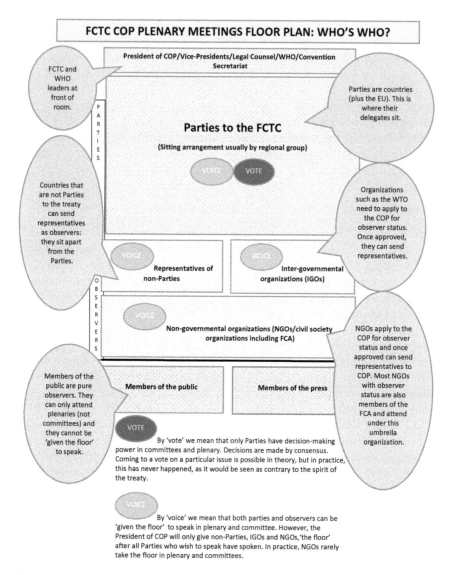

FCTC COP PLENARY MEETINGS FLOOR PLAN: WHO'S WHO?

President of COP/Vice-Presidents/Legal Counsel/WHO/Convention Secretariat

FCTC and WHO leaders at front of room.

Parties are countries (plus the EU). This is where their delegates sit.

PARTIES

Parties to the FCTC

(Sitting arrangement usually by regional group)

VOICE VOTE

Countries that are not Parties to the treaty can send representatives as observers: they sit apart from the Parties.

Organizations such as the WTO need to apply to the COP for observer status. Once approved, they can send representatives.

OBSERVERS

VOICE
Representatives of non-Parties

VOICE
Inter-governmental organizations (IGOs)

VOICE
Non-governmental organizations (NGOs/civil society organizations including FCA)

NGOs apply to the COP for observer status and once approved can send representatives to COP. Most NGOs with observer status are also members of the FCA and attend under this umbrella organization.

Members of the public are pure observers. They can only attend plenaries (not committees) and they cannot be 'given the floor' to speak.

Members of the public

Members of the press

VOTE
By 'vote' we mean that only Parties have decision-making power in committees and plenary. Decisions are made by consensus. Coming to a vote on a particular issue is possible in theory, but in practice, this has never happened, as it would be seen as contrary to the spirit of the treaty.

VOICE
By 'voice' we mean that both parties and observers can be 'given the floor' to speak in plenary and committee. However, the President of COP will only give non-Parties, IGOs and NGOs, 'the floor' after all Parties who wish to speak have spoken. In practice, NGOs rarely take the floor in plenary and committees.

Fig. 11.1 Floor plan for plenary meetings of an FCTC COP

Source: Adapted from an original diagram by Megan Wainwright

tobacco industry – manufacturing corporations, growers' organizations, producers and distributors. Coming in as a MoP was not a good means of gaining access to the COP for research purposes. Conference participants,[20] on seeing our distinctive day pass badges, were justifiably suspicious of who we might be, not a good way to establish trust and rapport with those ostensibly working to progress global tobacco control. Despite this, at our first COP, MoPs were permitted attendance at the back not only of the plenaries (Fig. 11.1) but also the meetings of the two Committees, A (treaty instruments and technical matters) and B (implementation, international cooperation and institutional matters, such as the budget). At COP5, however, after the opening plenary, MoPs were excluded from all meetings in which there were 'substantive issues to discuss', and at the following two COPs, MoPs found themselves excluded altogether. Fortunately we managed to change our designation at COP4 and subsequent COPs through affiliating with an NGO participating in the conference as part of the FCA. "Beware who you speak to and what conversations you have", said one FCA member concerned about the presence of tobacco industry representatives during the COP at an FCA meeting one evening, "they are everywhere and will be listening out for information". We had no way of assessing the validity of this somewhat paranoid-sounding statement. We went on, however, to become better versed about tobacco's infiltration of the places and spaces of global health diplomacy around tobacco control.

The nature of international law

International law cannot operate in quite the same way as the national laws of sovereign states in which fines, custodial sentences and other penalties can be used as punishment for their transgression. Short of economic sanctions and military action, there are few means of penalizing governments which ignore or flout an international agreement. However, a lot of informal pressure can be exerted on states that, like people, do not 'toe the line'. In this way, laws have agency over and above the punishments that can be meted out in their name. People may argue against them or oppose them, but ultimately the diplomatic goal is consensus and the production of legislation that imposes a growing coherence on people and states based on convention rather than force.

There are a number of characteristics that make the FCTC COPs distinctive as places for the creation of international law. Having entered the first plenary and joined fellow MoPs at the back of the hall, it was clear that the actions of tobacco as a global industry rather than tobacco *per se* were the primary focus of the debates. At the opening ceremony, the WHO's then Director-General, Dr Margaret Chan, pulled no punches in explaining how important she saw the FCTC and how she perceived the enemy:

> This is an epic battle between the protection of public health and the pursuit of corporate wealth. This is a ruthless pursuit of wealth, with no regard for the damage tobacco products cause to health. Protecting public health policy from interference by the tobacco industry is a cornerstone of the Framework Convention and vital to its implementation. Public

health has the evidence and the right values on its side. The tobacco industry has vast financial resources, lawyers, lobbyists, and no values whatsoever beyond the profit motive.

Margaret Chan went on to describe the civil society organizations present as a cornerstone of the FCTC. There was no guarantee that Party representatives would have much if any expert knowledge about tobacco control and the issues it faces.[21] Thus opinion-forming and monitoring progress was a key feature of the FCA's role. This included preparing a daily briefing sheet for conference delegates, one of the features of which were the "Orchid" and "Ashtray" awards. These were awards made by the FCA, based on intelligence received at their morning and evening meetings, to those countries or individuals whose actions or statements the FCA representatives felt either particularly favoured or undermined progress at the COP.

One of the interesting technologies the FCA employed, at least in earlier COPs, was the 'Death Clock', a large black clock with digital gold numbers (Fig. 11.2). Its upper display counted down the number of people who had died of a smoking-related illness since 1999, while the lower notched up the number of people around the world who had succumbed to tobacco during the period of the conference (one every six seconds in both cases). The 'Death Clock' was a powerful reminder of the need for dedication and haste in conducting the COPs activities, although at a later COP the decision was taken to dispense with it on the grounds it possible gave an overly pessimistic impression of the FCTC's prospects for success.

Another distinctive feature of the FCTC COPs that differs from other WHO meetings (such as the WHA) is the greater assistance given for representatives from low- and low-to-middle-income countries (LMIC)s to attend. The main way this happens is through the provision of funding, in the form of an economy airfare and daily (*per diem*) expenses, to permit every LMIC that is a Party to the Convention to send a representative. The WHO normally gives no such support for LMIC representatives to attend its meetings, and that the FCTC does so reflects the importance the FCTC Convention Secretariat accords their participation. However, at COP4 the decision was taken to reduce the threshold for travel support, and at COP5 this was reduced further still. Such measures resulted in some curious last minute largesse from countries that stood to gain most politically from such generosity (and had the power and resources to be able to do so). The Russian Federation, for example, ended COP5 offering to host the next COP in Moscow and, putting $3m on the table, agreed to fund the travel costs and per diem allowances of LMIC participants to COP6.

Despite these measures, however, participation by representatives from such countries has been low. They constituted nearly half of the 137 countries represented at COP4, for example, but only 10 per cent of total number of delegates.[22] The significance of this lies not in its implications for equivalence

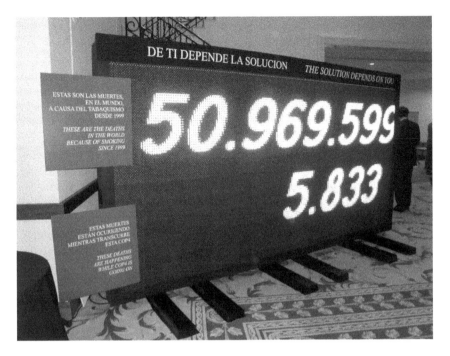

Fig. 11.2 The 'Death Clock' at COP4, November 2010
Source: Photo by the author

and equality between nations, since it would be naïve to argue there should or could be any sort of equality in numbers of delegates from different countries irrespective of size, wealth or geography, but in its practical consequences. Just as researchers need to practice CEE (above), it is impossible for a country represented by a single delegate to cover all the ground necessary at a COP. After the opening plenary, not only is a lone Party representative unable to split themselves in two to attend both of the Committees, but if a Committee Chair decides that a document under consideration is incompletely developed, or that continuing to work on a piece of legislation in a full Committee is an inefficient use of time, Working Groups are regularly organized to meet after hours. It is impossible for representatives from small delegations to attend everything. The number of such delegates was 39 at COP5 (out of 136 countries in attendance) and 41 at COP6. Not all of these were from LMICs, of course; some were representing wealthier countries that are small. However, across the first four COPs, nearly 40 per cent of LMICs were represented by a single person delegate compared to only 10 per cent of high-income countries.[23]

Challenging the relationship between health and trade

The first 'absence' we shall consider is the lack of consideration of what Brandt styles "the inevitable conflicts between public health restrictions and trade liberalization" in the text of the FCTC, something there was considerable debate about during the drafting process.[24] Some of the tensions this lacuna had created became clear during COP4, which was held at Punta del Este, Uruguay, in November 2010. The venue is significant because eight months before the COP started, Philip Morris International (PMI) filed a "Request for Arbitration" with the World Bank's International Centre for Settlement of Investment Disputes (ICSID) claiming Uruguay had violated four obligations in a Bilateral Investment Treaty between it and Switzerland.[25] Uruguay had introduced a law limiting tobacco companies to only one version of each brand in an attempt to stamp out unnecessary or misleading appellations such as 'Marlboro Lights' or 'Virginia Slims' (see Chapter 8). While other companies dealt with this regulation by simply giving new names to their different varieties, PMI objected, claiming the new law had forced the removal of seven of its eleven products from the Uruguayan market. The company also challenged the requirement that 80 per cent of all cigarette packs be covered with health warnings including pictures. The FCTC only recommended that 30 per cent of the pack be covered with a warning, and PMI claimed 80 per cent would cause a sense of repulsion both of the product and the company and, as such, was an unreasonable attack on their 'intellectual property', i.e. the brand and the company's right to market it. Switzerland was, quite conveniently, a non-Party to the FCTC and PMI had established a head office there.

A Uruguayan government representative with whom I spoke feared the lawsuit was likely to cost the country 3-4 million dollars to defend, money which was otherwise earmarked for smoking cessation and health promotion work. A multinational with a yearly turnover twice that of Uruguay's annual GDP, PMI hoped to create a 'chilling effect', i.e. fear of similar retributions discouraging governments of LMICs with possibly far larger potential cigarette markets from following Uruguay's lead.[26] However, filing this lawsuit eight months before Uruguay was due to host COP4 was possibly ill-timed. The Pan-American Health Organization lent Uruguay its support, and the Bloomberg Foundation (established by former New York mayor Michael Bloomberg), through the NGO Tobacco-Free Kids, gave the Uruguayan government half a million dollars to help fund its representation at the tribunal. COP4 also became a venue of support for Uruguay. The FCA's information booth offered a smorgasbord of reading materials, reports and paraphernalia including pins that said "Uruguay You Are Not Alone". In their plenary statements, many Party representatives emphatically stated what they saw as a moral obligation to support Uruguay's struggle. It became clear also that Uruguay's experience of intimidation by corporate tobacco was far from unique. At a lunchtime seminar on Day 2, for example, a delegate from Norway explained that his country's attempts to introduce a point-of-sale advertising ban in January 2010 had also been challenged by PMI, this time as a potential breach of the European Union (EU)'s free trade agreement.

The impending lawsuit thus shaped the debates and discussions that took place at COP4, as well as creating a highly significant outcome, the Punta del Este Declaration, proposed by Uruguay as an agenda item at the very start of COP4. This started with a general declaration on the importance of the FCTC in the face of tobacco industry interests, stating the need to continue to implement tobacco control policy and share information about tobacco industry interference. However, the forthcoming lawsuit brought by PMI was clearly alluded to in the statement that "Parties may adopt measures to protect public health, including regulating the exercise of intellectual property rights in accordance with national public health policies, provided that such measures are consistent with the TRIPS Agreement".[27] TRIPS stands for "Trade-Related aspects of Intellectual Property Rights" and was the point of law that PMI was hoping to test in bringing its suit against Uruguay.[28] To have included trade issues in the FCTC's original Articles when free trade, as previous chapters indicate, was regarded as an almost paramount international good, would have made the Convention's successful passage even more difficult than it was. The representative from the World Trade Organization (WTO) at COP4 helped clarify his own organization's position in the final plenary when he presented the WTO's trade agreements as a "toolbox" of rules available to help Parties take steps to protect public health. He did, though, argue that a balance needed to be struck between legitimate interests such as health and the need to avoid discriminating between partners or setting up unnecessary barriers to trade.

Rather than cowing Uruguay's tobacco-control efforts, PMI's attack seemed to have strengthened the country's reputation and status as a public health '*luchador*' (fighter) on the global stage, while cementing a sense of solidarity with its neighbours, and countries beyond, in becoming so.[29] In an open letter to the President and the Uruguayan Government at the end of the conference, the FCA wrote "The Government of Uruguay is demonstrating the priority it places on public health, and not only defending the health of its own population, but by defending its sovereign right, it is setting an example for the rest of the world".[30] While the status of the Declaration as an international legal document is somewhat opaque, it can be taken as clarifying "customary international law, particularly in respect of the sovereign powers of States to regulate in the public interest" (WHO 2012: 80). Another legal scholar and activist, Jonathan Liberman, comments that it "may be expected to be referred to by courts or tribunals in any proceedings brought against an FCTC Party under trade or investment agreements".[31] There is evidence that this is in fact happening, not only in international tribunals such as the ICSID, which found in Uruguay's favour in 2016, but in national courts too.[32]

Breaching symbolic boundaries

Despite the label, 'civil society' is not an inclusive term for all those non-governmental entities with an interest in the COP and its activities. Only international and inter-regional NGOs "whose aims and activities are in conformity with the spirit, purpose and principles of the Convention" are allowed to apply for observer status at the COPs.[33] Six organizations had indicated their desire to gain this status at COP4. Two of them were approved (the European Network for Smoking and Tobacco Prevention and the International Network of Women Against Tobacco). Three had their applications rejected, and one (the Human Rights and Tobacco Control Network) was deferred until the organization in question had fully established itself and conducted relevant activities that would support its application. Of the three rejected organizations, one (the Liga Italiana Anti Fumo) was told it had submitted inadequate documentation and that its activities appeared to be predominantly national rather than inter-regional or international, while two – the Global Acetate Manufacturers Association and the International Tobacco Growers' Association (ITGA) – were deemed to be involved in activities that "might not be in line with the aims and spirit of the Convention".

The ITGA, it is clear from the Master Settlement documents, is a front organization for the tobacco industry, funded to the tune of several million dollars per year.[34] After its rejection at COP4, representatives retired to a tent they had established in a supermarket car park across the road from the conference hotel, which they decorated with multilingual signs saying 'Don't Ruin Us' and 'We Defend Our Livelihoods'. From here they were able to distribute a daily green paper bulletin, *The Farmers' Voice*, to participants approaching the conference venue. This indicated their grievances, which were particularly with Articles 9 and 10 (concerning regulation of the contents and additives of tobacco products and disclosures regarding these), and Articles 17 and 18 (concerning support for economically viable alternatives to tobacco, and protecting the environment). Some of them attended the conference as MoPs, and on the third day their presence was established more forcefully with a demonstration at the entrance to the conference hotel. The Convention Secretariat Chair met the demonstrators in the conference hotel entrance and accepted a petition with 230,000 signatures expressing opposition to the Articles in question.

A similar issue arose at COP5 with the decisions about two applications for observer status from international organizations – one from the "South Centre", the other from Interpol, the international police network. The former was waved through without problem, but Interpol prompted disquiet amongst delegates on account of the organization having received 15 million Euros from PMI "to support the agency's global initiative to combat trans-border crime involving illicit goods, including tobacco products", as the PMI press release put it.[35] Since this was a direct contravention of Article 5.3 (above), Interpol's application for observer status was deferred.

The status of MoPs and how they should be handled remained a contentious issue at further COPs. According to some Party representatives they could not speak freely in sessions where MoPs were present for fear of subsequent recriminations. In consequence, MoPs have been increasingly excluded from the two Committees at which most of the substantive business of the COPs is conducted, and latterly the plenaries too. When these decisions have been taken at previous COPs (resulting in MoPs who were present having to undergo a 'walk of shame' out of the plenary session at COP6, for example), the layout of the conference venue has often meant MoPs could still hang around the corridors, lunch and coffee venues. At COP7, in Greater Noida (India), where MoPs were again permitted to attend only the first plenary session and were excluded from all other meetings that week, the security cordon around the venue made further infiltration impossible.

Such attempts at boundary creation, with the intention of creating tobacco-free spaces within the conference venue, goes beyond the vetting of observer organizations or the exclusion of MoPs, however. It is something of an international public secret that the government ministries of many nation states who are part of the FCTC still have strong links to the tobacco industry. Some Party delegations attend COPs with representatives of ministries that have a strong policy mandate to increase tobacco production or consumption in their country rather than reduce it, or who are strongly influenced by the tobacco industry in their country legislatures. Some delegations have first or business class air travel to the COPs funded through corporate tobacco sources. This all runs contrary to the protection from tobacco industry interests demanded by Article 5.3.

During COP5, the FCA acquired a copy of a letter from the Managing Director of BAT and others representing "the Tobacco Industry in Kenya" that had been sent to the Permanent Secretary of Foreign Affairs in Nairobi. It expressed disquiet that "it has come to the attention of our industry representatives...that the Kenya delegation has deviated from the agreed Kenya position". This position derived from an inter-ministerial committee that had apparently been held in Nairobi a month before the COP. This, the letter went on, "could have serious unintended consequences". The letter took particular exception to statements alleged to have been made at a side meeting that the tobacco industry was beating farmers who turned to alternative crops. "Taking into account the position of the tobacco industry in the economy, the industry takes great exception at the derogatory remarks made by the Kenya delegation at the Conference, in addition to the deviation from the agreed country position". Brazil also withdrew five members of its 19-person delegation who were felt to be too stridently anti-tobacco during COP5, including its representative from the National Health Surveillance Agency. Their names were contained in the 'provisional list' at the start of the COP, but they had disappeared from the final 'list of participants' dated 7th December 2012.

In other cases, membership of delegations included people who were only one step removed from tobacco industry representation, if that. The Vietnam delegation at COP5 contained two members, who were Secretary General and Interpreter of the Vietnam Tobacco Association respectively, an organization with strong links and staff crossover with companies such as BAT. Meanwhile, a member of the Italian delegation, listed in the COP5 participants' list as "Head of the Technical Secretariat of the Ministry of Agricultural, Food and Forestry Policies", was also easy to track down as the Secretary to the Italian Tobacco Producers' Association, as well as Secretary General of the European Federation of Tobacco Processors (FETRATAB). In this latter role, an article in the trade publication *Tobacco Journal International* revealed, he had chaired a two-day symposium at the World Tobacco Expo 2011 that included scientific discussions "on topics including whether ingredients can increase addictive qualities in tobacco products".[36]

To try and deal with situations like this, in an unprecedented step a month before the start of COP7 the Convention Secretariat sent out a 'Note Verbale' (an unsigned piece of third-person diplomatic correspondence) asking governments to consider the needs of Article 5.3 in selecting representatives to attend the COP. The Convention Secretariat followed through with an agenda item at COP7 headed "Maximizing transparency of Parties' delegations, intergovernmental organizations, nongovernmental organizations and civil society groups during sessions of the COP and meetings of its subsidiary bodies". The Thai delegation drafted a proposal making it mandatory for every participant to a COP to sign a Declaration of Interest (DoI) in advance. The Convention Secretariat's actions, and the DoI proposal, prompted indignant responses from some countries that saw such 'screening' applied to Representatives of Parties as a threat to state sovereignty. There was also a question about what to do with any information about a link to tobacco interests that was received by this process – would it be used to bar those who declared a connection with the tobacco industry, or was it simply a case of 'naming and shaming'? Despite efforts by some activists to get at least a DoI procedure agreed for media representatives (some of whom were known to represent the tobacco press and whose green badges occasioned the same degree of caution for some participants as the white badges of MoPs), the polarization generated by the issue meant that time ran out on the possibility of discussing even a truncated form of Thailand's proposal, and so no agreement was reached.

Tobacco's voices?

Like a mysterious smoke permeating all areas of the conference venues, tobacco's influence at the COPs thus remained real and pervasive, but far from clear. It was extraordinary to be at the governing body of global tobacco control treaty at COP7, for example, and hear country delegates claiming that "there is no evidence of tobacco industry interference" or "I don't think we have what is known as a tobacco epidemic in the world right now". Some suggested, contrary to Article 5.3, that tobacco and related industry interests might be legitimate stakeholders in the FCTC. There were also deliberate attempts made to slow progress on the key pieces of international legislation being discussed, either by invoking procedural issues or by raising a 'flag' and opening up an issue just at the point when the Chair of a committee thought s/he had achieved consensus and was moving to close it. Sometimes this happened just before lunch or the end of the day, giving Parties a chance to regroup or, in some cases, to consult with their governments at home and possibly return with a less flexible position.

At COP7, it subsequently transpired, more investigatory work regarding industry influence was going on behind the scenes than was apparent at the time. Journalists from Reuters were present, observing which companies sent representatives to the COP itself (BAT and JTI) and which did not (PMI). The report they produced used leaked PMI documents to demonstrate that the tactics observed during COP7, such as delaying and watering down decisions and encouraging the presence of delegates from ministries other than health who might be expected to have a more pro-tobacco stance, were all the result of tobacco industry lobbying. They also indicated some of the emergent differences between the transnational tobacco companies in how they handled COPs. Unlike its counterpart corporations, PMI stationed its representatives in a hotel about an hour's drive from the conference venue, from where they were able to monitor its progress and send a white VIP van to collect delegates who wanted to discuss issues of mutual benefit. One of these was the Director of the Vietnamese government department that deals with corruption, smuggling and trade fraud, who had attended the past three COPs.[37]

Even less could be done about restricting tobacco's voices outside the venues, however. Arriving at COP7 in India, delegates might have noticed posters plastering bus shelters and numerous three-wheeler autorickshaws. They featured an elderly man in typical North Indian peasant clothing, his hands clasped together in a beseeching prayer. "Protect our livelihood. I am a tobacco farmer", the caption read. "We appeal to the government to probe and expose the hidden agenda of agencies engaged in anti-tobacco campaigns" (Fig. 11.3). The posters were sponsored by the Federation of All India Farmer Associations (FAIFA), whose president claimed in an *Indian Express* article that "they [meaning tobacco control agencies] are creating an environment that facilitates the entry of global corporations to manipulate and earn profits from the lucrative Indian market". Such a conspiracy theory was incredible. In fact, FAIFA is an astroturf organization (Chapter 8) tapping into a broader global South fear that the actions of foreign-funded NGOs might be against national interests. Such pressure can have unfortunate consequences. Six months after COP7, the farmer appeared again on billboards in Delhi thanking the government for having "taken action against some NGOs". Two NGOs doing important work in the public health field that were receiving funding from

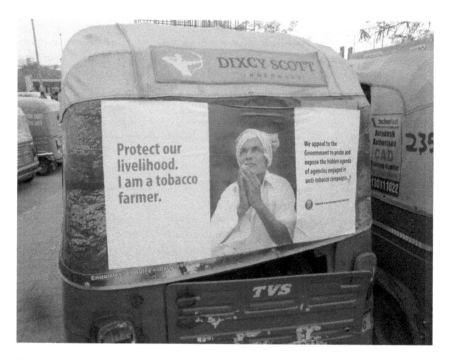

Fig. 11.3 Autorickshaw with tobacco livelihood poster, India, November 2016
Source: Photo by the author

the Bloomberg Foundation – an important philanthropic donor in the field of tobacco control – had their licences to receive foreign funds revoked, and staff in the organizations were laid off in consequence. A government spokesman said that such organizations were operating "against the national interest". In fact, it was tobacco interests that had prevailed over those of health in this instance.

E-cigarettes – new global problem or global solution?

E-cigarettes were barely invented when the FCTC was ratified, and they quickly became a 'disruptive innovation' for reasons explained in Chapter 9. The WHO's Tobacco Free Initiative (TFI) commissioned a group of US researchers to prepare a background paper for COP6 which was subsequently published in an academic journal,[38] and the TFI Programme Manager prepared a WHO report based to a considerable extent on the contents of the background paper.[39] This was problematic, because the paper in question said and interpreted things about e-cigarettes that a different group of tobacco-control researchers strongly opposed. As is often the case in scientific disputes of this kind, the arguments hinged around conflicting interpretations of the individual studies used and an over-selective use of different parts of the knowledge jigsaw. The background paper concluded that e-cigarettes should be subject to the same regulations as conventional cigarettes, with "at minimum" the same exclusions on their use in public spaces and the same restrictions on their advertising and promotion. Its critics argued against this, as long as any marketing promoted the devices as a stop-smoking tool while minimizing their appeal to non-smokers. Clearly e-cigarettes had already become different things to different people – the equivalent of a tobacco product, and an aid to help people stop smoking tobacco.

Another bone of contention that divided tobacco control was the potential attractiveness of e-cigarettes to young people, and whether they might be a gateway to tobacco smoking. The background paper claimed "youth are rapidly adopting e-cigarettes", but its critics cautioned that their use amongst non-smoking youngsters was very low "and there is currently virtually no regular use in children who have never smoked or never used tobacco".[40] Furthermore they pointed out how the arrival of e-cigarettes had coincided with a continuing reduction in youth smoking rates in the UK, France and the USA which made the 'gateway' hypothesis (Chapter 9) unlikely.[41] The disagreement revolved around how to interpret the meaning of having ever, regularly or never, used an e-cigarette. The authors of the background paper used a North Carolina survey that found only 12 per cent of young people who had ever used an e-cigarette had never smoked.[42] However, the paper's critics felt simply having tried one was not a convincing measure of use, reiterating how "other surveys confirm that to date, there have been hardly any instances of non-smokers becoming *regular* users of e-cigarettes".[43]

Further dissension concerned the intrinsic safety of e-cigarettes. The authors of the WHO background paper reminded readers that e-cigarettes were not free of toxins. But opponents argued that the difference between an e-cigarette and an ordinary cigarette in this regard is huge, with daily exposure to carcinogenic nitrosamines from cigarette use between 76 and 142 times higher than from an e-cigarette.[44] The only definitive evidence of toxicity came from studies in which cells had been washed with e-cigarette liquid – not the vapour that users actually inhale. While the background report's authors accepted that the indoor pollution caused by e-cigarettes is nothing like the smoke-filled bars and clubs of yesteryear, they argued that e-cigarettes do still cause some level of air pollution, contrary to the claims of some e-cigarette advertisements and users that they only produce "harmless water vapor".[45] However, e-cigarettes operate differently to ordinary cigarettes. They only give out vapour when being actively used (unlike the 'side-stream' smoke ordinary cigarettes continue to emit in a resting state), and the contents of that vapour are far less likely to be harmful to bystanders than cigarette smoke. While one study suggests nicotine levels amongst non-users sharing a room with e-cigarette users are comparable to those of passive smokers, opponents remind us that "it is not nicotine which is harmful in passive smoking, but the other smoke components".[46] Yet neither is nicotine completely harmless, particularly for certain sub-populations such as children, foetuses and those with heart disease.

The discord within tobacco control circles between opponents and supporters of e-cigarettes became more acute prior to COP6. In June 2014, 53 scientists wrote to Margaret Chan, the Director-General of the WHO. Their letter requested the WHO keep e-cigarettes separate from anti-tobacco legislation under the FCTC, arguing that e-cigarettes offered a new and increasingly popular way of encouraging smokers to quit. Two weeks later, a second letter, this time with 129 signatures, arrived in Chan's in-tray. The signatories to that letter argued that e-cigarettes were a means for the global tobacco industry to re-enter declining western markets through the development of apparently harmless but untested products. Meanwhile the mechanical safety of e-cigarettes had become the subject of media scrutiny. Stories abounded of e-cigarettes in both North America and Europe exploding while recharging,[47] while anecdotal reports – such as I had heard at a local alliance meeting in the UK (Chapter 10) – began of school-age children bringing e-cigarettes into school.[48]

ENDS and the FCTC – agreeing to disagree

Tobacco's shape-shifting into e-cigarettes (Chapter 9) required a corresponding shift of name within public health circles – to 'electronic nicotine delivery systems' (ENDS). Given the conflicting scientific viewpoints on what they were and what their harms might be, and the lack of decisive evidence on which any definitive attempts at global policy making could be made, provisional agenda item 4.4.2 "Electronic nicotine delivery systems, including electronic cigarettes"[49] at COP6 was set to be a contentious issue. The FCA's policy briefing on the matter argued that "it will be difficult to reach consensus at COP6 on specific regulatory approaches to ENDS".[50] It also pointed out that favoured regulatory approaches might differ according to a country's resource levels, with techniques that might be appropriate in a high-resource setting – involving, say, extensive testing of products and surveillance of marketing practices – might be entirely impractical in a low-resource one.[51] In the end, the approach adopted was one of 'agreeing to disagree'.[52]

Describing ENDS as "the subject of a public health dispute amongst bona fide tobacco-control advocates that has become more divisive as their use has increased",[53] Costa Rica at the start of COP6 proposed that Parties should "consider taking measures" to follow four regulatory objectives identified in the WHO's report namely to impede the uptake of ENDS by non-smokers, pregnant women and youth; to minimize potential health risks to ENDS users and non-users; to prohibit any kind of false, misleading or deceptive promotion of ENDS; and to protect tobacco control efforts from the tobacco industry that produces and sells ENDS. It proposed asking the WHO to monitor the use of ENDS amongst smokers and non-smokers and for the formation of an expert group to report back at COP7 with updates about the health impacts of ENDS, their efficacy for smoking cessation, and the regulatory options for achieving these objectives.

The extensive discussions of the ENDS issue and Costa Rica's draft decision reflected a variety of different approaches to regulating e-cigarettes: in the same way as tobacco products; to prohibit them; to treat them as either therapeutic products or general consumer items, or as a unique category altogether. China reflected the first of these in suggesting that Costa Rica's draft decision be reworded to regulate ENDS like other tobacco products. The Russian Federation, announced it was introducing measures prohibiting the production and sale of ENDS within its borders; others echoed this prohibitionist theme.[54]

The EU, which is permitted to speak as a bloc as well as individual countries at the COP, was more equivocal in its approach. In the EU's view, it was too early to make recommendations, let alone take a position at international level, since there was not yet enough experience to be able to determine which approach would ultimately deliver the best health outcomes. Panama brought up the question of what ENDS actually were, tobacco products or stop-smoking aids, arguing that there was the potential for great confusion over this. Rather than taking up any more time in general debate the Chair of Committee A asked interested Parties to form a working group to discuss Costa Rica's draft decision in detail and come back with a reworked version of it.

When the draft decision re-emerged from these deliberations two days later, two new clauses had been added. One invited Parties "to consider prohibiting or regulating ENDS, including as tobacco products, medicinal products, consumer products or other categories, as appropriate, taking into account a high level of protection for human health". The other urged Parties "to consider banning or restricting advertising, promotion and sponsorship of ENDS". In line with the FCA's prediction about different regulatory approaches being partly dependent on a country's resource levels, it was often (but not always) the LMICs that argued for treating ENDS like tobacco products or banning them altogether. The EU reflected the views and policies of some high-income countries in arguing that other regulatory approaches were possible. In the UK, for example, where (as we saw in Chapter 9) there had been little regulation of ENDS apart from as consumer products, a ban would have been impossible to implement, and the EU confirmed that position in COP6 on several occasions. Rumours abounded that Africa region countries disagreed with the newly revised draft decision, and had resolved to push for an outright ban. However, it turned out the only stalling that took place was over what title the Decision should have. After much debate, involving a huddled consultation at the back of the hall instigated by the Chair of Committee A, the cumbersome title "Electronic nicotine delivery systems, and Electronic non-nicotine delivery systems" (ENDS/ENNDS) was agreed on. Consensus reigned after further discussions but for the Russian Federation's insistence that it could not agree to including the option of regulating ENDS/ENNDS as consumer products. The report on item 4.4.2 notes the Russian Federation's dissent about regulating ENDS in this way.[55]

Respira Uruguay

Respira Uruguay came to COP3, but I didn't see it there. COP3 took place in Durban, South Africa, and an English-language version based on the 150 m^2 original exhibit located in the Espacio Ciencia ('Science Space'), in Uruguay's capital city, Montevideo, was a real talking point. Once COP3 was over, the exhibition transferred to Johannesburg but it is unclear what happened to it after that. So popular was it at COP3, though, that the Tobacco Free Kids initiative (funded by Bloomberg) paid for a presentation about it to take place at the 14th World Conference on Tobacco or Health. That's where I first became acquainted with Respira Uruguay. It uses a variety of different interactive and multisensory components to educate children, young people and other visitors about the health and other consequences of smoking, in an engaging and enjoyable way. Respira Uruguay was designed in collaboration with a leading campaign organization against tobacco in Uruguay, the Centro de Investigacion para la Epidemia del Tabaquismo (CIET). The resulting exhibition was officially opened by President Tabaré Vázquez in August 2007. It displays the results of a happy marriage between public health expertise and artistic inspiration. Whether or not it succeeds in what one commentator has called "museum experiences that change visitors",[56] Respira Uruguay has a distinctly transformative aim, to discourage its visitors, particularly its target audience of teenagers, from becoming or remaining smokers. It does so in a number of interesting ways.

Entering the exhibition (Fig. 11.4) has been described as "like slipping into the wide thoracic cavity of a large mammal, ribs open to the air and readily able to expand and contract with each breath. The inside of the rib cage is decorated with a picture of a young boy running joyfully in the open air, chasing a dandelion clock that has been scattered by the breeze – the image of the exhibition".[57] Once inside, the visitor is presented with four doors, each with a different enticing incentive or justification for starting to smoke. They could be voices inside our head. Translated into English, these are: "All your friends smoke so why not?", "You can easily stop again if you start", "It makes you look cool" and "You are old enough to decide for yourself" – all influential reasons given by young people for starting to smoke. Succumbing to one of these entreaties and pushing open a door, one enters a dark, low-ceilinged, somewhat claustrophobic room, very unlike

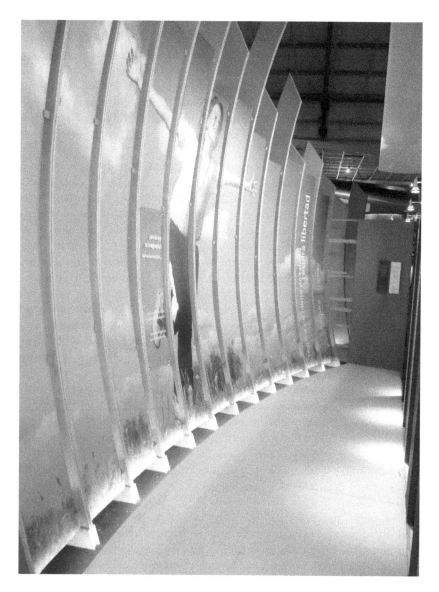

Fig. 11.4 "Like slipping into the wide thoracic cavity of a large mammal"
Source: Photo courtesy of Martha Cambre

the bright, open space outside. Like the 'Death Clock' display at COP4 (above), an illuminated digital clock computes the steadily increasing number of people in Uruguay who have died since the exhibition opened from a smoking-related disease, and the number of people in the world who have died from a smoking-related disease over a similar period (one every six seconds). The idea is to make the visitor think differently about the smoking life they have so glibly chosen. One might add irrevocably, because trying to leave is difficult. Only one of the four doors lets visitors out into the open air again, and it is heavy and hard to push open. Struggling to find a way out, the dangers of the smoker's path are further illuminated by a UV light playing tricks with fellow visitors' faces, illuminating their teeth and giving the appearance of ageing skin, simulating the effects of smoking on the body.

Other areas of the exhibition are equally interactive and multisensory. A rack of clothing aims to mimic the smell of cigarette smoke after a night out in a smoky atmosphere, compared with clothes that retain the pleasant smell of washing detergent (something of a biochemical challenge to effect). Elsewhere you can put your hand out to feel the relative strength of air that is expelled from non-smokers' and smokers' lungs. Roulette wheels compare the chances of getting a terminal illness as a smoker with those of a non-smoker. A financial implications section gives the costs of daily packet of cigarettes by week, month, year and decade, and suggests what you could otherwise buy with that money. In the fitness section you can step onto a treadmill and measure the effort required by a smoker compared to a non-smoker to walk up a steep hill while a video display features members of the Uruguayan football squad talking about the value of a healthy lifestyle; the resistance level is much higher on the smoker's treadmill. There is also an exhibit presenting the components of a cigarette in a particularly arresting way. A giant model of a cigarette is made out of clear, cutaway Perspex with objects from daily life representing some of the many components people may not realize are contained in their inhalations – rat poison (arsenic), moth balls (naphthalene) and battery juice (cadmium). It also reveals the shockingly high temperature of the burning end of cigarette, along its length and even where it makes contact with the smoker's lips.

A key point about Respira Uruguay is that it is intimately embedded within the local knowledge economy. Its further development, such as opportunities to construct appropriately adapted equivalents elsewhere in the world, has been partly hindered by the lack of evidence as to its effectiveness. Would effectiveness in the Uruguayan context translate into effectiveness elsewhere in the world? In 2012, I brought a group of six young people from the young persons' advocacy group W-WEST ('Why Waste Everything Smoking Tobacco) from Glasgow, UK, to see the exhibition for themselves, reflect on it and give feedback on its effectiveness and suitability for a different cultural context. Gaining their perspectives seemed crucial, and so they proved to be. However, it has not been possible to take the Respira Uruguay model forwards anywhere in the UK, despite our best intentions.

Uruguay has observed the fastest decline in smoking rates amongst young people age 16-24 of any country in Latin America – the size of the country and the relative paucity of educational venues such as Espacio Ciencia means that at least 10 per cent of its target audience (young people in Uruguay) visit the exhibition each year. This would be much less likely to happen in the UK and, even if it did, the notorious problem of attributing effectiveness to a specific intervention in a complex environment would still have to be addressed. The UK, for example, has moved from a situation of rising smoking rates amongst young people in the 1980s,[58] to a decline in the proportion of young people smoking during the first 16 years of the 21st century to 7 per cent amongst those aged 15, the lowest figure since records began. This has happened without a Respira Uruguay-type exhibition.[59] There was also the question of how such an exhibition would need to be adapted for UK audiences, and whether a travelling version would be necessary. The W-WEST group felt that, for an equivalent exhibition to be effective, it should focus not only on the health and personal benefits of not smoking, but should appraise visitors of the social, environmental and economic costs of producing and distributing tobacco, and corporate duplicity in doing so.[60]

It has not been possible to test out the effectiveness of the exhibition in a UK context. An equivalent has never been created, although small gestures to tobacco control are made in museums like the Thackray Medical Museum in Leeds, and the Wellcome Trust-funded 'Catch Your Breath' exhibit that will travel from Durham to London and Bristol in 2019. Like the disappearance of the English-language version in the South African context, the original Respira Uruguay has also been mislaid. The curator of the Espacio Ciencia reported in 2018 that Respira Uruguay moved out of the exhibition hall a few years previously – they didn't have enough cash to update it or transform it into a travelling exhibition as they had hoped to do. So Espacio Ciencia entered into an agreement with the departmental government of Rio Negro to install it in an old industrial complex that is now a UNESCO patrimony. Unfortunately at that point they had lost touch with its new curators and with what they planned to do with it. The 'failure of absence' we have observed in the eeriness of the COPs becomes the 'failure of presence' in the long-term future of an exhibit that aims to discourage young people from smoking. As we saw in Chapter 10, political and economic factors – inertia in funding and support – can be as potent as active tobacco industry interference in changing the reality of tobacco control in the 21st century.

Conclusion

The problem of preventing tobacco's infiltration, through corporate and other interests, into the work of the governing body of the world's first public health treaty, the FCTC, should not be a surprise. The Master Settlement documents revealed numerous other examples of corporate attempts to influence the outcome of international negotiations that might in some way or other have limited the distribution of their product. These include WTO negotiations,[61] newly emerging common markets in Central America,[62] and impact assessment legislation within the EU,[63] to name but a few. Tobacco control at the global level – the FCTC's remit – is already starting to have an impact in some countries which might previously never have had the strength or courage to wrestle with the corporate power of the tobacco multinationals. It has also had a galvanizing effect on certain aid and development budgets – the UK government, for example, gave £15 million to establish an FCTC2030 programme aimed at kick-starting tobacco control in 15 countries that had not previously achieved much in this field. The FCTC is also unique in its focus on both consumption *and* production issues. However, there are other tobacco control issues that a global focus and preoccupation with transnational tobacco corporations may overlook or find difficult to address.[64] I have highlighted health and trade, the influence of the tobacco industry despite attempts to keep it out of the processes of global health diplomacy, and the growth of ENDS, a shape-shifted form of nicotine inhalation, as three sources of disruption at the COPs I have attended. Respira Uruguay is an example of an exhibition for young people displayed at one COP but now no longer present at either its travelling or home venue.

The eerieness of the FCTC, then, derives from a 'failure of absence' in its attempts to create a 'tobacco-free space' that the COPs are supposed to exemplify, both physically and symbolically. The COPs appear to have become increasingly infiltrated by the tobacco industry over time. This can be partly attributed to the expanded membership of the FCTC (now comprising 181 states or 'Parties'). Some recent signatories such as Zimbabwe have a strong history of tobacco industry involvement in the country's politics (not to mention agriculture). Industry representatives have infiltrated COPs remotely too. Finally, the business of the COPs is subtly shifting from the kind of work done in Committee A, such as preparing and agreeing on Guidelines to support the different Articles, to Committee B's concern with how the FCTC is implemented on the ground. Implementation is far more challenging than writing texts, and has been differentially successful across the various Articles that comprise the FCTC.[65]

The approach to tobacco exemplified at the COPs may seem strange given the importance usually accorded to 'stakeholder participation' in the generation of policy. Participation, after all, is a key principle of contemporary governance concerned with how "those who are subject to laws and policies should participate in making them".[66] Participation in this sense revolves around the questions "Who participates? How do they communicate and make decisions? What is the connection between their conclusions and opinions on the one hand and public policy and action on the other?"[67] However, barring MoPs from most of the discussions at the COPs, and the selective admission of international organizations as "observers", reflects the need for boundaries and limitations to participation in order to prevent tobacco from having undue influence in such a forum.[68] Tobacco is well able to exert such agency, something that tobacco control has difficulty preventing. In the process, concepts such as 'participation', normally seen as an almost unadulterated moral good, become problematized.[69]

Previous chapters have shown how, for real progress to be made, tobacco needs to be pushed to the edge of the policy network. This chapter has shown furthermore that different ways of working may be relevant in different locales – Respira Uruguay is an exhibition that works in its national context, particularly where there are other forms of tobacco production and use to consider beyond the corporate domain that is the dominant focus of the FCTC. This chapter has shown how the FCTC, despite its best efforts to create a ritual space which is both symbolically and literally 'tobacco free', finds tobacco a spectral infiltrator of the rooms and hallways of COP venues in ways as pervasive as the smoke (or vapour?) that emanates from some of its products. In the final analysis, the ultimate and most powerful 'participant' of all in the global health diplomacy for tobacco control is not the Parties, NGOs, industry representatives, or researchers but, as Latour would wryly observe, tobacco itself, assuming we can agree what tobacco is. Perhaps the only way of solving this conundrum is a shift from a focus on tobacco control to tobacco elimination. The final chapter gives examples and reflections on the prospects for a world in which tobacco as we currently know it becomes a historical anomaly.

Notes

1 Fisher (2016: 61).
2 See for example Schatz (2009).
3 Six articles in the journal *Global Environmental Politics* (2014), 4(3) use this methodology, in the context of research into the UN Biodiversity treaty COP (see, for example, Campbell et al. [2014]).
4 Little (1995).
5 McCarthy (2002). The priority areas for the WHO in 1948 were malaria, tuberculosis, venereal diseases, maternal and child health, sanitary engineering and nutrition.
6 WHO (1970).
7 For a detailed exposition, see Wipfli (2015).
8 Mackay quoted in Reynolds and Tansey (2012: 28-29).
9 Nikogosian (2010).
10 Roemer et al. (2005) give a good witness account of this.
11 Roemer et al. (2005).
12 A statement attributed to Gro Harlem Brundtland is often repeated in tobacco control circles: "a cigarette is the only consumer product which, when used as directed, kills its consumer".
13 WHO Committee of Experts (2000: 244).
14 Kohrman and Benson (2011: 329).
15 Weishaar et al. (2012).

16 Mamudu and Glantz (2009). Grüning et al. (2012) discuss Germany; for China see Huang (2014). Assunta and Chapman (2006) demonstrate the Japanese government's success at diluting the language of the final text.

17 As well as its export earnings, tobacco growing provides employment for anything up to 40 per cent of Malawi's labour force. Many of these are tenant farmers and migrant labourers, including an estimated 78,000 children, who suffer severely from the socioeconomic, health and environmental impacts of growing tobacco in precarious situations (Otañez et al. 2009). Malawi remains one of the few countries in the world not to have ratified the FCTC today.

18 The FCTC has spawned a subsidiary treaty, the Illicit Tobacco Protocol (Joossens and Raw 2012). This entered into force on 25th September 2018. On some of the headwinds it faces, see Gilmore et al. (2018).

19 WHO (2003).

20 Members of the Public and Members of the Press are technically "Non-Participants".

21 See Lencucha et al. (2011, 2012).

22 Plotnikova et al. (2014).

23 Ibid.

24 Brandt (2007: 480); cf. Mamudu et al. (2011).

25 McGrady (2011).

26 See Russell et al (2015).

27 FCTC (2010b).

28 Indeed, it is an issue that has continued to exercise international law beyond the COP (WTO 2011).

29 For a fuller account of the generation of Uruguay's *luchador* ('fighter') status in global tobacco control see Russell et al. (2015), also Wipfli (2015: Chapter 6).

30 FCA (2010).

31 Liberman (2012: 217).

32 Zhou et al. (2018).

33 WHO (2006: 8).

34 Yach and Bettcher (2000).

35 *Business Wire* (2012).

36 Anon. (2012). Increasing the addictive properties of cigarettes is an ongoing industry interest. According to Connolly et al. (2007), nicotine content in a range of cigarettes increased by 1.78 per cent per year between 1998 and 2005.

37 Kalra et al. (2017).

38 Grana et al. (2013, 2014).

39 FCTC (2014b).

40 McNeill et al. (2014: 2128).

41 Bell and Keane (2014) make a similar argument about the 'gateway hypothesis'.

42 Ibid. (30).

43 McNeill, Etter et al. (2014: 2129), my emphasis.

44 Ibid. (2130).

45 Grana et al. (2014: 1983).

46 McNeill, Etter et al. (2014: 2131).

47 E.g. Byrne (2014); Eleftheriou-Smith (2014); Robinson (2014).

48 E.g. Hunt (2014).

49 FCTC (2014c).

50 FCA (2014: 1).

51 FCA (2014: 4).

52 Russell et al. (2018).

53 FCTC (2014d).

54 One Middle Eastern representative, for example, described ENDS as "dangerous and toxic".
55 FCTC (2014e: 76).
56 Soren (2009).
57 Macnaughton (2012).
58 Hughes (2003: 135) quotes figures of boys and girls smoking in Britain rising from 24 and 25 per cent respectively in 1982 to 28 and 33 per cent in 1986.
59 NHS Digital (2017).
60 The Florida Truth campaign focuses on similar issues – see Sly et al. (2001).
61 Holden et al. (2010).
62 Holden and Lee (2011).
63 Smith et al. (2010).
64 One of these, which space precludes discussing here, is the South Asian bidi (also spelt 'beedi') industry. The bidi is a hand-rolled leaf cigarette. Production is mainly as a cottage industry, predominantly employing women and children. It is thus organised in a very different way to the transnational tobacco corporations. See Srinivasulu (1997), Gopal (1999), Gupta and Asma (2008), Lal (2009), Lal and Wilson (2012), Roy (2011), Roy et al. (2012), Majumder and Patel (2017), Centre for Health and Social Justice (2017) and Sharma (2018), among others.
65 Chung-Hall et al. 2018.
66 Fung (2006: 66).
67 Ibid. (67).
68 "Undue influence" means "any improper or wrongful constraint, machination, or urgency of persuasion, by which one's will is overcome and one is induced to do or forbear an act which one would or would not do if left to act freely" (Heckler and Russell 2008a: 18).
69 As an example, think of Arnstein (1969)'s "ladder of citizen participation" where increasing degrees of participation are associated with increased devolvement of power to citizens.

Chapter 12

'Imagine a world without tobacco'

Fifty years ago, the title of this chapter would have been regarded as incredible, almost unthinkable, culturally speaking, by people in many parts of the world. There many aspects to life which are impossible to imagine being otherwise; this book has shown how tobacco infiltrated its 'new world' home in the 16th century and shaped it in ways that stretched cognition and made the prospect of its lack strain credulity. Thanks to the shape-shifting acumen and agency of tobacco, its ability to change minds and bodies, to shape a global industry and public health responses, the UK in the 1960s recorded roughly 70 per cent of men and 40 per cent of women regularly smoking tobacco, a product which was "omnipresent, accepted, established".[1]

Since then, however, for large swathes of the population in the UK at least, smoking is no longer the norm. Tax increases on tobacco products made cigarettes 27 per cent less affordable in real terms between 2006 and 2016.[2] From a situation where the tobacco industry was a core player in the tobacco policy network (Chapter 8), most other important stakeholders in the field of tobacco and tobacco control – government ministries, the media and large sections of the general public – accept the social harms occasioned by tobacco and the need to protect others from tobacco smoke. Public places and private cars are subject to smoke-free legislation and most households have informal smoke-free rules. Legally marketed cigarettes are sold in plain packages from behind closed cabinets. Consequent on these and other measures, and the changing perspectives about tobacco amongst young people in particular, in the UK smoking rates have dropped to 21 per cent for men and 16 per cent for women, and the smallest proportion of children and young people are taking up smoking since records began.

This chapter looks to the future. For all I and others have said about the 'biochemical grip', the strength of the hybrid bonds between people and tobacco, it is clearly possible for such bonds to be broken or, more easily, for them not to be forged in the first place. Because of this, the invitation to imagine a world without tobacco is now being extended to us by what has become a global movement for tobacco control. This chapter will look at how and where these imaginings are framed, and by whom. I shall present some findings and reflections from my own ethnographic research working with the supporters of tobacco-free utopias. I shall focus particularly on Bhutan and Aotearoa/New Zealand – Bhutan for a fascinating history involving the imaginary amalgam of two different substances, opium and tobacco, Aotearoa for its less advanced but equally strong policy intention to be 'tobacco free' by 2025.

Just as the last chapter portrayed the eeriness of global tobacco control, given the difficulties of absenting tobacco from global health policy decision making, this chapter will make a play for considering spectres of a different sort as tobacco disappears, an eeriness created by what Fisher calls "a failure of presence". There is, I will argue, a need to take heritage and legacy issues seriously as we remember the world as it was.[3] Meanwhile, the shape-shifting continues, not only of e-cigarettes but of tobacco's corporate vectors. At least one major tobacco corporation is making fantastical new plans, and the promise of tobacco offering a cure for the Ebola virus offers further challenges to the prospect of its imminent demise.

'Endgame scenarios' and their discontents

In order to turn a future without tobacco from an imaginary utopia to a possible reality, various 'endgame scenarios' are proposed. A special issue of the journal *Tobacco Control* offers a number of these, including outright prohibition (or, at least abolition),[4] giving control of the markets to non-profit organizations with a harm reduction mandate, reducing the nicotine content of cigarettes, and developing what the New Zealanders call, metaphorically, a "sinking lid" for tobacco supply.[5] Singapore is offering a "tobacco free generation" law, prohibiting the sale of tobacco products to individuals born after a certain year.[6] However, countries such as these, and others that seek to emulate them, will not come close to realizing their ambitious proposals in the first half of the 21st century without a much more consistent and sustained set of tobacco-control efforts.[7]

There are places where we can see endgame scenarios being implemented even now. The Himalayan kingdom of Bhutan was the first nation to outlaw smoking completely. Other countries have declared their policy intentions for smoke- or tobacco-free futures by 2025 (New Zealand and Ireland), 2034 (Scotland) and 2040 (Finland). The *Lancet* medical journal is also campaigning for a tobacco-free world by 2040, with five leading researchers (including Derek Yach, who will appear again later) arguing that "a tobacco-free world by 2040 where tobacco is out of sight, out of mind, and out of fashion – yet not prohibited" is achievable. However such a feat will be impossible, they say, without "strengthened UN leadership, full engagement of all sectors, and increased investment in tobacco control".[8] Whether or not this utopian vision is fulfilled, the FCTC gives countries increasing confidence and guidance about introducing tougher controls on tobacco. 'End game scenarios' – different ways of imagining a world without tobacco – are now regularly discussed. What was once unimaginable is moving into the realm of possible futures in many societies, reflected in the names of organizations like 'Tobacco Free Futures' and 'ASPIRE 2025: Research for a Tobacco Free Aotearoa'.[9]

"Why not prohibit it then altogether if it's so bad for you?" some people ask about tobacco, but prohibition has an unfortunate pedigree and a more sophisticated approach might work better.[10] The notion of 'endgame scenarios' probably crystalized with the publication of the *Lancet* special issue. Yet one operates within a moral compass. Movements for change in any global system have consequences that may be unforeseen – for (exploited) child labourers in the tobacco fields of Malawi or bidi-rollers in the slums of South India, for example, (victimized) smokers on the streets of Vancouver, or (wealthy) executives of tobacco transnational corporations in Geneva, not to mention ageing artists in Los Angeles. One person's utopia can often be another's dystopia. One only needs to think of colonialism or Nazi visions of world domination to be brought up starkly against this truth. As one writer on utopian philosophies puts it, "the 'other' – Jew, foreigner, heretic – has often had a difficult time in utopia".[11] A tobacco-free future makes tobacco hybridity similarly difficult and 'other', at least for some.

The Himalayan Kingdom of Bhutan – a long history banishing demon tobacco

Bhutan is a predominantly Buddhist country sandwiched in the foothills of the Himalayas between China and India. Prohibitions on the sale and use of tobacco were included in its Penal Code in 2004 and were further refined and developed in the Tobacco Control Act which Parliament approved in 2010. This Act banned the cultivation, harvesting, production, sale and purchase of tobacco and tobacco products, making Bhutan the first country in living memory to have attempted such a comprehensive policy. The Act initially permitted individuals to import up to 200 cigarettes, 200 bidis (South Asian leaf cigarettes), 30 cigars and 50 grams of "other" tobacco products for their personal use in non-public places, subject to payment of appropriate duties and taxes. These numbers were amended and increased somewhat in 2012, but the sale and distribution of tobacco within the country remains prohibited. The Act gives the police powers to enter people's homes if they suspect illegal tobacco is being consumed; consumers who are unable to provide customs receipts for their product can be jailed for up to five years, as can shopkeepers selling tobacco. A thriving smuggling operation from India has made enforcement of this Act problematic, however.[12]

This legislation follows a long history of disquiet about tobacco amongst Tibetan Buddhist leaders. Tobacco offends Buddhist ideals of non-attachment and (some authors claim) produces 'erroneous cognition'. Bhutan was unified by a Tibetan lama, Zhabdrung Ngawang Namgyal (1594-1651), a descendant of the founder of the Drukpa spiritual lineage. He came to Bhutan with his followers in 1616, age 22, to escape a dispute over who was the reincarnation of the 4th Gyalwang Drukpa or spiritual leader of Tibet.[13] Visions of the guardian deities of Bhutan led to him found a new monastery in western Bhutan, where he spent three years in religious retreat between 1620 and 1623. After this he constructed a fortified monastery (or Dzong) three miles south of what is now Bhutan's capital, Thimpu. Namgyal was responsible for the first prohibition of tobacco in Bhutan.[14] His proclamation talks of

> the evil nourishment called tobacco, which is one of the many arrangements by demons *bdud*. . .Not only does it suppress the supports of the body, speech and mind, by pollution, it causes the decline of the gods above, agitation of the *btsan* spirits of the middle sphere and harms the spirits *klu*. . .of the world below. This substance makes a long eon of diseases, wars and famines arise in this sphere of the World of Destruction.[15]

It is a proclamation that reflects various concerns about tobacco by religious and political leaders in Bhutan and Tibet at the time.[16] They argued strongly that it pollutes the relationship between humans and supernatural forces, which then bring epidemics, climatic disaster and poor harvests. The fifth Dalai Lama of Tibet (1617-1682), in an influential book of *vinaya* rules composed in 1669, suggested the plant derived from the menstrual blood of a female demon.

> Given the circumstances of its creation, the evil demons *'byung po* enter the heart of those who inhale its smoke and there is a little help from the need [to smoke it]; it gives rise to many diseases and other things. Thus is should be strictly prohibited and as with *chang* [Tibetan liquor] it should be included among those items which [cause] heedlessness.[17]

Disturbed spirits were extremely challenging to the fifth Dalai Lama at this time, so it is hardly surprising that he sought to prevent the circulation of substances such as tobacco which might make people susceptible to them. At the end of the same year in which he wrote the *vinaya*, he constructed a special crypt as a home for the disturbed spirit of Drakpa Gtaltsen, a fellow reincarnate and rival scholar who had died under mysterious circumstances at a time of considerable political turmoil. Despite numerous offerings, these measures failed, and the spirit, who came to be called "Dolgyal", was bring- ing disease and death to both people and cattle, as well as being responsible for climatic disturbances such as hailstorms. Only after coordinated efforts across 11 district capitals, involving 70 monasteries and culminating in an elaborate ritual burning, was the "perfidious spirit" overcome. In his auto-biography the fifth Dalai Lama wrote, "indirectly these *'byung-po*...were delivered to the peaceful state of being, released from having to experience the intolerable suffering of bad states of rebirth due to their increasingly negative actions". However, the Wikipedia entry concerning these events records "the unification of Tibet having occurred at least in part on account of scapegoating the departed spirit of a controversial but popular rival *lama* was not to be without eventual historic consequence".[18]

Two hundred and fifty years later, the 13th Dalai Lama issued a decree against cigarettes, aiming to outlaw them within five years. According to this decree, cigarettes had been entering Tibet "since the year of the wood-dragon" (1914). The Dalai Lama clearly considered them a great danger. The decree begins with the suggestion that an oracle had advised that the water which had started leaking from the throats of the sea-monster carvings on the roof of Lhasa's central temple was caused by "the widespread leaves of the evil tobacco plant in this dharma-field of Tibet, which appeared through black and evil aspiration". The 13th Dalai Lama then went on to reiterate the origin myth about tobacco described by his predecessor, as well as prophecies (that preceded the arrival of tobacco) concerning its drying effects on the "veins of enlightened mind". [19] The first hereditary monarch of Bhutan, Ugyen Wangchuk, made similar comments in his promulga-tion banning the "most filthy and noxious herb, called tobacco" in 1916.

Charles Bell, writing about Tibet in 1928, describes the strength of the authorities' opposition to tobacco. Monks that indulged only did so in secret. Small pipes were more common amongst lay people; snuff was used and tolerated across all the social strata although it was previously more tolerated in monasteries than was then the case. He asked one of the Dalai Lama's Secretaries why smoking was prohibited, and was told: "When people indulged in smoking, there was a serious outbreak of illness. Further inquiry showed that Spirits of Tibet disliked the smell and caused the illness. So smoking was forbidden".[20] Heinrich Harrer, writing of his experiences in Tibet during and after the Second World War, described how the authorities

> consider tobacco smoking to be a vice and control it very closely and, though one can buy any sort of cigarette in Lhasa, there is no smoking in offices, in the streets, or at public ceremonies. When the monks take control in Fire-Hound-Year they even forbid the sale of cigarettes. That is why all Tibetans are snuff takers. The laity and the monks use their own preparation of snuff, which they find stimulating. Everyone is proud of his own mixture, and when two Tibetans meet, the first thing they do is to take out their snuffboxes and exchange a pinch of snuff.[21]

Since this time, however, Tibet has come under Chinese domination while Bhutan has maintained its independence. It is also noteworthy as the first country in the world to make 'Gross National Happiness' rather than 'Gross National Product' its watchword. The views of the government concerning tobacco fit into this approach. At the fourth Conference of the Parties for the WHO's Framework Convention on Tobacco Control the Health Minister, L. K. Dukpa, explained that making the sale or distribution of tobacco a criminal offence was "not aimed at penalizing the people but to help them live happier and healthier lives in a harmonized society".[22] Bhutan is an example of a country in which religion, myth and culture have been strong forces against tobacco use. Because of its small size and relative isolation, it has also never been a target of transnational tobacco companies.[23] The 2010 Tobacco Act, the geography, and politico-religious history of Bhutan conspire to fit with existing knowledge and attitudes in a "culturally compelling" way.[24]

Tobacco Taliban

Bhutan is not the only jurisdiction in which serious attempts have been made to imagine a world without tobacco by going down a prohibitionist route. In the first decade of the new millennium, the unsavoury post-war metaphor 'Nicotine Nazis' shifted to 'Tobacco Taliban', particularly in the UK.[25] There is no easily tobacconized title to make out of the Islamic State of Iraq and the Levant (ISIL). News reports from ISIL strongholds during their rule indicated a strong commitment to tobacco control, measures taken in the context of a more general larger terrorization and brutalization of the populace. One escapee from the clutches of ISIL spoke of "a boy who had been caught smoking being tortured with electric shocks. He didn't stop crying. 'Don't you know it's forbidden?' they shouted at him".[26] In Fallujah, another stronghold, cigarette and shisha pipe smoking was forbidden, with a punishment of 80 lashes, and execution for repeated violations.[27] In the city of Raqqa, ISIL burnt confiscated boxes of Marlboro cigarettes, and the severed head of a murdered ISIL official was found in eastern Syria with a cigarette in his mouth and a note on the corpse nearby saying: "This is not permissible". The group's severe interpretation of Sharia law declared smoking a form of "slow suicide" and therefore forbidden in areas they controlled.[28] Imperial Tobacco, which, like ITC in India (Chapter 9), changed its name to Imperial Brands in 2016, ostensibly to broaden its consumer base, attributed 40 per cent of an overall 5 per cent decline in its global tobacco sales in 2014 to the deteriorating situation in ISIL held areas.[29]

   As Chapter 9 and earlier chapters have demonstrated, the Islamic world has a long history of opposition to tobacco use and the tobacco industry perceived this as a threat to its expanding markets in North Africa, the Middle East and Asia.[30] Like the Anglo-American world of the 20th century, it has started targeting women in more liberal jurisdictions – a woman without a headscarf advertises Gauloises Blondes under a heading "Freedom Always" in Qatar. But even the Islamic State's terror proved weaker than desire for tobacco: in September 2014, the group relented in the face of popular anger and allowed shops in Raqqa to sell cigarettes again.[31]

Destination Aotearoa/New Zealand

I was keen to see for myself a country that had intentions to become tobacco free. Having seen so many examples of tobacco worlds, what would a tobacco-free world look like? I went to Aotearoa, the Maori name for New Zealand, for two weeks in February 2014 because (unlike Bhutan) I was able to get some help with my travel costs through a travel grant administered by my University. Two weeks may seem like an inordinately short period of time to undertake any kind of research that is attempting to encompass the policy making and experience of a whole country, but it is amazing what a heavy carbon footprint, the internet and serendipity can do to facilitate what might once have taken much longer to achieve. My initial contacts were with people working for ASPIRE 2025, the academic partnership that is helping the government achieve its goal through tobacco-control research.

However, as my preparations for the trip went on, it became apparent that there were other conversations to be had about the agency of tobacco in New Zealand apart from those concerning the country's ambitious plans to banish it. I always like to read novels of the country I am visiting and I remembered one about New Zealand – *The Bone People* – from its debut in 1985; it won the Booker prize the following year. In looking for the name of its author via Wikipedia, I was astonished to find that Keri Hulme had "worked as a tobacco picker in Motueka after high school. She began studying for an honours law degree at the University of Canterbury in 1967, but left after four terms and returned to tobacco picking".[32]

The wonders of the internet are such that an ignorant Antipodean like me might only have realized that tobacco once grew in New Zealand on arrival, if s/he realized it at all. Surfing the web in preparation for my visit, I not only found out well in advance that there was a history of tobacco growing in New Zealand, but was able to download substantial amounts of information about it as well as incorporating Motueka, the town where Keri Hulme once worked, into my travel plans. Through the kind offices of a local newspaper editor I managed to track Keri Hulme herself down to a village on the west coast of South Island, through an article which in December 2011 had reported Hulme's intention of leaving 'McMansion Okarito' (her village home) and shifting to Otago.[33] The editor suggested she would be best contacted via her next door neighbours. I decided instead to write her a letter in advance, something which itself seems an increasingly rare wonder in our internet-connected world.

Again by chance, the internet version of the *Greymouth Star* newspaper had a recent news item about shops in the town stopping the sale of tobacco.[34] Nothing similar appeared to have happened in the UK apart from a Scottish supermarket that was reported to have decided to stop selling tobacco products.[35] Meanwhile, entering 'tobacco growing Motueka' as a search phrase on Google revealed the creation of an exhibition at the town's local history museum and a recent talk by the former manager of the Rothman's tobacco factory about the company's history in the town to the Motueka Historical Association.[36] This proved the basis for a valuable internet correspondence with the secretary of the Motueka Historical Association, Coralie Smith, who gave me all sorts of useful information in advance including details of a fascinating book, *The Golden Harvest*, about the history of tobacco growing in the area.[37] Searching 'tobacco' on websites of institutions like the National Library and Te Papa, the National Museum of New Zealand, yielded other intriguing artefacts, such as a 3D Viewmaster reel titled 'Tobacco Harvest Motueka' at Te Papa. I thus had plenty of material in advance to guide my passage into and through this particular tobacco world.

Parliament debates

One of my first direct experiences of Aotearoa's moves towards excluding tobacco was following a debate about the country's plain packaging bill from the visitors' gallery of the parliament building in Wellington, the capital, on February 11th 2014. Members of the Ministry of Health's tobacco control team had told me about the debate that afternoon, and I was enthusiastic about seeing democracy in action. Anthropology is often seen as a route into dealing with 'the ethnic minority' issues, and smoking rates in New Zealand certainly demonstrate high levels of ethnic inequality linked to poverty and deprivation. Members of ASPIRE 2025 and my interlocutors in the Health Ministry were well aware of how strongly this tracks back to the 'early colonial exchange' as well as contemporary cultural practices. Similar to *guanxi* in China (Chapter 8), cigarettes continue to be an important marker of Maori hospitality. Change is occurring, however, and in the five years from 2006 to 2013, Maori smoking rates are reported to have declined from 42.2 per cent to 32.7 per cent, although this is a lower rate of decline than the population as a whole, which went from 21 per cent to 15 per cent. Smoking rates amongst Maori women remain particularly high.[38] The Maori Select Committee and Maori politicians have been particularly dedicated in establishing tobacco control, rather like the disadvantaged nations of the 'global South' that had been at the forefront of pushing for the strongest versions of the FCTC (Chapter 11). They had played an important part in organizing the legislation that was being discussed in the chamber.

Unfortunately jet lag quickly got the better of me – I found myself being prodded awake by a security guard, who was very pleasant about it. Members of parliament surely fall asleep all the time during debates, but it is probably against the rules to permit a visitor to do so. The debate picked up a little at that point, however, when John Banks started to speak on behalf of his far right ACT party.[39] He was one of the few not supporting the bill's onward passage to a select committee, although he said he was "opposed with a lower case narrative". His criticisms with the bill were that it was an "exercise in rain dancing". Invocations of 'fate' over 'agency', of 'determinism' over 'free will', are always strong polarities amongst those opposed to tobacco control[40] – fateful inevitabilities (such as the notion there will be tobacco) square against such apparent opposites as the individual's right to choose. The tobacco control people I spoke with were happy with the bill overall, although they expressed disappointment that it contained a clause delaying implementation until after the conclusion of World Trade Organization hearings (on plain packaging) against Australia. This is seen by legal experts as deliberate stalling by the tobacco industry, an attempt at creating a 'chilling effect' (Chapter 11) on other countries even though their likelihood of success is small.

Keri Hulme reminisces

Six days later I was sitting in the book-bound central room of Keri Hulme's octagonal house in the tiny village of Okarito talking tobacco (and other things). The previous night there had been a performance by a guitar and double bass duo called The Tattletale Saints in the village hall. "Keri Hulme will be there", our host at the guest house where we were staying had said confidently, based on the fact she had noticed Keri's car outside the hall. A woman near the back was clearly enjoying the concert, clapping along with the music in a somewhat disjointed fashion, a bottle of wine under her chair. I approached her at the end of the performance and introduced myself (from my letter) as "Andrew". "Andrew!" she exclaimed (for this is Keri Hulme), "you must come to my house tomorrow, but I must go out first to get in supplies". There was no indication from this exchange that she hadn't a clue who I was.

A notice on the gate of Keri Hulme's house guarded her privacy by stating that unless you had made prior arrangements, you should stay away. Confident in the knowledge that I had indeed made a plan with her in advance, next day I approached the house via the thick vegetation in her garden and walked up the steps onto her verandah. There was a light behind her front door, but no reply. I returned in the evening and had a conversation mediated by the door. This was when I realized that she hadn't received my letter, although less surprising was that the night before was a hazy memory. But Keri generously invited me in nonetheless. A path of sorts ran through the shelves and piles of books and other literary debris to two chairs which she cleared of further books to enable us to sit down. My wife Jane was with me, and considering we were two pahekas[41] showing up out of the blue, Hulme's hospitality was incredibly kind. She explained how wool packing and tobacco picking had been the two things she did in her "youth". At that time, in 1968, tobacco picking was a rather alternative existence to the conventions of New Zealand at that time. Although it was hard work, with 6.00 a.m. starts, "what the leaf required, you had to do", as she put it. The tobacco growers' ethos had been that the workers were part of their family. Keri had regularly returned to two families in the Upper Moutere valley during the picking season. A piece she wrote about her experiences was called 'Of Green and Golden Days', but she had never published it because of potentially incriminating stories it contained about people who might subsequently have assumed different personas to the carefree, libidinous characters they had been in their youth. She was surprised though, to hear that tobacco as a commercial crop was finished in Motueka, so I had the impression she had not kept in particularly close touch with her erstwhile fellow pickers or the families who had employed her.

Tobacco-free shops

The Director of ASPIRE 2025 had passed on email correspondence to me concerning a retailer in Wanganui on North Island who had decided to stop selling cigarettes. This seemed to parallel the item in the *Greymouth Star* about three shopkeepers ("dairy owners") who had decided to do the same thing. The ASPIRE 2025 researchers had conducted research into the views of retailers in general about the prospect of going 'smoke free',[42] but not of the experience of people who had actually 'taken the plunge' and done so. I exchanged drafts of a questionnaire that a smoke-free coordinator had prepared in an attempt to survey the retailers she knew of who had made this decision, and I offered to pilot it for her during our passage through Greymouth, a port town midway between Okarito and Motueka.

It was strange to arrive unannounced at shops in a strange town with a research agenda such as this, but our timings and itinerary were hard to predict. Merv 'n' Kips' Dairy had been mentioned in the *Greymouth Star* article, but the proprietor was a 'tea lady' at the local hospital on Tuesday afternoons and her nephew was hard at work refurbishing the shop, so there wasn't much opportunity to discuss tobacco. According to the article, though, the decision to stop selling tobacco here had been an economic one – cigarettes were becoming unprofitable. Our next destination was the Santa Fe Dairy. The owner was probably the first retailer in New Zealand to stop selling tobacco. A former fisherman, he had moved into the Dairy and Takeaway business after having given up running an all-night restaurant with business partners, because of its effects on his sleep patterns. He had found keeping a stock of cigarettes and tobacco on the premises a big outlay, and had resented being "a tax collector for the government", as he put it. A 'point-of-sale' display ban had been the last straw in his decision making about tobacco. Although he used to smoke he had given up 20 years earlier while fishing, since the seafarer's life frequently made it impossible to maintain dry hands for a smoke. His "manager" (i.e. his wife) still smoked "like a steam train" (he said), but that had not been a factor in his decision to stop selling tobacco products.

Munchies on Marsden was our final stop. When the owner was not working there, she was a consultant gynaecologist although it was her partner, a smoker without plans to quit, who had been the driver for making the premises tobacco free when they took over the shop two months earlier. This was "a bit of a punt", she said, because the former owners appeared to have made quite a lot out of money out of the sale of tobacco. However, the capital cost of tobacco was more than the combined total of all the other stock in the store, and since the return on this capital was very low, they couldn't see the point in being so tied up in just one product. Furthermore, the shop was just across the road from a sports centre, a high school and primary school. A shop selling tobacco products in the midst of such a complex didn't seem quite right. They were working with the school to lift a long-term ban on students coming to the shop during school hours and one of the 'levers' they were keen to use to make this happen was going tobacco-free.

People's responses to the questionnaire revealed a number of other highly significant issues. For example, Munchies reported coming under "huge pressure from the tobacco people who almost threatened us that we would lose customers left right and centre if we didn't have cigarettes". Intimidation like this made quitting the sale of cigarettes seem an even bigger step to take as they set up their new premises. Other comments concerned the reactions – positive and negative – from people in the local community to going tobacco free. I felt I had made a contribution to the fulfilment of the utopian vision of a tobacco-free world – or at least to research into retailers who had taken the decision to stop selling it. I was also conscious of similarities and differences with other parts of the country. For example, none of the shops in Grey-mouth had any signs in the window indicating they no longer sold 'smokes', unlike the shop in Wanganui which had featured a sign in the window saying "Smoke free dairy – smokes are not sold here". Nor had the occurrence of a smoking-related illness in a partner or family member figured in anyone's narratives about why they had decided to stop selling tobacco products, again different to the Wanganui report, where the owner's mother had died of lung cancer and he had decided on emotional as well as economic grounds to give up selling the product which had killed her.

Motueka – tobacco heritage town

Coralie Smith had very kindly arranged for me to meet with Geoff, the former manager of the Rothman's tobacco factory, at the Motueka Historical Museum. Geoff had brought some photographs of his years in the industry and we spent a memorable morning as the two of them reminisced about tobacco's past – particularly the things Geoff had known about like climate, labour, machinery, soils, manufacturing and crop diseases.[43] *The Golden Harvest* had proved to be an impressive social history, with some of the more conflictual issues, such as growers' grievances against companies and differences of opinion amongst growers, ably handled. Geoff described it as a "well researched and accurate" book, but added

> it's just a shame that the anecdotal things that happened during the life of this industry, they've never been recorded in that sense – there were some really hard case characters and a lot of funny things happened. . .[the book]'s more, I won't say 'dry' because it's anything but, but it's a factual record. But [what I'm talking about]. . .is outside that, it's people who were involved in the industry, their personal experiences.

CS: There have been several attempts to write such a book, you know. . .

GT: But unfortunately all those folk have died

CS: And there have been some recordings, of growers, but more the growers, not the workers – it's really the workers' stories [we need] and some of the growers, you know, their experiences with the workers. . .mostly I think the workers came for a good time rather than to make money!

GT: People used to, in the days of what we called the "Six O'Clock Swill", licensed premises had to close at six o'clock, and you had literally thousands of seasonal employees here because on any one tobacco farm there would be 20-30 people involved, 25 people involved in lighting a kiln, people in the paddock, it was so labour intensive. They used to close the pubs at six o'clock and we'd get sort of a hard core element. People used to come across from Nelson and line up along the street outside the Swan, which has since disappeared – that was the name of the hotel – and watch them come out and all the fights, and that – an entertainment centre!

CS: And the taxi business flourished because they had several taxis – there's one that struggles now – and you could wait hours for a taxi to take you and then of course they were going miles, they might be going half an hour's drive to get these workers back, you know.

GT: I actually boarded with one [a taxi driver] – this is back in the late 50s, early 60s, and I'd go three weeks and not see him because he'd be working 'til two, three, four o'clock in the morning then sleep during the day, and I'm at work and off he'd go, you know, and it was just a repeat. . .They would do a thousand miles in two days and not go outside the district.

Geoff and Coralie's memories are like Keri Hulme's "green and golden days" – nostalgia for a unique horticultural context in which memorable human characters as well as valuable plants could flourish. Both alerted me to the importance of recognizing and respecting past heritage while looking forwards to a future in which tobacco has become *persona non grata*. Their evocation of the past is buoyed up by material artefacts such as the disused tobacco kilns that still dot the countryside. Their nostalgia reflected the views of the inhabitants, many of whom were 'tobacco-people' and had something to do with tobacco over the many years it grew in the region. As Coralie described it in a subsequent email, the tobacco crop "brought money to the whole province but particularly Motueka; people are reluctant to let it go and are very defensive of it, seeing it as their livelihood not a health problem".

Aotearoa/New Zealand had done more to respect its tobacco heritage than many jurisdictions where tobacco had become a thing of the past that lived on in the architecture and furnishings of the present. Jacques Derrida, whose philosophy has been described as centred on tobacco,[44] cautions us to remember how spectres from the past – the intellectual and material legacy of, in this case, a world which was formerly tobacconized – insinuate themselves into what is present and real.[45] We may seek to exorcize tobacco,[46] but failure to honour its past makes it more likely that it will be troublesome in the present – maybe in the form of tobacco corporations who take over nurturing a tobacco 'heritage' in order to make further mischief in the future.

Adventures in stereoscopy

The ViewMaster reel at the national museum, Te Papa, provided an interesting twist to my two-stranded research into tobacco and tobacco control in Aotearoa/New Zealand. It was a disc of seven pairs of small transparencies taken in 1964 for stereoscopic viewing through a ViewMaster machine. Titled 'Tobacco Harvesting in Motueka', it was one of 237 discs by F.R. Lamb that the museum acquired in 2009.[47] The careful preservation of this artefact meant it was impossible for me to see it during my short time in Wellington since the transition time out of the museum's cold storage archive to room temperature was two days. However, I noticed another of F.R. Lamb's reels had been uploaded onto the Te Papa website and the curator kindly agreed to do the same thing for reel 182, CT.059383 so that they can now be seen online.[48] The sleeve had additional information. Lamb stuck a newspaper clipping to its back cover, indicating 1964 was a record year for tobacco production in New Zealand – there were 521 more acres under tobacco cultivation than the year before. One of the photographs, of a "tobacco inspector", is probably his wife – Coralie Smith (when I asked who the picture might be) said she was "too well dressed" to be anything other than a visitor.

Given my sense of tobacco's role in world history, Lamb's artefact in the Te Papa museum with its 3-D views of tobacco harvesting seemed particularly significant. The ViewMaster was invented in 1939 in the USA. It consists of a plastic stereo viewer that takes circular disks with seven pairs of colour stereo images. Based on the advice of a local photo-historian, the photography curator at Te Papa, had previously believed F.R. Lamb might have held a license to produce his images, but the Wikipedia entry concerning the history of View-Master technology revealed that, while most ViewMaster disc photographs were commercially produced, in 1952 Sawyer's Inc. had produced a ViewMaster Personal Stereo Camera which allowed anyone to take their own 3D pictures. Lamb's photographs were probably an example of these: the sleeves of the Lamb discs described their contents as a 'personal reel mount', and each of the 237 reels in the museum's collection appeared unique. The cameras had been manufactured in the USA for ten years, after which Sawyer Europe had continued with a View Master Mark II. As a result of my research into this historical artefact, the curator changed the website entry about the reels to indicate that "a special stereo camera was marketed from 1952 which allowed anyone to create their own disks. Lamb was possibly the only person in New Zealand who did so".

I became increasingly fascinated by the history of artistic perspective – the creation of 3-dimensional effects on 2-dimensional surfaces using linear structures that take the eye to a horizontal 'vanishing point'. They started with the experiments of Giotto in the 13th century, a good few centuries before tobacco appeared on the European scene. I wonder, however, whether artistic perspective might have contributed to a growing sense of curiosity that encouraged explorers such as Columbus to find out what lay beyond the vanishing point in the first place.[49] Contemporary British artist David Hockney, who, as it happens is rarely to be seen without a cigarette in his hand, argues persuasively that a transformation took place around 1420-30 with the development (probably in Flanders) of a concave mirror-lens, a device for drawing which could project an image of a scene onto a canvas or any flat surface.[50] Hockney has spent his whole life experimenting with and challenging the vanishing point approach to perspective, in the process becoming a particular champion of reverse perspectivism. This puts the viewer back in the centre of things (think cosmological perspectivism), with infinity opening up and multiplying around him (or her) rather than closing down in linear fashion towards a single vanishing point. It is tempting to attribute some of Hockney's interest in expanding rather than narrowing perspectives to the lifetime he has spent with tobacco as his ever-constant companion.

Robert Macfarlane reminds us of a ghost story by M.R. James, 'A View from a Hill'.[51] In it, an English pastoral idyll is transformed by being viewed through a pair of binoculars in which a wooded hilltop transforms into a view of a gibbet with a hanging body. Another form of binocular viewing, stereoscopy, reached its zenith in the 19th century. The stereoscope was a forerunner of the ViewMaster. By taking advantage of the binocular vision of two eyes both machines turn photographs placed at eye's width from each other three-dimensional.[52] Fig. 12.1 is an example of English stereoscopic photograph salvaged from my maternal grandmother's house. The picture in

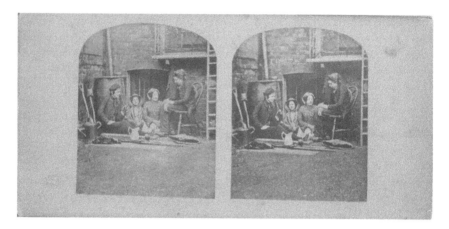

Fig. 12.1 A stereoscopic Victorian family group (c. 1875)
Source: Author's private collection

can be looked at three dimensionally. The eerie presence that jumps out at me on looking at the Victorian family group featured in it is the pipe the lad is smoking.

People in Aotearoa/New Zealand are spontaneously seeking to represent and preserve tobacco's heritage – its tangible and non-tangible legacy, whether it is kilns, factories, memories or ViewMaster reels, at the same time as aspiring to eradicate its presence in the future. Just as the workings of the FCTC are haunted by tobacco due to a 'failure of absence', so Aotearoans are attempting to tackle the converse form of eeriness – 'failure of presence' – seriously. It is necessary to respect a legacy, if one is to keep it in check. The material objects and landscape of the museum and Motueka help to do this.

Back in the UK, a friend who had engaged with her partner's decision to stop smoking by framing his final pouch of rolling tobacco and associated paraphernalia under glass, as a record for posterity (Fig. 12.2). He has not smoked since.

Foundation for a Smoke-Free World

By COP7, it was apparent that the major tobacco companies were all moving into the e-cigarette (ENDS) business.[53] They are also organizing 'vapers' into campaigner 'front' groups in much the same way that they had previously organized tobacco smokers into pro-smoking astroturf organizations and sock puppet groups (Chapter 9). "The tobacco industry's integration with e-cigarette manufacturers is not altruistic", the President of the UK Faculty of Public Health

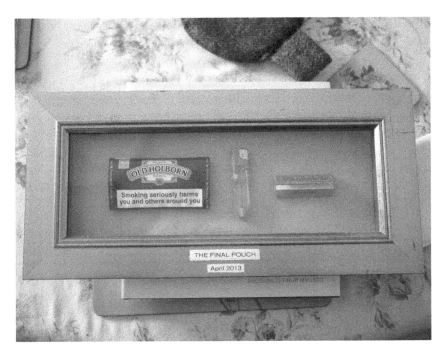

Fig. 12.2 The Final Pouch
Source: Photo by Mary Robson

wrote in a *British Medical Journal* editorial weeks before he was forced to resign due to an abusive late-night social media exchange with ENDS users.[54] Motives become key. Does the industry see ENDS as an alternative to the production of ordinary cigarettes, or are they getting into the market to sink it? The 13 per cent increase in cigarette consumption worldwide in the past decade would suggest the industry feels confident in the long-term health of its main product, if not its users. Or does it?

On September 17th 2017 a tax-exempt corporation was registered in the USA – Foundation for a Smoke-Free World (FSFW). The funder, to the tune of 80 million US dollars a year for 12 years, was Philip Morris International (PMI). In an extraordinary press release, PMI announced that, having "built the world's most successful cigarette company…we've made a dramatic decision…We're building PMI's future on smoke-free products that are a much better choice than cigarette smoking. Indeed, our vision – for all of us at PMI – is that these products will one day replace cigarettes". "Why are we doing this?" the declaration goes on, "because we should…and because we can".[55]

The pronouncement put those working in the tobacco control world into something of a tailspin. Creating the Foundation is an innovation every bit as disruptive as e-cigarettes, the technology that had made such a dramatic statement 'culturally thinkable'. In something of a publicity coup, the FSFW had appointed Derek Yach, the former head of the WHO's Tobacco Free Initiative, as its CEO. A key architect of the FCTC, with its Article 5.3 obliging Parties to protect their public health policies from tobacco industry interests (Chapter 11), Yach had started to advocate for harnessing commercial interests to achieve public health objectives[56] – after leaving the WHO, Yach took up an appointment with the food and drink manufacturer PepsiCo. Reprising the ontological argument made in Chapter 8, a *Lancet* editorial commenting on Yach's latest move argues that, while his influence at PepsiCo may have been benign – helping the company to improve its range of health products and pushing for reductions in salt, sugar and fat in them – "unlike food...tobacco has zero health benefits – only harms". Furthermore, there can be little certainty that PMI is serious in its aspirations, and the likelihood that the Foundation will achieve its objectives "are poor".[57] This, after all, is the company responsible for the recent Be Marlboro campaign (Chapter 9), and for attempting to sue the Government of Uruguay for implementing anti-smoking legislation (Chapter 11). One researcher, writing for a tobacco trade journal in 2015, reports a PMI executive as saying "combustible cigarettes are likely to remain at the core of PMI's business for years".[58] Whatever might happen in high-income countries, one executive told another researcher with access to corporate opinions "emerging markets will be a solid combustible cigarette consuming base for many, many years to come...cigarettes are extremely cheap"; another found it "really hard...to imagine a bunch of very low-income individuals...wanting to switch, or even caring, if they can afford cigarettes". Yet the decline in cigarette sales, which as a proportion of total global tobacco sales fell below 90 per cent for the first time in several decades, is also surely a significant.[59]

The creation of the FSFW has been as disruptive an innovation, in research and policy terms, as the e-cigarette. There is general agreement within tobacco control that the Foundation is an industry corporate social responsibility move that lacks credibility and is in breach of the FCTC's Article 5.3.[60] The World Conference on Tobacco or Health (WCTOH), for example, a key tobacco-control conference that takes place once every three years, was quite specific on both its registration and eligibility pages that "affiliations (current and/or during the past five years) with tobacco entities, including the PMI-funded FSFW, will make an individual ineligible to attend or present at the conference".[61] Then came an general invitation, from the Brocher Foundation on the shores of Lake Geneva, for researchers to attend a fully funded Summer Academy in Population-level Bioethics in May 2018, "Ethics and Nicotine: moral dimensions of harm reduction within global tobacco control". Derek Yach was listed as one of the "confirmed speakers". Whether this counts as an 'affiliation' or not is unclear, as is who might be funding this apparently bona fide venture. A naïve researcher through deliberate or inadvertent liaison with a potential 'tobacco entity' such as this might well find themselves blocked not only from attending the WCTOH but also publication in most international public health journals.

The FSFW offers a challenge to tobacco control that tobacco control experts still need to debate. The *Lancet* editorial argues that "boycotting the Foundation, as WHO suggests, is a mistake".[62] Is Yach's view one of consolidation and, perhaps, compromise with the industry, at least one of its transnational corporations, acceptable? What are the economic implications of imagining a world without tobacco if the only corporations producing it are wound down or depleted? Isn't PMI's stance simply (and laudably) brand stretching out of tobacco altogether? If so, will it even happen?

Biopharming – tobacco's final reprieve?

E-cigarettes and the FSFW, from tobacco's point of view, are all very well but their ontological status and unspecified (and dubious) futures, make another shape-shifting turn worth considering. Tissue from tobacco plants, genetically modified, cultured as crystalline blobs known as callus (Fig. 12.3) and nurtured to make tobacco plants can produce therapeutic antibodies for diseases such as HIV and Ebola. This kind of molecular farming (or 'pharming') enables the production of "medically useful proteins like antibodies, vaccines and hormones".[63] Tobacco, being so easy to grow and harvest, is ideal for a process called 'biopharming'. Also, being a non-food plant, there is no risk of gene transfer into the food chain, a fear that campaigners (including the food industry) have had about the genetic engineering of some of the other plants favoured for biopharming such as maize, tomatoes and rice. The first small-scale clinical trials of the tobacco HIV antibody indicate it is safe, and further testing will establish whether or not it is effective. 'Plantibodies' could revolutionize medical treatment, reducing costs dramatically, but concerns over the safety and the ethics of large-scale production have slowed progress. If these trials are successful, perhaps greenhouses will turn into pharmaceutical factories.[64]

E-cigarettes are controversial in public health terms. But finding a cure for the Ebola virus is different. Ebola is a devastating infectious condition, which promises 50 per cent of its victims a horrifying end essentially bleeding to death. ZMapp is one of a number of potential wonder drugs produced through biopharming. Genetically engineered plant viruses (harmless to humans and animals) are injected into plants, causing them to synthesize large numbers of antibodies. In the case of the Ebola virus, a species called *Nicotiana benthamiana* has been used to produce high concentrations of three different antibodies which are harvested, homogenized, purified and used to

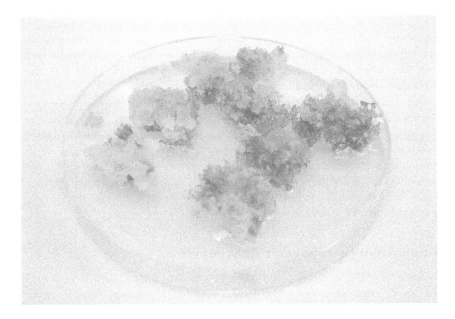

Fig. 12.3 Callus *Nicotiana tabacum*
Source: Photo by Wikimedia user Igge (Creative Commons License BY-SA 3.0)

treat patients infected with the deadly disease. The antibodies have been produced at Kentucky Bioprocessing, a unit of Reynolds American (which as we saw in Chapter 8 is 42 per cent owned by British American Tobacco). ZMapp is not a miracle cure – some of those treated with ZMapp have still died, but in a situation where other options are lacking, it provides a glimmer of hope in a sea of despair. Could it be the final chapter in attempts by tobacco to shed its negative image as a recreational drug and agent of death by becoming a pharmaceutical factory?

Interrogating tobacco

What, then, is tobacco? Asking this, rather than the more obvious 'what do we know about it?' question, extending the reach of tobacco across time and space, has hopefully helped to widen perspectives on how tobacco can be multiply conceived, formed and performed in the world today. Taking Salmond's view of 'things' (Introduction) and taking it as an invitation to explore the many manifestations of tobacco past and present, it is extraordinary how tobacco has commandeered virtually all Salmond's forms during the course of this book. At the very least, the argument has hopefully been one that tobacco is more than 'just a plant'. It has been the mainstay of shamanic dreaming in Amazonian rainforests, the fledgling settlement and subsequent plantation slavery of colonial North America, Enlightenment coffee shops and taverns, gentlemen's clubs in Victorian London, the battlefields of Europe during the First and Second World Wars. The cigarette has been a fetish object, an aberration of late 19th and 20th century capitalism, the subject of tobacco control opprobrium. Tobacco has transformed lives, for good as well as bad, with much artistic creativity and scientific advancement from the 17th century onwards having taken place under its influence. The stories derive only from the successful in this partnership, in the main; less is heard from those who do not live to tell the tale. Tobacco's hybrid bonds have become so strong they can perhaps only be dislodged through more than just smoking cessation, health education and lobbying work; what is needed is to comprehend and, possibly, undermine the place of tobacco in the wider flows of product and meaning. The discourse in and around (and, in a few cases, by) tobacco has shifted, and needs to shift further, if the intention is to invoke perspectives that re-story this erstwhile commodity as exploitative, parasitic, addictive and damaging.[65]

So is it possible to imagine a world without tobacco? Not without its disadvantages outweighing its benefits for individuals, and not without a radical overhaul of the power of the tobacco corporations and a better sense of how they see their global future. There is evidence that the notion of a world without tobacco is already taking hold in some parts of the globe. Here is a school student talking in a US school about how he sees the future of tobacco farming:

> I believe that within the next few years, raising tobacco will be a thing of the past for most farmers, including my papaw. It is difficult to make a profit raising tobacco and much harder to sell. Many tobacco warehouses have closed, and farmers are not getting contracts with the tobacco companies. The companies that are still open are thinking about making farmers change the way they sell the tobacco they raise. Most farmers in the past have had what is known as 'little bales' of tobacco that weigh 80 to 100 lbs.; tobacco warehouses are now deciding whether to move to big bales of tobacco, which can't be moved by hand. The big bales range from 300 to 400 lbs., so most little farmers would have to buy and build new stripping rooms, and buy a tractor or bobcat, just to raise something that they have raised their whole life.[66]

Yet at the same time, tobacco production and marketing is increasing in resource-poor countries such as Malawi, where corporations can capitalize on low wages and less stringent regulations. And while the proportion of those who use tobacco may decrease, numerically use of tobacco is likely to rise, with concomitant increases in the numbers dying from their habit. This is a global health problem.

Conclusion

When it arrived, into a very different Europe than exists today, tobacco took on a subaltern role while simultaneously extending its agency to a phenomenal extent. This book has taken an agentive view to counteract the addictive grip of a mutually constituted ideology that was only too happy to perpetuate the notion – the myth, if you like – of tobacco as a passive commodity. Yet in emphasizing a materialist view of the importance of tobacco in human affairs, I have argued for the need to think about the imaginary – the perspective lens – through which tobacco is presented and, in some cases, presents itself. One perspective offers tobacco as a gift to responsible adults free to consume it and who continue to choose to do so. Another sees it as a necessary and sometimes 'satisfying' part of their existence, which may or may not be the same as addiction. The third is tobacco control tackling addiction as part of a whole set of demand and supply issues simultaneously on many fronts. This has been an extraordinary aspect of 21st century life in many, but by no means all, countries. The final perspective presented in this chapter brings the material and imaginary together to recognize tobacco as an exploitative, deceitful and damaging presence, a 400-year game we should be bringing to an end.

Tobacco occurs within wider networks of material, relational and cultural significance. Earlier chapters demonstrated that tobacco has always been a controversial actant in human affairs. Yet in the contemporary world, tobacco stands as not only more powerful but also more opposed than ever before. The three key hybrids here identified – 'tobacco-persons', 'tobacco corporations' and 'tobacco control' – may look sequential, but there are as many commonalities in the historical threads as there are in the contemporary threads traversing the tobacco universe. To use a different metaphor, both historical depth and contemporary breadth are essentially two sides of the same coin – that coin in question being tobacco. Yet tobacco is multivalent. What was left behind in South America on that fateful transit at the end of the 15th century? What came along but was unacknowledged, a 'failure of absence' that contributed to the Enlightenment and human (largely male) creativity?

Tobacco can usefully be thought of as a spectral presence, its past permeating not only the present but, equally sinisterly, the future. It can also be thought of as a parasite, as Richard Craze did three years before it killed him. Looking at tobacco as a multiple reality substance opens the door to fresh perspectives on the plant and its people. Looking askance, sideways, fleetingly, out of the corner of our eyes, what strange objects might be glimpsed, shimmering on the borderlands of comprehension and perception, hidden in plain sight? This book has attempted to turn an everyday commodity into an uncommon object, in the process glimpsing the strength of its more-than-human agency, power, and relationships: an entity that is simultaneously dense, desirable and deadly, shape-shifting and world-creating. When it speaks, it should be with a voice that is less than benign.

Notes

1 Thompson (2012: vii).
2 NHS Digital (2017: 33).
3 Fisher (2016: 61).
4 Proctor (2011) makes 'the case for abolition' his major work; however his focus, as shown in Chapter 9, is on cigarettes rather than the outright abolition of tobacco (see also Proctor 2013).
5 On putting non-profit organizations in charge of the market, see Borland (2013) and Callard and Collishaw (2013). On nicotine reduction strategies, see Benowitz and Henningfield (2013). A "sinking lid" on tobacco supply is proposed by Wilson et al. (2013), by which is meant an end to tobacco use through the imposition of increasing limits on the amount of commercial tobacco released for legal sale, the remaining portion being released to licensed suppliers by auction.
6 Berrick (2013).
7 Malone (2016).
8 Beaglehole et al. (2015: 1011).
9 Aotearoa is the indigenous Maori name for the country. It literally translates as "land of the long white cloud" (Marshall, 2013).
10 The prohibition era against alcohol in the USA is the oft-quoted example of this – see, for example, Hall (2010).Of course, it could be pointed out that tobacco is already partially prohibited – where juvenile smoking is prohibited, for example, or through smoke-free public places legislation.
11 Claeys (2011: 186-7).
12 Givel (2011).
13 It is reported that the 4th Gyalwang Drukpa prophesied that he would have two incarnations to propagate further his spiritual teachings. In accordance with this prophecy, two incarnations were discovered. But it was not to Zhabdrung Ngawang Namgyal's advantage that his rival incarnate was supported by the Tsang Desi, the most powerful ruler of Tibet.
14 As we saw in Chapter 3, many other countries around the world attempted to ban the spread of tobacco around this time (e.g. Turkey 1611; Japan 1616; Mughal India 1617; Persia during the reign of Abbas (1587-1629); Sweden 1632; Denmark 1632; Russia 1634; China c. 1637; Manchuria 1638; Vatican 1642; Germany 1649).
15 Translation by Berounský (2013: 10). I am grateful to Robin Wright for this reference.
16 Berounský argues that Tibetan writers see tobacco and opium as related. "Besides the rather well-known fact that opium was frequently sold in a form mixed with tobacco in China and India, the Chinese expression *yān* (煙) designates both tobacco and opium. Opium was known much earlier than tobacco, and is called nowadays in Tibetan *nyal thag / nyal tha* ('lie down-tobacco') or *tha mag nag po* ('black tobacco')" (ibid: 18-19). Various texts refer to tobacco as a plant with flowers of five colours corresponding to the five poisons – pride (yellow), ignorance (blue), hatred (white), lust (red) and slander (black). According to Sangye Lingpa (a Buddhist seer and sage writing in the 14th century, before the spread of tobacco), the name of the poison, which appears in five kinds and colours, is Black Hala *(ha la nag po)* (ibid: 17, 18). As Berounský adds, "the plant renowned for the great variation of colours of its blossoms, including that of almost black (mentioned by Sangye Lingpa), is the opium poppy (*Papaver sominferum*)",
17 Berounský, D. (2013: 14). A 20th century Tibetan author gives a fuller account of the myth. As she approached death the demoness issued a curse to humanity:

"May my bodily remains be hidden undamaged. One day, from within its womb will grow a flower, which will be unlike any other. To bodies and minds an incomprehensible pleasure and bliss will come by smelling its odour. [The body and mind] will be intoxicated by bliss, which would exceed that of sexual intercourse between males and females. It will become widespread and eventually most of the people...will use it involuntarily" (ibid: 15). This myth reverberates strongly with the South American Yanomami myth of the origin of tobacco in its recognition that the desire for and pleasure deriving from tobacco can be better than sex (Chapter 2).

18 Wikipedia (2014a). Students and supporters of Drakpa Gyaltsen argued that it was not his spirit at all, but that of the 5th Dalai Lama's minister Desi Sönam Chöpel, that was causing the trouble (see Wikipedia (2014b).

19 Berounský (2013: 29, 30).

20 Bell (1928: 243).

21 Harrer (1982: 177).

22 FCTC (2010a).

23 Ugen, S. (2003).

24 Panter-Brick et al. (2006) discuss the importance of innovations in public health being "culturally compelling".

25 Schneider and Glantz (2008: 295).

26 Espinoza (2015).

27 Anon. (2015).

28 Winsor (2015).

29 Sheffield and Jameson (2015).

30 Petticrew et al. (2015).

31 Dyer (2015).

32 Wikipedia (2014c).

33 *Otago Daily Times* (2011).

34 *Greymouth Star* (2014).

35 *Edinburgh Evening News* (2012). Nine further stores owned by the same retailer have subsequently followed suit. See Harrison (2012).

36 Smith (2012).

37 O'Shea (1997). In return I sent Coralie an article by Benson (2010) about tobacco growers in North Carolina for comparative purposes. She agreed with my tentative suggestion that former growers in New Zealand (where the final tobacco harvest took place in 1995) might share or have once shared similar perspectives, and certainly sentiments – pride, defensiveness, denialism – to those expressed by growers in the US article.

38 I am grateful to Monique Leerschool for sending me a useful video about Maori smoking history: Cantobacco (2011).

39 On ACT's principles, see ACT (n.d.a). John Banks has been charged with breaching electoral finance laws by asking for a donation from John Dotcom to be provided in two separate $25,000 amounts so that it could remain anonymous. He was forced to resign as leader of his party, had indicated his intention not to stand at the next election, but resigned his seat on June 13th 2014 (see ACT n.d.a) .

40 Like Geertz (1984)'s views on abortion expressed in his lecture 'anti anti-relativism', we could regard such people as being 'anti anti-tobacco'.

41 *Paheka* is a Maori term for white person.

42 Jaine et al. (2014).

43 These interestingly don't feature heavily in Pete Benson's book (2012) or article (2010), both of which are more concerned with politics, citizenship, affect and tobacco corporations.

44 Ziser (2013: 194fn71).
45 Derrida (2006).
46 For an example, see Russell (2017). On tobacco industry sponsored heritage sites, see Benson (2012).
47 The others contain photographs of Christchurch and South Island scenes in the 1950s and 1960s, including images of a wedding, a street parade, floral displays, small town scenes, rivers, autumn trees, and so on. According to the curator of photography at the museum, "most of his images are quite mundane, consisting of scenic photos of the South Island – the sort that keen amateurs might have taken during their holidays".
48 See Museum of New Zealand, Te Papa Tongarewa (n.d.)
49 It is of course indulgent speculation to suggest that more-than-human tobacco might have played a role in this process.
50 Hockney (2001).
51 Macfarlane (2015).
52 Around 1635 (the time of the first wave of tobacco's European surge), the Florentine painter Jacopo Chimenti da Empoli (1554-1640) did a pair of drawings which show he was well aware of the principle involved. However, he lacked the opportunities for reproduction and hence commercial exploitation offered by photography some 240 years later.
53 Grana et al. (2013: 2).
54 Ashton (2014).
55 See PMI (n.d.).
56 See for example Yach (2008).
57 Anon. (2017).
58 Tuinstra (2015: 16). A BAT representative said almost exactly the same thing.
59 MacGuill (2017).
60 Daube, Moodie and McKee (2017). Yach certainly misquotes Article 5.3 in his defence of the Foundation. It is not saying that the goal of industry is to 'interfere in public policy' but, rather, that governments should act to protect such policies from the commercial and other vested interests of the tobacco industry (Chapter 11).
61 See, for example, World Conference on Tobacco or Health (2018).
62 Anon. (2017).
63 McLusky (2013).
64 Ibid.
65 An alternative subtitle for this book might have been 'shape-shifting substance from South America'.
66 Ethan Smith in Kingsolver (2011: 170).

Bibliography

Abbott, E. (2010) *Sugar: A Bittersweet History*. London: Duckworth.

ACT (n.d.a) Principles. http://www.act.org.nz/?q=principles [Accessed 23rd June 2014].

ACT (n.d.b) John Banks. http://www.act.org.nz/posts/author/john-banks [Accessed 23rd June 2014].

Addison (1716) *The Free-Holder; Or Political Essays*. London: printed for D. Midwinter and J. Tonson.

Adler I. (1912) *Primary Malignant Growths of the Lung and Bronchi: A Pathologic and Clinical Study*. New York: Longmans, Green and Company.

Adshead, S.A.M. (1992) *Salt and Civilization*, London: Macmillan.

Aitken, C., T.R. Fry, L. Grahlmann and T. Masters (2008) Health perceptions of home-grown tobacco (chop-chop) smokers. *Nicotine and Tobacco Research*, 10(3): 413–16.

Albert And Mary Lasker Foundation (2018) http://www.laskerfoundation.org/about [Accessed 23rd October 2018].

Alford, B.W.E. (1973) *W.D.and H.O.Wills and the Development of the U.K. Tobacco Industry 1786–1965*. London: Methuen.

Alis, M.M. and Dwyer, D.S. (2009) Estimating peer effects in adolescent smoking behavior: a longitudinal analysis. *Journal of Adolescent Health*, 45: 402–08.

Allen, S.L. (2001) *The Devil's Cup: Coffee, the Driving Force in History*. London: Canongate.

Alston, L.J., R. Dupré and T. Nonnenmacher (2002) Social reformers and regulation: the prohibition of cigarettes in the United States and Canada, *Explorations in Economic History*, 39: 425–45.

Anderson, B.T., B.C. Labate, M. Meyer, K.W. Tupper, P.C.R. Barbosa, C.S. Grob, A. Dawson and D. McKenna (2012) Statement on ayahuasca. *International Journal of Drug Policy*, 23: 173–75.

Anon. (1630) *Wine, Beere, Ale, and Tobacco. Contending for Superiority. A Dialogue*. Printed at London: By T[homas] C[otes] for Iohn Groue, and are to be sold at his shop at Furniuals Inne Gate in Holborne.

Anon. (1675) *The Women's complaint against tobacco, or, An excellent help to multiplication: pespicuously [sic] shewing the annoyance that it brings to mankind and the great deprivation of comfort and delight to the female sex, with a special and significant order set forth by the women for suppressing the general use thereof amongst their husbands, they finding that tobacco is the only enemy to pleasure and procreation as they now plainly make it appear in this their declaration*. London, pamphlet.

Anon. (1725) The Triumph of Tobacco over Sack and Ale, in *A Collection of Old Ballads*, vol. 3. London: J. Ambrose Philips, pp.154–56.

Anon. (1732) On a Snuff-Box, By a Country Parson, in *The Scarborough Miscellany*. London.

Anon. (1736) The Convert to Tobacco, A Tale. In *A Collection of Merry Poems*. London: printed and sold by T.J. Cooper.

Anon. (1858) A Screw of Tobacco. *Chamber's Journal*, 239 (July 31st): 71–3.

Anon. (1875) Minor Notices, *The Examiner*, 10th April (3506): 415-7.

Anon. (1888a) Amusing Breach of Promise Case. *Oamaru Mail*, 10 (4234), October 9th: 4.

Anon. (1888b) Prizes for Ill-Doing. *New York Times*, December 25th: 8.

Anon. (2006) Obituary: Richard Craze: prolific writer and unconventional publisher who specialised in promoting unknown authors. *The Times*, 9th September (issue 68801): 77.

Anon. (2012) Gathering in Munich. *Tobacco Journal International*, http://www.tobaccojour nal.com/Gathering_in_Munich.50984.0.html [Accessed 16th November 2012].

Anon. (2015) Day-to-day life in the 'Islamic State' – where any breach of restrictive, divinely inspired rules is savagely punished. *The Independent*, 27th June.

Anon. (2017) Tobacco control: a Foundation too far? *Lancet*, 390: 1715.

Antonopoulos, G.A. and A. Hall (2016) The financial management of the illicit tobacco trade in the United Kingdom. *British Journal of Criminology*, 56(4): 709–28.

Appadurai, A. (1986) Introduction: commodities and the politics of value. In A. Appadurai (ed.) *The Social Life of Things*. Cambridge: Cambridge University Press.

Apperson, G.L. (1914) *The Social History of Smoking*. Reprinted by Biblio Bazaar.

Arbuckle, J. (1719) *Snuff: A Poem*. Glasgow: James McEuen.

Armstrong, C. (2007) *Writing North America in the Seventeenth Century: English Representations in Print and Manuscript*. London: Routledge.

Arnstein, S. (1969) A ladder of citizen participation. *Journal of the American Institute of Planners*, 35(4): 216–24.

Asch, R.G. (2014) *Sacral Kingship Between Disenchantment and Re-enchantment: The French and English Monarchies 1587–1688*. New York: Berghahn.

ASH (Action on Smoking and Health) (2008) *Beyond Smoking Kills: Protecting Children, Reducing Inequalities*. London: ASH.

ASH (2016a) *Smoking Statistics: Who Smokes and How Much*. London: ASH. http://ash.org. uk/wp-content/uploads/2016/06/Smoking-Statistics-Who-Smokes-and-How-Much. pdf [Accessed 10th November 2018].

ASH (2016b) Use of electronic cigarettes (vapourisers) among adults in Great Britain, May. http://www.ash.org.uk/files/documents/ASH_891.pdf [Accessed 28th June 2018].

ASH (2017a) Standardized tobacco packaging. London: ASH. http://ash.org.uk/informa tion-and-resources/briefings/ash-briefing-on-standardised-tobacco-packaging-2 [Accessed 28th June 2018].

ASH (2017b) Key dates in the history of anti-tobacco campaigning. London: ASH. http:// ash.org.uk/information-and-resources/briefings/key-dates-in-the-history-of-anti-tobacco-campaigning [Accessed 28th June 2018].

Ashton J.R. (2014) Regulation of electronic cigarettes: a familiar clash between commercial politics and public health. *British Medical Journal*, 349(7974): g5484.

Association of Social Anthropologists (2014) ASA14: Anthropology and enlightenment conference. http://www.theasa.org/conferences/asa14/theme.shtml [Accessed 26th October 2018].

Assunta, M. (2002) BAT flouts tobacco-free World Cup policy. *Tobacco Control*, 11: 277–78.

Assunta, M. and S. Chapman (2004) Industry sponsored youth smoking prevention programme in Malaysia: a case study in duplicity. *Tobacco Control*, 13 (SupplII): ii37–ii42.

Assunta, M. and S. Chapman (2006) Health treaty dilution: a case study of Japan's influence on the language of the WHO Framework Convention on Tobacco Control, *Journal of Epidemiology and Community Health*, 60: 751–6.

Baba, A., D.M. Cook, T.O. McGarity and L.A. Bero (2005) Legislating 'Sound Science': the role of the tobacco industry. *American Journal of Public Health*, 95: S20–S27.

Bachinger, E., M. McKee and A. Gilmore (2008) Tobacco policies in Nazi Germany: not as simple as it seems. *Public Health*, 122: 497–05.

Baer, G. (1992) The one intoxicated by tobacco: Matsigenka shamanism. In J. Matteson-Langdon and G. Baer (eds) *Portals of Power: Shamanism in South America*. Albuquerque: University of New Mexico Press, pp. 79–100.

Bage, R. (1792) *Man as He Is: A Novel in Four Volumes*. London: Minerva Press.

Bakan, J. (2004) *The Corporation: The Pathological Pursuit of Profit and Power*. New York: Free Press.

Bal, D.G., K.W. Kizer, P.G. Felten, H.N. Mozar and D. Niemeyer (1990) Reducing tobacco consumption in California: development of a statewide anti-tobacco use campaign. *Journal of the American Medical Association*, 264(12): 1570–4.

Baluška, F., S. Mancuso, D. Volkmann and P. Barlow (2009) The 'root-brain' hypothesis of Charles and Francis Darwin, *Plant Signaling and Behavior*, 4(12): 1121–7.

Baptist, E.E. (2014) *The Half Has Never Been Told: Slavery and the Making of American Capitalism*. New York: Basic Books.

Barbira Freedman, F. (2010) Shamanic plants and gender in the healing forest. In E. Hsu and S. Harris (eds) *Plants, Health and Healing: On the Interface of Ethnobotany and Medical Anthropology*. Oxford: Berghahn, pp. 130–58.

Barbira Freedman, F. (2015) Tobacco and shamanic agency in the upper Amazon: historical and contemporary perspectives. In A. Russell and E. Rahman (eds) *The Master Plant: Tobacco in Lowland South America*. London: Bloomsbury, pp. 63–86.

Barclay, W. (1614) *Nepenthes, or The vertues of tabacco*. Edinburgh: Printed by Andro Hart, and are to be sold at his shop on the north side of the high street, a litle beneath the Crosse.

Barrie, J.M. ([1890] 1925) *My Lady Nicotine*. London: Hodder & Stoughton.

Baudelaire, C. ([1857] 1993) *Fleurs du Mal [Flowers of Evil]*, Oxford: Oxford University Press.

Baum, F. and M. Fisher (2014) Why behavioural health promotion endures despite its failure to reduce health inequities. *Sociology of Health and Illness*, 36(2): 213–25.

Bayer, R. (2008) Stigma and the ethics of public health: not can we but should we. *Social Science and Medicine* 67(3): 463–72.

Beaglehole, R., R. Bonita, D. Yach, J. Mackay and K.S. Reddy (2015) A tobacco-free world: a call to action to phase out the sale of tobacco products by 2040. *Lancet*, 385: 1011–18.

Beaumont, J. (1602) The metamorphosis of tabacco. In A.B. Grosart (1869) (ed.) *The Poems of Sir John Beaumont*, Blackburn: The Fuller Worthies' Library.

Bednarz, J.P. (2004) Marlowe and the English literary scene. In P. Cheney (ed.) *Cambridge Companion to Christopher Marlowe*, Cambridge: Cambridge University Press, pp. 90–105.

Beenstock, J., F.F. Sniehotta, M. White, R. Bell, E.M. Milne and V. Araujo-Soares (2012) What helps and hinders midwives in engaging with pregnant women about stopping smoking? A cross-sectional survey of perceived implementation difficulties among midwives in the northeast of England. *Implementation Science*, 7(36).

Belfast Forum (2010) various contributors, Greenshield stamps and cigarette coupons, http://www.belfastforum.co.uk/index.php?topic=29660.0 [Accessed 28th August 2015].

Bell, C. (1928) *The People of Tibet*, Oxford: Oxford University Press.

Bell, K. (2011) Legislating abjection? Secondhand smoke, tobacco control policy and the public's health. *Critical Public Health*, 21(1): 49–62.

Bell, K. (2012) Whither tobacco studies? *Sociology Compass*, 7(1): 34–44.

Bell, K. (2014) Science, policy and the rise of 'thirdhand smoke' as a public health issue. *Health, Risk and Society*, 16(2): 154–170.

Bell, K. and S. Dennis (2013) Editors' introduction: towards a critical anthropology of smoking: exploring the consequences of tobacco control. *Contemporary Drug Problems*, 40(1): 3–20.

Bell, K. and H. Keane (2012) Nicotine control: e-cigarettes, smoking and addiction. *The International Journal of Drug Policy*, 23(3): 242–247.

Bell, K. and Keane H. (2014) All gates lead to smoking: the 'gateway theory', e-cigarettes and the remaking of nicotine. *Social Science and Medicine*, 119: 45–52.

Bell, K., A. Salmon, M. Bowers, J. Bell and L. McCullough (2010) Smoking, stigma and tobacco 'denormalisation': further reflections on the use of stigma and a public health tool. *Social Science and Medicine*, 70: 795–9.

Bell, R., S. Glinianaia, Z. van der Waal, A. Close, E. Moloney, S. Jones, V. Araújo-Soares, S. Hamilton, E. Milne, J. Shucksmith, L. Vale, M. Willmore, M. White and S. Rushton (2017) Evaluation of a complex healthcare intervention to increase smoking cessation in pregnant women: interrupted time series analysis with economic evaluation. *Tobacco Control*, doi:10.1136/tobaccocontrol-2016-053476.

Bellamy, L. (2007) It-narrators and circulation: defining a subgenre. In M. Blackwell (ed.) *The Secret Life of Things: Animals, Objects, and It-Narratives in Eighteenth-Century England*. Lewisburg: Bucknell University Press, pp. 117–46.

Benedict, C. (2011a) *Golden-Silk Smoke: A History of Tobacco in China 1550-2010*. Berkeley: University of California Press.

Benedict, C. (2011b) Between state power and popular desire: tobacco in pre-conquest Manchuria, 1600-1644. *Late Imperial China*, 32(1): 13–48.

Bennet, S. (2009) Review of Goodfellow (2008) 'Pharmaceutical intimacy: sex, death, and methamphetamine'. *Opticon1826*, (7): 1–3.

Bennett, H.S. (1949) Shakespeare's stage and audience. *Neophilologus*, 33(1): 40–51.

Bennett, J. (2004) The force of things: steps towards an ecology of matter. *Political Theory*, 32(2): 347–72.

Bennett, J. (2010) *Vibrant Matter: A Political Ecology of Things*. Durham: Duke University Press.

Benowitz, N.L. and J.E. Henningfield (2013) Reducing the nicotine content to make cigarettes less addictive. *Tobacco Control*, 22(s1): i14–i17.

Benson, P. (2010) Tobacco talk: reflections on corporate power and the legal framing of consumption. *Medical Anthropology Quarterly*, 24(4): 500–21.

Benson, P. (2012) *Tobacco Capitalism: Growers, Migrant Workers, and the Changing Face of a Global Industry*. Princeton: Princeton University Press.

Benson, P. and S. Kirsch (2010) Capitalism and the politics of resignation. *Current Anthropology*, 51(4): 459–86.

Bentley, R. (1692) *Matter and Motion Cannot Think, or A Confutation of Atheism from the Faculties of the Soul*. London: Printed for Thomas Parkhurst at the Bible and Three Crowns in Cheapside and Henry Mortlock at the Phoenix in St Paul's Church-Yard.

Benzoni, G. (1565) *La Historia del mondo nuovo*. Venice: Appresso Francesco Rampazetto.

Berlant, L. (2007) Slow death (sovereignty, obesity, lateral agency). *Critical Inquiry*, 33(4): 754–80.

Bernays, E. (1923) *Crystallizing Public Opinion*. New York: Liveright.

Berounský, D. (2013) Demonic tobacco in Tibet. *Mongolo-Tibetica Pragensis*, 13(2): 7–34.

Berrick, A.J. (2013) The tobacco-free generation proposal. *Tobacco Control*, 22(s1): i22–i26.

Berridge, V. (2007) *Marketing Health: Smoking and the Discourse of Public Health in Britain, 1945-2000*. Oxford: Oxford University Press.

Berridge, V. (2013) *Demons: Our Changing Attitudes to Alcohol, Tobacco, and Drugs*. Oxford: Oxford University Press.

Bevan, T.F. (1890) *Toil, Travel, and Discovery in British New Guinea*. London: Kegan Paul, Trench, Trubner & Co.

Black, D. (2014) Where bodies end and artefacts begin: tools, machines and interfaces. *Body and Society*, 20(1): 31–60.

Blaut, J.M. (1993) *The Colonizer's Model of the World: Geographical Diffusionism and Eurocentric History*. London: Guilford Press.

Bloch, M. (2012) *Anthropology and the Cognitive Challenge*. Cambridge: Cambridge University Press.

Bonell, C., Farah Jamal, G. J. Melendez-Torres and S. Cummins (2015) 'Dark logic': theorising the harmful consequences of public health interventions. *Journal of Epidemiology and Community Health*, 69: 95–8.

Borland, R. (2013) Minimising the harm from nicotine use: finding the right regulatory framework. *Tobacco Control*, 22(s1): i6–i9.

Brabec de Mori, B. (2011) Tracing hallucinations: contributing to a critical ethnohistory of ayahuasca usage in the Peruvian Amazon. In B.C. Labate and H. Jungaberle (eds) *The Internationalization of Ayahuasca*. Zurich: Lit-Verlag, pp. 23–48.

Brabec de Mori, B. (2015) Singing white smoke: tobacco songs from the Ucayali Valley. In A. Russell and E. Rahman (eds) *The Master Plant: Tobacco in Lowland South America*. London: Bloomsbury, pp. 89–106.

Brady, M. (2002) Historical and cultural roots of tobacco use among Aboriginal and Torres Strait Islander people. *Australian and New Zealand Journal of Public Health*, 26(2): 120–24.

Brady, M. (2013) Drug substances introduced by the Macassans: the mystery of the tobacco pipe. In M. Clark and S.K. May (eds) *Macassan History and Heritage: Journeys, Encounters and Influences*. Canberra: Australian National University E-Press, pp. 141–57.

Bragg, M. (2007) We tend to forget that life can only be defined in the present tense (interview of Dennis Potter). Great interviews of the 20th century series. *The Guardian*, September 12th. http://www.guardian.co.uk/theguardian/2007/sep/12/greatinterviews [Accessed 29th November 2011].

Braine T. (2007) Mexican billionaire invests millions in Latin American health. *Bulletin of the World Health Organization*, 85(8): 574–76.

Brandt, A.M. (2007) *The Cigarette Century: The Rise, Fall, and Deadly Persistence of the Product that Defined America*. New York: Basic Books.

Bratby, R. (2014) Edward Elgar (1857-1934) Variations on an Original Theme 'Enigma', Op.36. In I. Stephens (ed.) *Royal Liverpool Philharmonic Orchestra 2013/2014 Season Concert Programme*. Liverpool: RLPO.

Breen, T.H. (1973) George Donne's 'Virginia Reviewed': a 1638 plan to reform colonial society. *William and Mary Quarterly*, Third Series, 30(3): 449–66.

Breen, T.H. (1985) *Tobacco Culture: The Mentality of the Great Tidewater Planters on the Eve of Revolution*. Princeton: Princeton University Press.

Briggs, A. (1983) *A Social History of England*. London: Weidenfeld and Nicolson.

British Lung Foundation (2016) *The Battle for Breath: The Impact of Lung Disease in the UK*. London: British Lung Foundation.

Brook, T. (2004) Smoking in Imperial China. In S. Gilman and Z. Xun (eds) *Smoke: A Global History of Smoking*. London: Reaktion, pp. 84–91.

Brook, T. (2008) *Vermeer's Hat: The Seventeenth Century and the Dawn of the Global World*. London: Bloomsbury.

Brookhenkel (2009) Turning Tables. *Thing Theory* (blog) https://thingtheory2009.word press.com/2009/06/22/turning-tables-2.

Browne, I.H. (1736) *A Pipe of Tobacco: In Imitation of Six Several Authors*. London: W. Bickerton.

Browne, J. (1842) *Tobacco Morally and Physically Considered in Relation to Smoking and Snuff Taking*. Driffield: B. Fawcett.

Brownell, K.D. and K.E. Warner (2009) The perils of ignoring history: big tobacco played dirty and millions died. how similar is big food? *The Milbank Quarterly*, 87(1): 259–94.

Buckley, J.H. ([1952] 2012) *The Victorian Temper: A Study in Literary Culture*. London: Routledge.

Bunton, R. and Coveney, J., (2011). Drug's pleasures. *Critical Public Health*, 21(1): 9–23.

Buñuel, L. (1984) *My Last Breath*, trans. A. Israel. London: Jonathan Cape.

Burch, T., N. Wander and J. Collin (2010) Uneasy money: the Instituto Carlos Slim de la Salud, tobacco philanthropy and conflict of interest in global health. *Tobacco Control*, 19: e1–e9.

Burckhardt, J. ([1860] 1958) *The Civilization of the Renaissance in Italy*, 2 vols, trans. S.G.C. Middlemore. New York: Harper.

Burke, K. (1935) *Permanence and Change: An Anatomy of Purpose*. New York: New Republic.

Burrows, D.S. (1984) Strategic Research Report. R.J. Reynolds 29th February, Legacy Library document http://legacy.library.ucsf.edu/tid/tqq46b00 [Accessed 11th November 2018].

Business Wire (2012) Philip Morris International Provides 15 Million Euro Contribution to INTERPOL to Fight Trafficking in Illicit Goods, June 21st, https://www.businesswire.com/news/home/20120620006558/en/Philip-Morris-International-15-Million-Euro-Contribution [Accessed May 2018].

Byatt, A.S. (2006) Donne and the embodied mind. In A. Guibbory (ed.) *The Cambridge Companion to John Donne*. Cambridge: Cambridge University Press.

Byrne P. (2014) Video: Watch e-cigarette EXPLODE and set fire to barmaid in busy pub. *Mirror Online*, April 8th. http://www.mirror.co.uk/news/weird-news/video-watch-e-cigarette-explode-set-3388651 [Accessed 21st October 2014].

California Department of Health Services, Tobacco Control Section (1998) *A Model for Change: The California Experience in Tobacco Control*. Sacramento: CDHS, TCS.

Callard, C.D. and N.E. Collishaw (2013) Supply-side options for an endgame for the tobacco industry. *Tobacco Control*, 22(s1): i10–i13.

Campbell, L.M., C. Corson, N.J. Gray, K.I. MacDonald and J.P. Brosius (2014) Studying global environmental meetings to understand global environmental governance: Collaborative event ethnography at the tenth Conference of the Parties to the Convention on Biological Diversity. *Global Environmental Politics*, 14(3): 1–20.

Campbell, T. (2005) *The Politics of Despair: Power and Resistance in the Tobacco Wars*. Lexington: University Press of Kentucky.

Cantobacco (2011) Māori Tobacco Video http://www.youtube.com/watch?v=9LF7qoJdEXc [Accessed 28th February 2014].

Carel, H. (2016) *Phenomenology of Illness*. Oxford: Oxford University Press.

Carr, A. (1985) *The Easy Way to Stop Smoking*. London: Arcturus Publishing.

Carr, E.H. (1961) *What is History?* New York: Alfred A. Knopf.

Carter, K.C. (1985) Koch's postulates in relation to the work of Jacob Henle and Edwin Klebs. *Medical History*, 29(4): 353–74.

Cartier, J. ([1545] 1580) *A shorte and briefe narration of the two navigations and discoveries to the northweast partes called Newe Fraunce.* London: H. Bynneman.

Cassanelli, L.V. (1986) Qat: changes in the production and consumption of a quasilegal commodity in northeast Africa. In A. Appadurai (ed.) *The Social Life of Things: Commodities in Cultural Perspective.* Cambridge: Cambridge University Press, pp. 236–58.

CDC (Centers for Disease Control and Prevention) (2017) Quitting smoking among adults – United States, 2000-2015. *Morbidity and Mortality Weekly Report*, 65(52): 1457–64.

Centre for Health and Social Justice (2017) *Ground realities of Beedi Workers in Tamil Nadu.* New Delhi: Centre for Health and Social Justice.

Chapman, S. (2014) E-cigarettes: the best and the worst case scenarios for public health. *British Medical Journal*, 349 (7974): g5512.

Charlton, A. (2005) Tobacco or health 1602: an Elizabethan doctor speaks. *Health Education Research*, 20(1): 101–11.

Chesterton, G.K. (1917) The nightmare of Dr. Saleeby. *The Living Age*, 292: 373–75.

Chignell, A.K. (1915) *An Outpost in Papua* (2nd ed.) London: Smith, Elder and Co.

Chung-Hall, J., L. Craig, S. Gravely, N. Sansone and G.T. Fong (2018) Impact of the WHO FCTC over the first decade: a global evidence review prepared for the Impact Assessment Expert Group. *Tobacco Control*, Epub ahead of print [Accessed 14th June 2018] doi:10.1136/tobaccocontrol-2018-054389.

Chute, A. (1595) *Tabaco. The distinct and severall opinions of the late and best Phisitions that have written of the divers natures and qualities thereof.* London: Printed by Adam Islip.

Claeys, G. (2011) *Searching for Utopia: The History of an Idea.* London: Thames & Hudson.

Clark, S., D. Swan and C. Ogden (2000) in *The Tobacco Industry and the Health Risks of Smoking*, House of Commons, London, https://publications.parliament.uk/pa/cm199900/cmselect/cmhealth/27/2702.htm [Accessed 23rd October 2018].

Clucas, S. (2009) Thomas Harriot's *A briefe and true report*: knowledge-making and the Roanoke Voyage. In K. Sloan (ed.) *European Visions: American Voices.* London: British Museum Research Publication 172, pp. 17–24.

Coates, P. (2007) *American Perceptions of Immigrant and Invasive Species: Strangers on the Land.* Berkeley: University of California Press.

Cohen, J.E. (2001) Universities and tobacco money: some universities are accomplices in the tobacco epidemic. *British Medical Journal*, 323(7303): 1–2.

Coleridge, S.T. (1966) *Collected Letters*, E.L. Griggs (ed.) Oxford: Clarendon Press.

Collins, W. (1874) *The Moonstone: A Novel.* London: Harper and Brothers.

Connolly, G.N., H.R. Alpert, G.F. Wayne and H. Koh (2007) Trends in nicotine yield in smoke and its relationship with design characteristics among popular US cigarette brands, 1997-2005. *Tobacco Control*, 16(5): e5.

Connor, S. (2011) Exclusive: Smoked out: Tobacco giant's war on science. Philip Morris seeks to force university to hand over confidential health research into teenage smokers. *The Independent*, September 1st. https://www.independent.co.uk/news/science/exclusive-smoked-out-tobacco-giants-war-on-science-2347254.html [Accessed 22nd June 2018].

Connor, S. (2011) *Paraphernalia: The Curious Lives of Magical Things.* London: Profile Books.

Courtwright, D. (2001) *Forces of Habit: Drugs and the Making of the Modern World.* Cambridge, MA: Harvard University Press.

Cowan, B. (2005) *The Social Life of Coffee: The Emergence of the British Coffeehouse.* New Haven: Yale University Press.

Cowlishaw, S. and S.L. Thomas (2018) Industry interests in gambling research: Lessons learned from other forms of hazardous consumption. *Addictive Behaviors,* 78: 101–6.

Cowper, W. (1995) Epistle to the Rev. William Bull. In J.D. Reid and C. Ryskamp (eds) *Poems of William Cowper, Vol. 2, 1782–1785.* Oxford: Oxford University Press.

Cox, H. (2000) *The Global Cigarette: Origins and Evolution of British American Tobacco 1880–1945.* Oxford: Oxford University Press.

Craze, R. (2003) *The Voice of Tobacco: A Dedicated Smoker's Diary of Not Smoking.* Great Ambrook: White Ladder Press.

Creighton, S. (2008) Black People in the North East. *North East History,* 39: 11–24.

Crosby, A.W. (2003) *The Columbian Exchange: Biological and Cultural Consequences of 1492* (30th Anniversary Edition). Westport: Praeger.

Crosby, A.W. (2004) *Ecological Imperialism: The Biological Expansion of Europe, 900–1900* (2nd ed.) Cambridge: Cambridge University Press.

Cunningham, R. (1996) *Smoke and Mirrors: The Canadian Tobacco War.* Ottawa: International Development Research Centre.

Darwin, C. (1880) *The Power of Movement in Plants.* London: John Murray.

Dash, M. (2000) *Tulipomania: The Story of the World's Most Coveted Flower and the Extraordinary Passions it Aroused.* London: Indigo.

Daube, M. (2012) Waiting for the domino effect. *Bulletin of the World Health Organization,* 90: 876–77.

Daube, M., R. Moodie and M. McKee (2017) Towards a smoke-free world? Philip Morris International's new Foundation is not credible. *The Lancet,* 390: 1722–24.

Davey Smith, G. and M. Egger (1996) Smoking and health promotion in Nazi Germany. *Journal of Epidemiology and Community Health,* 50(1): 109–10.

Davey Smith, G., S. Ströbele and M. Egger (1995) Smoking and death: public health measures were taken more than 40 years ago. *British Medical Journal,* 310: 396.

Davies, K.G. (1974) *The North Atlantic World in the Seventeenth Century.* Minneapolis: University of Minnesota Press.

Davies, S. (1991) *The Historical Origins of Health Fascism.* London: Forest.

Davis, M. (2006) *City of Quartz: Excavating the Future in Los Angeles.* London: Verso.

Davison, C., S. Frankel and G. Davey Smith (1992) The limits of lifestyle: re-assessing 'fatalism' in the popular culture of illness prevention. *Social Science and Medicine,* 34(6): 675–85.

de Bry, T. (1592) *Americae Tertia Pars.* Francofurti ad Moenum: Sigismundi Feierabendii.

De Grazia, V. (2005) *Irresistible Empire: America's Advance Through Twentieth-Century Europe.* Cambridge: Harvard University Press.

de Oviedo y Valdés, G.F. (1535) *La Historia general de las Indias.* Seville: Juam Cromberger.

Deacon, J. (1616) *Tobacco Tortured, or, The Filthie Fume of Tobacco Refined.* London: Richard Field.

Dear, M.J. and J.R. Wolch (1987) *Landscapes of Despair: From Deinstitutionalization to Homelessness.* Princeton: Princeton University Press.

Dekker, T. (1609) *The guls horn-booke,* (1st ed.) 1609 (1 vol.). Imprinted at London: Nicholas Okes for R. S[ergier?].

Delphia, C.M., M.C. Mescher, G. Felton and C.M. De Moraes (2006) The role of insect-derived cues in eliciting indirect plant defenses in tobacco, *Nicotiana tabacum. Plant Signaling and Behavior,* 1(5): 243–50.

Dennis, S. (2006) Four milligrams of phenomenology: an anthro-phenomenological exploration of smoking cigarettes. *Popular Culture Review* 17(1): 41–57.

Dennis, S. (2011) Smoking causes creative responses: on state antismoking policy and resilient habits. *Critical Public Health*, 21(1): 25–35.

Dennis, S. (2013) Golden chocolate olive tobacco packaging meets the smoker you thought you knew: the rational agent and new cigarette packaging legislation in Australia. *Contemporary Drug Problems*, 14: 71–97.

Dennis, S. (2016) *Smokefree: A Social, Moral and Political Atmosphere.* London: Bloomsbury.

Dennis, S. and H. Alexiou (2018) More than smoke and mirrors: thinking through smokers' relations with cigarette packets. *Journal of Material Culture*, 23(4): 459–71.

Department of Health (1998) *Smoking Kills: A White Paper on Tobacco.* London: HMSO/

Department of Health and Social Care (1999) *Saving Lives: Our Healthier Nation.* London: HMSO.

Derrida, J. (1981) Plato's Pharmacy. In *Dissemination,* trans. B. Johnson. London: The Athlone Press, pp. 61–172.

Derrida, J. (2006) *Specters of Marx: The State of the Debt, the Work of Mourning, and the New International,* trans. Peggy Kamuf. London: Routledge.

DeSantis, A.D. (2003) A couple of white guys sitting around talking: the collective rationalization of cigar smokers. *Journal of Contemporary Ethnography,* 32(4): 432–66.

Descola, P. ([1986] 1993) *In the Society of Nature: Native Cosmology in Amazonia.* Cambridge, Cambridge University Press.

Desjarlais, R. (1997) *Shelter Blues: Sanity and Selfhood among the Homeless.* Philadelphia: University of Pennsylvania Press.

Devall, W. and G. Sessions (1985) *Deep Ecology: Living as if Nature Mattered.* Salt Lake City: Gibbs M. Smith.

Devine, T.M. (1975) *The Tobacco Lords: A Study of the Tobacco Merchants of Glasgow and their Trading Activities c. 1740–90.* Edinburgh: John Donald.

Diamond, J. (1997) *Guns, Germs and Steel: A Short History of Everybody for the Past 13,000 Years.* London: Jonathan Cape.

Dickens, C. (1842) *American Notes for General Circulation.* Paris: Buadry's European Library.

Dickson, S.A. (1954) *Panacea or Precious Bane: Tobacco in Sixteenth Century Literature.* New York: New York Public Library.

DiClemente C.C., J. Prochaska, S.K. Fairhurst, W.F. Velicer, M.M. Velasquez and J.S. Rossi (1991) The process of smoking cessation: an analysis of precontemplation, contemplation, and preparation stages of change. *Journal of Consulting and Clinical Psychology,* 59(2): 295–304.

Dobson, M and S.W. Wells (2001) (eds) *The Oxford Companion to Shakespeare.* Oxford: Oxford University Press.

Dole, G.E. ([1964] 1973) Shamanism and political control among the Kuikuru. In D. R. Gross (ed.) *Peoples and Cultures of Native South America.* New York: Doubleday, pp. 294–307.

Donne, J. (1896) *The Poems of John Donne.* E.K. Chambers (ed.) London: Lawrence and Bullen.

Don't Be The 1 (2014) Michelle's Story. http://www.dontbethe1.tv/real-story-michelle. php [Accessed 11th November 2018].

Douglas, A. ([1993] 2007) Britannia's rule and the it-narrator. In Blackwell, M. (ed.) *The Secret Life of Things: Animals, Objects, and It-Narratives in Eighteenth-Century England.* Lewisburg: Bucknell University Press, pp. 147–61.

Dresser, M. (2001) *Slavery Obscured: The Social History of the Slave Trade in an English Provincial Port.* London: Continuum.

Dunhill, M. (1979) *Our Family Business*, London: The Bodley Head.

Dunhill Medical Trust (2018) About us. http://dunhillmedical.org.uk/about [Accessed 1st May 2018].

Durden, R.F. (1975) *The Dukes of Durham, 1865–1929.* Durham, NC: Duke University Press.

Dwyer, J (1993) Introduction – 'A Peculiar Blessing': social converse in Scotland from Hutcheson to Burns. In J. Dwyer and R.B. Sher (eds) *Sociability and Society in Eighteenth Century Scotland.* Edinburgh: The Mercat Press, pp. 1–22.

Dyer, O. (2015) Tobacco industry sought to prevent Islamic fatwas against smoking. *British Medical Journal*, 28(350): h2281.

Echeverri, J.A. (2015) Cool tobacco breath: the uses and meaning of tobacco among the People of the Centre. In A. Russell and E. Rahman (2015) (eds) *The Master Plant: Tobacco in Lowland South America*, London: Bloomsbury, pp. 107–29.

Edem, R. (2014) To vape or not to vape, that is the question. *The Collegian*, September 18th. http://www.kstatecollegian.com/2014/09/18/to-vape-or-not-to-vape-that-is-the-question [Accessed 19th September 2014].

Edinburgh Evening News (2012) Store stops selling cigarettes to dodge tax. June 11th. http://www.edinburghnews.scotsman.com/news/store-stops-selling-cigarettes-to-dodge-tax-1-2349046 [Accessed 12th September 2014].

Eleftheriou-Smith L.-M. 2014. Exploding E-cigarette 'caused fire' in house where elderly man found dead, October 21st. http://www.independent.co.uk/news/uk/home-news/exploding-ecigarette-caused-fire-in-house-where-elderly-man-found-dead-9657142.html [Accessed 14th October 2014].

Elliot, R. (2012) Smoking for taxes: the triumph of fiscal policy over health in postwar West Germany, 1945-55. *Economic History Review*, 65(4): 1450–74.

Elliot, R. (2015) Inhaling democracy: cigarette advertising and health education in post-war West Germany, 1950s-1975. *Social History of Medicine*, 28(3): 509–31.

Elliott, J. (2007a) *Empires of the Atlantic World: Britain and Spain in America, 1492–1830.* New Haven: Yale University Press.

Elliott, J. (2007b) The Iberian Atlantic and Virginia. In P.C. Mancall (ed.) *The Atlantic World and Virginia, 1550–1624.* Chapel Hill: University of North Carolina Press.

Engell, J. (1981) *The Creative Imagination: Enlightenment to Romanticism.* Cambridge: Harvard University Press.

English, A.C. (1905) Assistant Resident Magistrate's Report for Rigo District of the Central Division, British New Guinea. *Annual Report for the Year Ending 30th June, 1905*, Appendix C: 22-4.

Erskine, T. ([1739] 1870) Smoking Spiritualized (poem). In T. Erskine *Gospel Sonnets; Or, Spiritual Songs.* Glasgow: John Pryde, pp. 339–40.

Espinoza, J. (2015) 'I survived Jihadi John's threats to cut my throat', *Sunday Times*, 15th March: 4.

Fausto, C. (2004) A blend of blood and tobacco: shamans and jaguars among the Parakanã of Eastern Amazonia. In N.L. Whitehead and R. Wright (eds) *In Darkness and Secrecy: The Anthropology of Assault Sorcery and Witchcraft in Amazonia.* Durham: Duke University Press, pp. 155–78.

Fay, J. (2008) *Theaters of Occupation: Hollywood and the Reeducation of Postwar Germany.* Minneapolis: University of Minnesota Press.

FCA (Framework Convention Alliance) (2010) Open Letter to the Uruguayan President and Government. Framework Convention Alliance. http://www.fctc.org/images/stories/Letter%20Support%20Uruguay_EN.pdf [Accessed May 2018].

FCA (2014) *Electronic Nicotine Delivery Systems*. FCA Policy Briefing, Geneva: FCA.

FCA (2016) *Beginner's Guide to the FCTC Conference of the Parties* (2nd ed.) Ottawa: FCA.

FCTC (Framework Convention on Tobacco Control) (2010a) Conference of the Parties to the WHO Framework Convention on Tobacco Control. Fourth Session, Punta del Este, Uruguay, 15-20 November. *Verbatim Records of Plenary Meetings*. FCTC/COP/4/REC/2. Geneva: WHO.

FCTC (2010b) FCTC/COP4(5) *Punta del Este Declaration on the Implementation of the Framework Convention on Tobacco Control*, 19 November.

FCTC (2014a) Prevention and control of electronic nicotine delivery systems, including electronic cigarettes. FCTC/COP/6/A/Conf.Paper No. 7, 14 October.

FCTC (2014b) Electronic Nicotine Delivery Systems: Report by WHO. FCTC/COP/6/10, 21 July.

FCTC (2014c) Provisional agenda (annotated). FCTC/COP/6/1 Rev.2 (annotated), 13 October.

FCTC (2014d) [Prevention and control of] electronic nicotine delivery systems, including electronic cigarettes. FCTC/COP/6/A/Conf.Paper No.7 Rev.1, 17 October.

FCTC (2014e) Report of the sixth session of the Conference of the Parties to the WHO Framework Convention on Tobacco Control. http://apps.who.int/gb/fctc/PDF/cop6/FCTC_COP6_Report-en.pdf [Accessed 19th December 2014].

Feinhandler, S.J., H.C. Fleming and J.M. Monahon (1979) Pre-Columbian tobaccos in the Pacific. *Economic Botany*, 33: 213–26.

Feldman, S. (2007) Clouded judgement. *New Humanist*, 122(4): 30–33.

Fellowes, E.H. (1967) *English Madrigal Verse 1588–1632*, revised and enlarged by Frederick W. Sternfeld and David Greer (3rd ed.). Oxford: Clarendon Press.

Fisher, M. (2009) *Capitalist Realism: Is There No Alternative?* Ropley: John Hunt Publishing.

Fisher, M. (2016) *The Weird and the Eerie*. London: Repeater Books.

Fleischacher, S. (2013) *What is Enlightenment?* London: Routledge.

Flint, C. ([1998]/2007) Speaking objects: the circulation of stories in eighteenth-century prose fiction. In M. Blackwell (ed.) *The Secret Life of Things: Animals, Objects, and It-Narratives in Eighteenth-Century England*. Lewisburg: Bucknell University Press, pp. 162–86.

Fluharty, M., A.E. Taylor, M. Grabski and M.R. Munafò (2017) The association of cigarette smoking with depression and anxiety: a systematic review. *Nicotine and Tobacco Research*, 19(1): 3–13

Flynn, D. (1995) *John Donne and the Ancient Catholic Nobility*, Bloomington: Indiana University Press.

Folsom, S.W.B. (2006) *The Highway War: A Marine Company Commander in Iraq*. Washington, DC: Potomac Books.

Fotiou, E. (2014) On the uneasiness of tourism: considerations on shamanic tourism in Western Amazonia. In B.C. Labate and C. Cavnar (eds) *Ayahuasca Shamanism in the Amazon and Beyond*. Oxford: Oxford University Press, pp. 159–81.

Foust, C.M. (1992) *Rhubarb: The Wondrous Drug*. New Haven: Yale University Press.

Fox, A. (2008) Socio-cultural factors that foster or inhibit alcohol-related violence. In *Alcohol and Violence: Exploring Patterns and Responses*. International Center for Alcohol Politics, pp. 1-28. http://ec.europa.eu/health/ph_determinants/life_style/alcohol/Forum/docs/alcohol_lib18_en.pdf [accessed 11th November 2018].

Fox, G. (2015) *The Archaeology of Smoking and Tobacco*. Gainesville: University Press of Florida.

Frazer, J.G. (1920) *The Golden Bough* (2nd ed.). London: Macmillan.

Fresh Smoke Free North East (2011) Every breath. http://www.freshne.com/everybreath [Accessed 18th November 2011].

Fresh Smoke Free North East (2012) About us. http://www.freshne.com/About-Us [Accessed 5th July 2012].

Fresh Smoke Free North East (2018a) Fresh position statement on e-cigarettes. http://freshne.com/in-the-news/pr/item/2194-statement-ecigs [Accessed 15th June 2018].

Fresh Smoke Free North East (2018b) Minister and Shadow Public Health Minister praise work to cut smoking in the North East. http://freshne.com/in-the-news/pr/item/2197-minister-shadow-minister-praise-fresh [Accessed 15th June 2018].

Fung, A. (2006) Varieties of participation in complex governance. *Public Administration Review*, 66(s1): 66–75.

Furst, P.T. (1991) Nicotine addiction and shamanic ecstasy. Review of J. Wilbert (1986) 'Tobacco and shamanism in South America'. *History of Religions*, 30(3): 319–21.

Garcia, A. (2010) *The Pastoral Clinic: Addiction and Dispossession along the Rio Grande*. Berkeley: University of California Press.

Gardiner, E. (1610) *The Triall of Tabacco*. London: Matthew Lownes.

Garzón, P.C. and F. Keijzer (2011) Plants: adaptive behaviour, root-brains, and minimal cognition. *Adaptive Behavior*, 19(3): 155–71.

Gately, I. (2001) *Tobacco: A Cultural History of How an Exotic Plant Seduced Civilization*. London: Simon & Schuster.

Gay, P. (1966) *The Enlightenment: An Interpretation. Vol. 1: The Rise of Modern Paganism*. New York: Alfred A. Knopf.

Gayle, D. (2015) Durham police stop targeting pot smokers and small-scale growers. *The Guardian*, 22nd July. http://www.theguardian.com/society/2015/jul/22/durham-police-stop-targeting-pot-smokers-and-small-scale-growers [Accessed 23rd July 2015].

Geertz, C. (1963) *Agricultural Involution: The Process of Ecological Change in Indonesia*. Berkeley: University of California Press.

Geertz, C. (1984) 'Anti anti-relativism', *American Anthropologist*, 86(2): 263–78.

Geismar, H. (2011) 'Material culture studies' and other ways to theorize objects: a primer to a regional debate. *Comparative Studies in Society and History*, 53(1): 210–18.

Gell, A. (1998) *Art and Agency: An Anthropological Theory*. Oxford: Oxford University Press.

Gerard, J. (1597) *The Herball or Generall Historie of Plantes*. London: John Norton.

Gilmore, A.B., G. Fooks, J. Drope, S. Aguinaga Bialous and R. Rose Jackson (2015) Exposing and addressing tobacco industry conduct in low-income and middle-income countries. *Lancet*, 385: 1029–43.

Gilmore, A.B., A.W.A. Gallagher and A. Rowell (2018) Tobacco industry's elaborate attempts to control a global track and trace system and fundamentally undermine the Illicit Trade Protocol. *Tobacco Control*, Epub ahead of print: July 2nd 2018, doi:10.1136/tobaccocontrol-2017-054191.

Givel, M.S. (2011) History of Bhutan's prohibition of cigarettes: implications for neo-prohibitionists and their critics. *International Journal of Drug Policy*, 22: 306–10.

Glantz, S. (1996) Editorial: preventing tobacco use – the use access trap. *American Journal of Public Health*, 86(2): 156–158.

Global Environmental Politics (2014) Special Issue 4 (3).

Gokhale, B.G. (1974) Tobacco in seventeenth century India. *Agricultural History*, 48(4): 484–92.

Goldgar, A. (2007) *Tulipmania: Money, Honor, and Knowledge in the Dutch Golden Age.* Chicago: University of Chicago Press.

Goodman, J. (1993) *Tobacco in History: The Cultures of Dependence.* London: Routledge.

Gopal, M. (1999) Disempowered despite wage work: women workers in the beedi industry. *Economic and Political Weekly*, 34 (16/17):WS12–WS20.

Gow, P. (1994) 'River People: shamanism and history in Western Amazonia', in N. Thomas and C. Humphrey (eds) *Shamanism, History and the State*. Michigan: University of Michigan, pp. 90–113.

Gow, P. (2015) Methods of tobacco use among two Arawakan-speaking peoples in southwestern Amazonia: a case study of structural diffusion. In A. Russell and E. Rahman (2015) (eds) *The Master Plant: Tobacco in Lowland South America*. London: Bloomsbury, pp. 45–61.

Graham, H., (1987). Women's smoking and family health. *Social Science and Medicine*, 25(1): 47–56.

Grammeniati, B. (2011) *Filippo d'Agliè's Ballets (1604–1667)*. Bloomington: Authorhouse.

Grana R., N. Benowitz and S.A. Glantz (2013) *Background Paper on E-cigarettes (Electronic Nicotine Delivery Systems)*. Geneva: WHO Tobacco Free Initiative.

Grana R., N. Benowitz and S.A. Glantz (2014) E-cigarettes: a scientific review. *Circulation* 129: 1972–86.

Gray, S. (2008a) *The Smoking Diaries*. London: Granta.

Gray, S. (2008b) *The Last Cigarette: The Smoking Diaries Vol. 3*. London: Granta.

Greaves, L. (1996) *Smoke Screen: Women's Smoking and Social Control*. London: Scarlet Press.

Greenblatt, S. (2011) *The Swerve: How the Renaissance Began*. London: Bodley Head.

Gregory, J. (2003) Vegetarianism and the anti-tobacco movement (United Kingdom), in J.S. Blocker, D.M. Fahey and I.R. Tyrrell (eds) *Alcohol and Temperance in Modern History: An International Encyclopedia*, Vol. 1, pp. 633–35.

Grehan, J. (2006) Smoking and 'early modern' sociability: the great tobacco debate in the Ottoman Middle East (seventeenth to eighteenth centuries). *The American Historical Review*, 111(5): 1352–77.

Greymouth Star (2014) Shops Kick Tobacco Habit. http://www.greystar.co.nz/content/shops-kick-tobacco-habit [Accessed 6th January 2014].

Grieve, G. (2017) Why tabbing is a real drag. *Scottish Field*, 116(6): 72–3.

Griffin, D. (2004) Philips, John (1676-1709). *Oxford Dictionary of National Biography*, Oxford: Oxford University Press. https://doi.org/10.1093/ref:odnb/22123 [Accessed 11th November 2018].

Grüning, T., H. Weishaar, J. Collin and A.B. Gilmore (2012) Tobacco industry attempts to influence and use the German government to undermine the WHO Framework Convention on Tobacco Control. *Tobacco Control*, 21: 30–38.

Guasco, M. (2014) *Slaves and Englishmen: Human Bondage in the Early Modern Atlantic World*. Philadelphia: University of Pennsylvania Press.

Gupta, P.C. and S. Asma (2008) (eds) *Bidi Smoking and Public Health*. New Delhi: Ministry of Health and Family Welfare, Government of India.

Haapanen, L (2003) Tobacco industry. In P Knight (ed.) *Conspiracy Theories in American History*. Santa Barbara, CA: ABC-CLIO. http://ezphost.dur.ac.uk/login?url=http://search.credoreference.com/content/entry/abcconspir/tobacco_industry/0   [Accessed 11th November 2018].

Habermas, J. (1989) *The Structural Transformation of the Public Sphere: An Inquiry into a Category of Bourgeois Society*. Cambridge, MA: MIT Press.

Hackshaw, A., J.K. Morris, S. Boniface, J.L. Tang and D. Milenković (2018) Low cigarette consumption and risk of coronary heart diseae and stroke. *British Medical Journal*, 360: j5855.

Hadfield, A. (2006) Literary contexts: predecessors and contemporaries. In A. Guibbory (ed.) *The Cambridge Companion to Donne*. Cambridge: Cambridge University Press, pp. 49–64.

Hahn, B. (2011) *Making Tobacco Bright: Creating an American Commodity, 1617–1937*. Baltimore: Johns Hopkins University Press.

Hall, M. (2011) *Plants as Persons: A Philosophical Botany*. Albany: State University of New York Press.

Hall, W. (2010) What are the policy lessons of National Alcohol Prohibition in the United States, 1920-1933? *Addiction*, 105(7): 1164–73.

Hallé, F. (2002) *In Praise of Plants*. Portland: Timber Press.

Hanewinkel, R. and B. Isensee (2006) One for every 113 inhabitants: cigarette vending machines in Germany. *International Journal of Epidemiology*, 35(4): 1104–05.

Hannah, L. (2006) The Whig fable of American Tobacco, 1895-1913. *Journal of Economic History*, 66(1): 42–73.

Haraway, D. ([1985] 1991) A cyborg manifesto: science, technology, and socialist-feminism in the late 20th Century. In D. Haraway, *Simians, Cyborgs, and Women: The Reinvention of Nature*. New York: Routledge, pp. 149–81.

Haraway, D. (2003) *The Companion Species Manifesto: Dogs, People, and Significant Otherness*. Chicago: Prickly Paradigm Press.

Haraway, D. (2008) *When Species Meet*. Minneapolis: University of Minnesota Press.

Haraway, D., N. Ishikawa, S.F. Gilbert, K. Olwig, A.L. Tsing and N. Bubandt (2016) Anthropologists are talking – about the Anthropocene. *Ethnos*, 81(3): 535–64.

Hargreaves, K., A. Amos, G. Highet, C. Martin, S. Platt, D. Ritchie and M. White (2010) The social context of change in tobacco consumption following the introduction of 'smokefree' England legislation: a qualitative, longitudinal study. *Social Science and Medicine*, 71: 459–66.

Hariot, T. ([1590] 1972) *A Briefe and True Report of the New Found Land of Virginia*. New York: Dover Publications [author's name spelt 'Harriot'].

Harley, D. (1993) The beginnings of the tobacco controversy: Puritanism, James I, and the royal physicians. *Bulletin of the History of Medicine*, 67(1): 28–50.

Harrer, H. ([1953] 1982) *Seven Years in Tibet*. New York: Tarcher.

Harris, B. (2011) The intractable cigarette 'filter problem'. *Tobacco Control*, 20 (Suppl 1): i10–i16.

Harris, J.G. (1998) *Foreign Bodies and the Body Politic: Discourses of Social Pathology in Early Modern England*. Cambridge: Cambridge University Press.

Harris, M. (1974) *Cows, Pigs, Wars and Witches: The Riddles of Culture*. New York: Random House.

Harris, R. (1991) Foreword. In S. Davies *The Historical Origins of Health Fascism*. London: Forest.

Harrison, J. (2012) Sainsbury's ends sale of cigarettes, 12th November. http://www.heralds cotland.com/news/home-news/sainsburys-ends-sale-of-cigarettes.19395477?page=8 [Accessed 12th September 2014].

Harvey, D. (2005) *A Brief History of Neoliberalism.* Oxford: Oxford University Press.

Harvey, M., S. Quilley and H. Beynon (2002) *Exploring the Tomato: Transformations of Nature, Society and Economy.* Cheltenham: Edward Elgar Publishing.

Hastings, G. (2012a) Why corporate power is a public health priority. *British Medical Journal,* 345: e5124. doi: 10.1136/bmj.e5124.

Hastings, G. (2012b) *The Marketing Matrix: How the Corporation Gets Its Power – And How We Can Reclaim It.* London: Routledge.

Hays, T.E. (1991) 'No tobacco, no hallelujah': missions and the early history of tobacco in Eastern Papua. *Pacific Studies,* 14(4): 91–112.

Hays, T.E. (2003) 'They are beginning to learn the use of tobacco', in W. Jankowiak and D. Bradburd (eds) *Drugs, Labor, and Colonial Expansion.* Phoenix: University of Arizona Press.

Health Canada (1999) *New Directions for Tobacco Control in Canada: A National Strategy.* http://publications.gc.ca/collections/Collection/H39-505-1999E.pdf [Accessed 11th November 2018].

Heckler, S. and A. Russell (2008a) Confronting collaboration: dilemmas in an ethnographic study of health policy makers. *Anthropology in Action,* 15(1): 14–21.

Heckler, S. and A. Russell (2008b) Emotional engagement in strategic partnerships: grassroots organising in a tobacco control partnership in the North East of England. *Evidence and Policy,* 4(4): 331–54.

Heikkinen, H., Patja, K. and Jallinoja, P. (2010) Smokers' accounts on the health risks of smoking: why is smoking not dangerous for me? *Social Science and Medicine,* 71(5): 877–83.

Heimann, J. and S. Heller (2018) *Alcohol and Tobacco: 100 Years of Stimulating Ads.* Köln: Taschen.

Henare, A., M. Holbraad and S. Wastell (2007) (eds) Introduction. In A. Henare, M. Holbraad and S. Wastell (eds) *Thinking Through Things: Theorising Artefacts Ethnographically.* London: Routledge, pp. 1–31.

Henry, J.Q.A. (1906) *The Deadly Cigarette; Or, the Perils of Juvenile Smoking.* London: R.J. James.

Hess, H. (1996) The other prohibition: the cigarette crisis in post-war Germany. *Crime, Law and Social Change,* 25: 43–61.

Heywood, V.H. (1993) *Flowering Plants of the World (updated edition).* Oxford: Oxford University Press.

Hill, C. ([1972] 1975) *The World Turned Upside Down: Radical Ideas During the English Revolution.* Harmondsworth: Penguin.

Hill, D. and Carroll T. (2003) Australia's national tobacco campaign. *Tobacco Control,* 12 (suppl 2): ii9–ii14.

Hillyard, P. and Tombs, S. (2007) "From 'Crime' to Social Harm?" *Crime, Law and Social Change,* 48, (1-2): 9–25.

Hilton, M. (1998) Retailing history as economic and cultural history: strategies for survival by specialist tobacconists in the mass market. *Business History,* 40(4): 115–37.

Hilton, M. (2000) *Smoking in British Popular Culture.* Manchester: Manchester University Press.

Hirayama, T. (1981) Non-smoking wives of heavy smokers have a higher risk of lung cancer: a study from Japan. *British Medical Journal,* 282(6259): 183–185.

HM Revenue and Customs (2010) Government and industry take a significant step in the fight against tobacco smuggling. https://www.wired-gov.net/wg/wg-news-1.nsf/print/Government+and+industry+take+a+significant+step+in+the+fight+against+tobacco+smuggling+15072010130700 [Accessed 22nd June 2018].

HM Revenue and Customs (2017) Excise Notice 476: Tobacco Products Duty. https://www.gov.uk/government/publications/excise-notice-476-tobacco-products-duty/excise-notice-476-tobacco-products-duty [Accessed 28th June 2018].

HM Revenue and Customs (2018) Guidance: Tobacco Products Duty. https://www.gov.uk/guidance/tobacco-products-duty [Accessed 28th June 2018].

Hobhouse, H. (1999) *Seeds of Change: Six Plants that Transformed Mankind.* London: Papermac.

Hobsbawn, E. and T.O. Ranger (1992) *The Invention of Tradition.* Cambridge: Cambridge University Press.

Hoby, E. (1613) *A Counter-Snarle for Ishmael Rabshacheh, a Cecropidan Lycaonite.* London: Printed by G. Eld and Thomas Snodham for Nath. Butter, by the authoritie of superiours.

Hochschild, A. R. (2003). *The Managed Heart: Commercialization of Human Feeling* (20th Anniversary edition). Berkeley: University of California Press.

Hockney, D. (2001) *Secret Knowledge: Rediscovering the Lost Techniques of the Old Masters.* London: Thames & Hudson.

Hodder, I. (2014) The entanglements of humans and things: a long-term view. *New Literary History*, 45(1): 19–36.

Hogg, S., S.E. Hill and J. Collin (2016) State-ownership of tobacco industry: a 'fundamental conflict of interest' or a 'tremendous opportunity' for tobacco control? *Tobacco Control*, 25: 367–72.

Holbraad, M. (2011) *Can the Thing Speak?* Open Anthropology Cooperative Press, Working Papers Series #7.

Holbraad, M., M.A. Pedersen and E. Viveiros de Castro (2014) The politics of ontology: anthropological positions. Theorizing the Contemporary, *Cultural Anthropology*, January 13th. https://culanth.org/fieldsights/462-the-politics-of-ontology-anthropological-positions [Accessed 11th November 2018].

Holden C., K. Lee, A. Gilmore, G. Fooks and N. Wander (2010) Trade policy, health, and corporate influence: British American Tobacco and China's accession to the World Trade Organization. *International Journal of Health Services*, 40: 421–41.

Holden, C. and K. Lee (2011) 'A major lobbying effort to change and unify the excise structure in six Central American countries': how British American Tobacco influence tax and tariff rates in the Central American Common Market. *Globalization and Health*, 7(15).

Hong, Y.-S. (2002) Cigarette butts and the building of socialism in East Germany. *Central European History*, 35(3): 327–44.

Hornsby, R. and D. Hobbs (2007) A zone of ambiguity: the political economy of cigarette bootlegging. *British Journal of Criminology*, 47 (4): 551–71.

hotukdeals (2009-12) (various contributors) 'What Pontins Cigarette House was you in?' http://www.hotukdeals.com/misc/what-pontins-cigarette-house-was-you-459339 [Accessed 28th August 2015].

Huang, Y. (2014) China's position in negotiating the Framework Convention on Tobacco Control and the revised international health regulations. *Public Health*, 128(2): 161–166.

Hughes, J. (2003) *Learning to Smoke: Tobacco Use in the West.* Chicago: University of Chicago Press.

Hugh-Jones, S. (2009) The fabricated body: objects and ancestors in Northwest Amazonia. In F. Santos-Granero (ed.) *The Occult Life of Things*, Tucson: University of Arizona Press, pp. 33–59.

Humair, J.-P.; N. Garin, E. Gerstel, S. Carballo, D. Carballo, P.-F. Keller and I. Guessous (2014) Acute respiratory and cardiovascular admissions after a public smoking ban in Geneva, Switzerland. *PLoS ONE*, 9(3): e90417.

Hunt, H. 2014. No smoke without fire! Kids are caught puffing on e-cigarettes in school, school. *Liverpool Echo*, March 31st, http://www.liverpoolecho.co.uk/news/liverpool-news/liverpool-kids-smoking-e-cigarettes-school-6895830 [Accessed 10th October 2014].

Hunt, K. and H. Sweeting (2014) You have been QUALIFIED for a smokeless e-cig starter kit. *Journal of Epidemiology and Community Health*. Published online first 29 April, doi: 10.1136/jech-2014-203879.

Hunter, D. (2009) Leading for health and wellbeing: the need for a new paradigm. *Journal of Public Health*, 31(2): 202–04.

Hunter, M. (2010) *Love in the Time of AIDS: Inequality, Gender and Rights in South Africa*. Bloomington: Indiana University Press.

Imperial Tobacco (2011) Homepage. http://www.imperial-tobacco.com [Accessed 18th September 2011].

Ingold, T. (1996) Culture, perception and cognition. In J. Howarth (ed.) *Psychological Research: Innovative Methods and Strategies*. London: Routledge, pp. 99–119.

Ingold, T. (2000) *The Perception of the Environment: Essays on Livelihood, Dwelling and Skill*. London: Routledge.

Ingold, T. (2013) Dreaming of dragons: on the imagination of real life. *Journal of the Royal Anthropological Institute*, 19(4): 734–52.

Isenberg, N., 2004. Cinematic smoke: from Weimar to Hollywood. In S. Gilman and Z. Xun (eds) *Smoke: A Global History of Smoking*. London: Reaktion, pp. 248–64.

Isherwood, C. ([1976] 2012) *Christopher and His Kind*. London: Vintage.

Israel, J. (2006) *Enlightenment Contested: Philosophy, Modernity, and the Emancipation of Man 1670-1752*. Oxford: Oxford University Press.

Israel, J. (2010) *A Revolution of the Mind. Radical Enlightenment and the Intellectual Origins of Modern Democracy*. Princeton: Princeton University Press.

Israel, J. (2011) *Democratic Enlightenment: Philosophy, Revolution, and Human Rights 1750–1790*, Oxford: Oxford University Press.

Jaine, R., M. Russell, R. Edwards, G. Thomson (2014) New Zealand tobacco retailers' attitudes to selling tobacco, point-of-sale display bans and other tobacco control measures: a qualitative analysis. *New Zealand Medical Journal*, 127(1396): 53–66.

Jankowiak, W. and D. Bradburd (1996) Using drug foods to capture and enhance labor performance: a cross-cultural perspective. *Current Anthropology*, 37 (4): 717–20.

Jenness, D. and A. Ballantyne (1920) *The Northern d'Entrecasteaux*. Oxford: Clarendon Press.

Jerome, J.K. ([1926] 1984) *My Life and Times*. New York: Harper and Brothers.

Jit, M., P. Aveyard, P. Barton and C.A. Meads (2010) Predicting the life-time benefit of school-based smoking prevention programmes. *Addiction*, 195(6): 1109–16.

Johnson, S. (1779) *Prefaces . . . to the Works of the English Poets, Vol. 4*. London: For H. Hughs; For C. Bathurst, et al.

Johnson, S. (1947) John Donne and the Virginia Company. *ELH*, 14(2): 127–38.

Jones, H. (1724) *The Present State of Virginia*. London: Printed for J. Clarke.

Jonson, B. ([1610] 1732) *The Alchemist: A Comedy*. London: J. Walthoe, G. Conyers, J. Knapton, R. Knaplock, D. Midwinter and others.

Jonson, B. ([1616] 1919) *Every Man in His Humour*, Percy Simpson (ed.) Oxford: Clarendon Press.

Joossens, L. and M. Raw (1998) Cigarette smuggling in Europe: who really benefits? *Tobacco Control*, 7: 66–71.

Joossens, L. and M. Raw (2012) From cigarette smuggling to illicit tobacco trade. *Tobacco Control*, 21: 230–34.

Joossens, L., A.B. Gilmore, M. Stoklosa and H. Ross (2016) Assessment of the European Union's illicit trade agreements with the four major transnational tobacco companies. *Tobacco Control*, 25: 254–60.

Kalra, A., P. Bansal, D. Wilson and T. Lasseter (2017) Reuters Investigates – The Philip Morris Files. Part 1: Treaty Blitz. https://www.reuters.com/investigates/special-report/pmi-who-fctc [Accessed 14th June 2018].

Kane, R.J. (1931) Anthony Chute, Thomas Nashe, and the first English work on tobacco. *Research in English Studies*, 7(26): 151–59.

Karban, R., I.T. Baldwin, K.J. Baxter, G. Laue and G.W. Felton (2000) Communication between plants: induced resistance in wild tobacco plants following clipping of neighboring sagebrush. *Oecologia*, 125: 66–71.

Karban, R., M. Huntzinger and A.C. McCall (2004) The specificity of eavesdropping on sagebrush by other plants. *Ecology*, 85(7): 1846–52.

Karhausen, L.R. (2011) *The Bleeding of Mozart: A Medical Glance on his Life, Illnesses and Personality*. Bloomington: Xlibris Corporation.

Kezar, D. (2003) Shakespeare's addictions, *Critical Inquiry*, 30(1): 31–62.

Kiernan, V.G. (1991) *Tobacco: A History*. London: Hutchinson Radius.

Kim, K. (2017) *'Hands Up': Female Call Centre Workers' Labour, Protest and Health in the Seoul Digital Industrial Complex, Korea*. PhD thesis, Durham University. http://etheses.dur.ac.uk/12236 [Accessed 11th November 2018].

Kim, K. (2018) Creating polluted spaces and bodies: labor control in a call center and the stigma of female smoking. *Korean Anthropology Review*, 2: 73–107.

King James 1st (1604) *A Counterblaste to Tobacco*. London: Imprinted by Robert Barker.

King, B. (2016) Attacking the source of a 6 million deaths per year epidemic: tobacco industry divestment. http://blogs.bmj.com/tc/2016/10/20/attacking-the-source-of-a-6-million-deaths-per-year-epidemic-tobacco-industry-divestment/?q=w_tc_blog_sidetab [Accessed 11th November 2018].

Kingsolver, A.E. (2011) *Tobacco Town Futures: Global Encounters in Rural Kentucky*. Long Grove: Waveland Press.

Kinoshita, A., A.R. Skinner, N. Guidon, E. Ignacio, G. Daltrini Felice, C. de A. Buco, S. Tatumi, M. Yee, A.M. Graciano Figueiredo and O. Baffa (2014) Dating human occupation at Toca do Serrote das Moendas, Sao Raimundo Nonato, Piauí-Brasil by electron spin resonance and optically stimulated luminescence. *Journal of Human Evolution*, 77: 187–95.

Kipling, R. ([1886] 1994) The Betrothed. In *The Collected Poems of Rudyard Kipling*. Ware: Wordsworth Poetry Library, pp. 51–2.

Kipling, R. (1926) In the interests of the Brethren. In R. Kipling, *Debits and Credits*. London: Macmillan.

Kisluk-Grosheide, D.O. (1988) Dutch tobacco boxes in the Metropolitan Museum of Art: a catalogue. *Metropolitan Museum Journal*, 23: 201–31.

Klein, D. (2010) The Sultan's envoys speak. The ego in 18th-century Ottoman sefâretnâmes on Russia, in R. Elger and Y. Köse (eds) *Many Ways of Speaking about the Self: Middle Eastern (Oriental) Ego-documents in Arabic, Persian, and* Turkish (14*th*-20*th Century)*. Weisbaden: Harrowitz Verlag, pp. 89–103.

Klein, H.S., S.L. Engerman, R. Haines and R. Shlomowitz (2001) Transoceanic mortality: the slave trade in comparative perspective. *William and Mary Quarterly*, 58(1): 93–118.

Klein, R. (1993) *Cigarettes Are Sublime*. Durham: Duke University Press.

Knapp, J. (1988) Elizabethan tobacco. *Representations*, 21: 26–66.

Knapp, J. (1992) *An Empire Nowhere: England, America, and Literature from* Utopia to The Tempest. Berkeley: University of California Press.

Knutson, R. Lander (2001) *Playing Companies and Commerce in Shakespeare's Time*. Cambridge: Cambridge University Press.

Koehler, M. (2012) *Poetry of Attention in the 18*th* Century*. London: Palgrave.

Kohn, E. (2007) How dogs dream: Amazonian natures and the politics of transspecies engagement. *American Ethnologist*, 34(1): 3–24.

Kohn, E. (2013) *How Forests Think: Toward an Anthropology Beyond the Human*. Berkeley: University of California Press.

Kohrman, M. (2007) Depoliticizing tobacco's exceptionality: male sociality, death, and memory-making among Chinese cigarette smokers. *The China Journal*, 58: 85–109.

Kohrman, M. (2008) Smoking among doctors: governmentality, embodiment, and the diversion of blame in contemporary China. *Medical Anthropology*, 27(1): 9–42.

Kohrman, M. (2017) Curating employee ethics: self-glory amidst slow violence at the China Tobacco Museum. *Medical Anthropology*, 36: 47–60.

Kohrman, M. and P. Benson (2011) Tobacco. *Annual Review of Anthropology*, 40: 329–44.

Kollewe, J.and J. Glenza (2017) British American Tobacco to acquire Reynolds as activists decry merger. *The Guardian*, July 19th. https://www.theguardian.com/business/2017/jul/19/british-american-tobacco-reynolds-merger-cigarettes [Accessed 28th October 2017].

Kopenawa, D. and B. Albert (2013) *The Falling Sky: Words of a Yanomami Shaman*. Harvard: Harvard University Press.

Krarup T.M. and A. Blok (2011) Unfolding the social: quasi-actants, virtual theory, and the new empiricism of Bruno Latour. *Sociological Review*, 59(1): 42–63.

Kulikoff, A. (1986) *Tobacco and Slaves: The Development of Southern Cultures in the Chesapeake, 1680-1800*. Chapel Hill: University of North Carolina Press.

Kurlansky, M. (1999) *Cod: A Biography of the Fish that Changed the World*. London: Vintage.

Kurlansky, M. (2003) *Salt: A World History*. New York: Vintage.

Lacan, J. (1996) *The Seminar of Jacques* Lacan *1959–1960: The Ethics of Psychoanalysis* (Book VII). New York: W.W. Norton.

Lal, P. (2009) Bidi: a short history. *Current Science*, 96(10): 1335–37.

Lal, P.N. and N.C. Wilson (2012) The perverse economics of the bidi and tendu trade. *Economic and Political Weekly*, 47(2): 77–80.

Lamb, C. ([1822] 1985) Confessions of a drunkard. In A. Phillips (ed.) *Charles Lamb: Selected Prose*. Harmondsworth: Penguin Books.

Landsman, M. (2005) *Dictatorship and Demand: the Politics of Consumerism in East Germany*. Cambridge: Harvard University Press.

Lange, P (2015) Lung-function trajectories leading to Chronic Obstructive Pulmonary Disease. *New England Journal of Medicine*, 373: 111–22.

Langmore, D. (1981) *European Missionaries in Papua, 1874-1914: A Group Portrait.* PhD thesis, Australian National University.

Larkin, K.T. (2010) *'A Taste of the Great, Wide World': The Cigarette, Public Health and Consumer Culture From the Third Reich to the Federal Republic.* PhD thesis, Department of History, Stony Brook University.

Latour, B. (1993) *We Have Never Been Modern.* New York: Harvester Wheatsheaf.

Latour, B. (1999) *Pandora's Hope: Essays on the Reality of Science Studies.* Cambridge, MA: Harvard University Press.

Latour, B., (2005) *Reassembling the Social: An Introduction to Actor-Network Theory.* Oxford, Oxford University Press.

Latour, B., I. Stengers, A. Tsing and N. Bubandt (2018) Anthropologists are talking – about capitalism, ecology, and apocalypse. *Ethnos*, 83(3): 587–606.

Laufer, B. (1924) *The Introduction of Tobacco into Europe.* Chicago: Field Museum of Natural History, Department of Anthropology, Leaflet Number 19.

Lavack, A. (1999) Denormalization of tobacco marketing in Canada. *Social Marketing Quarterly*, 5(3): 82–85.

Lee, K., A. Gilmore and J. Collin (2004) Breaking and re-entering: British American Tobacco in China 1979-2000. *Tobacco Control*, 13: 88–95.

Lefferts, P.M. (1988) *Subtilitas* in the tonal language of *Fumeux fume. Early Music*, 16(2): 176–183.

Lencucha R., A. Kothari and R. Labonté (2011) The role of non-governmental organizations in global health diplomacy: negotiating the Framework Convention on Tobacco Control. *Health Policy and Planning* 26: 405–12.

Lencucha R., A. Kothari A and R. Labonté (2012) Enacting accountability: networked governance, NGOs and the FCTC. *Global Health Governance* 5(2): 1–17.

Leonardi-Bee J., M.L. Jere and J. Britton (2011) Exposure to parental and sibling smoking and the risk of smoking uptake in childhood and adolescence: a systematic review and meta-analysis. *Thorax*, 66: 847–55.

Lévi-Strauss, C. ([1964] 1992) *Introduction to a Science of Mythology*, vol. 1: *The Raw and the Cooked*, trans. J. and D. Weightman. London: Penguin Books.

Lévi-Strauss, C. ([1966] 1973) *Introduction to a Science of Mythology*, vol. 2: *From Honey to Ashes*, trans. J. and D. Weightman. London: Jonathan Cape.

Lewis, S. (2014) Presentation: E-cigarettes: enlightened approach or new social and public health threat? ASA Decennial Conference, Edinburgh, June.

Lewis, S. and A. Russell (2011) Being embedded: a way forward for ethnographic research. *Ethnography*, 12(3): 398–416.

Lewis S. and Russell A. (2013) Young smokers' narratives: public health, disadvantage and structural violence. *Sociology of Health and Illness*, 35(5): 246–60.

Lewy, J. (2006) A sober Reich? Alcohol and tobacco use in Nazi Germany. *Substance Use and Abuse*, 41(8): 1179–95.

Li, C., W. Teng, Q. Shi and F. Zhang (2007) Multiple signals regulate nicotine synthesis in tobacco plant. *Plant Signaling and Behavior*, 2(4): 280–81.

Liberman, J. (2012) Four COPs and counting: achievements, underachievements and looming challenges in the early life of the WHO FCTC Conference of the Parties. *Tobacco Control*, 21: 215–20.

Lickint, F. (1939) *Tabak und Organismus.* Stuttgart: Hippokrates-Verlag.

Lien, M. (2015) *Becoming Salmon: Aquaculture and the Domestication of a Fish.* Berkeley: University of California Press.

Linton, J. (1998) *The Romance of the New World: Gender and the Literary Formations of English Colonialism.* Cambridge: Cambridge University Press.

Little, P.E. (1995) Ritual, power and ethnography at the Rio Earth Summit. *Critique of Anthropology*, 15: 265–88.

Livingstone, D. and C. Livingstone (1866) *Narrative of an Expedition to the Zambesi and its Tributaries; And of the Discovery of the Lakes Shirwa and Nyasa, 1858-1864.* New York: Harper.

Locke, J. (1690) *An Essay Concerning Humane Understanding.* 1st ed. London: Thomas Bassett.

Londoño-Sulkin, C. (2012) *People of Substance: An Ethnography of Morality in the Colombian Amazon.* Toronto: University of Toronto Press.

Long, A.A. and D.N. Sedley (1987) *The Hellenistic Philosophers*, Vol. 1: *Translations of the Principal Sources with Philosophical Commentary.* Cambridge: Cambridge University Press.

Loureiro, M. L., A. Sanz-de-Galdeano and D. Vuri, (2010) Smoking habits: like father, like son, like mother, like daughter? *Oxford Bulletin of Economics and Statistics*, 72: 717–43.

Lowell, J.R. (1904) A winter-evening hymn to my fire. In B. Carman, J.V. Cheney, C.G.D. Roberts, C.F. Richardson, F.H. Stoddard and J.R. Howard (eds) *The World's Best Poetry*, Vol. 1. Philadelphia: John D. Morris & Co.

Lukes, S. (1973) *Individualism.* Oxford: Oxford University Press.

Lundbäck, B., A. Lindbert, M. Lindström and K. Larsson (2003) Not 15 but 50% of smokers develop COPD? Report from the obstructive lung disease in Northern Sweden studies. *Respiratory Medicine*, 97: 115–22.

Lynch, D. (1998) *The Economy of Character: Novels, Market Culture and the Business of Inner Meaning.* Chicago: University of Chicago Press.

McCallum, C. (2014) Cashinahua perspectives on functional anatomy: ontology, ontogenesis, and biomedical education in Amazonia. *American Ethnologist*, 41(3): 504–17.

McCarthy, M. (2002) A brief history of the World Health Organization. *The Lancet*, 360 (9340): 1111–12.

Macaulay, T.B. (1849) *The History of England from the Accession of James II*, vol. 1. London: printed for Longman, Brown, Green, and Longmans.

McCusker, J.J. and R.R. Menard (1985) *The Economy of British America 1607-1789.* Chapel Hill: University of North Carolina Press.

Macfarlane, A. (1978) *The Origins of English Individualism.* Oxford: Blackwell.

Macfarlane, R. (2015) The eeriness of the English countryside. *The Guardian*, April 10th. https://www.theguardian.com/books/2015/apr/10/eeriness-english-countryside-robert-macfarlane [Accessed 26th April 2018].

McGeachie, M., K.P. Yates, X. Zhou, F. Guo, A.L. Sternberg, M.L. Van Natta et al. (2016) Patterns of growth and decline in lung function in persistent childhood asthma. *New England Journal of Medicine*, 374: 1842–52.

McGonigle, I.V. (2013) Khat, chewing on a bitter controversy. *Anthropology Today*, 29(4): 4–7.

McGrady, B. (2011) *Philip Morris v. Uruguay*: The Punta del Este Declaration on the Implementation of the WHO Framework Convention on Tobacco Control. *European Journal of Risk Regulation*, 2(2): 254–60.

MacGregor, W. (1892) Despatch reporting administrative visits to Tagula and Murua, etc. British New Guinea. *Annual Report from 1st July, 1890, to 30th June, 1891*, Appendix I: 31-2.

McGuill, S. (2017) Latest Research: What the 2017 Edition Tobacco Data is telling us. *Euromonitor*, https://blog.euromonitor.com/2017/06/latest-research-tobacco-2017-edition-data.html [Accessed 26th April 2018].

Mackay, J. and M. Eriksen (2002) *Tobacco Atlas*, 1st ed. Geneva: World Health Organization.

McLusky (2013) Farm to pharmacy. *Biomedical Picture of the Day*, May 16th. http://www.bpod.mrc.ac.uk/archive/2013/5/16 [Accessed 28th April 2018].

Macnaughton, J. (2012) The Smoking Interest Group in Uruguay: visiting 'Respira Uruguay' (blog). http://centreformedicalhumanities.org/the-smoking-interest-group-in-uruguay [Accessed 14th November 2014].

Macnaughton, J., S. Carro-Ripalda and A. Russell (2012) 'Risking enchantment': how are we to view the smoking person? *Critical Public Health*, 22(4): 455–69.

McNeill, A., J.-F. Etter, F. Konstantinos, P. Hajek, J. le Houezecs and H. McRobbie (2014) A critique of a World Health Organization commissioned report and associated paper on electronic cigarettes. *Addiction*, 109: 2128–34.

McNeill, A., B. Iringe-Koko, M. Bains, L. Bauld, G. Siggens and A. Russell (2014) Countering the demand for, and supply of, illicit tobacco: an assessment of the 'North of England Tackling Illicit Tobacco for Better Health' programme. *Tobacco Control*, 23: e44–e50.

Maitland, T. (1871) The fleshly school of poetry: Mr. D.G. Rossetti. *The Contemporary Review*, 18: 334–50.

Majumder, B. and J. Patel (2017) Livelihood security of home-based beedi-rolling workers in Uttar Pradesh. *Economic and Political Weekly*, 52(14): 65–71.

Malcolm, C. and N. Goodman (2011) *Making Smoking History in Wrekenton*. Gateshead: Gateshead Council. http://www.freshne.com/Uploads/file/Alliances/Gateshead/Wrekenton%20Smoking%20History%20Report%202011.pdf [Accessed 3rd July 2012].

Malinowski, B. ([1922] 2002) *Argonauts of the Western Pacific: An Account of Native Enterprise and Adventure in the Archipelagos of Melanesian New Guinea*. London: Routledge.

Malone, R. (2016) The race to a tobacco endgame. *Tobacco Control*, 25: 607–8.

Mamudu H. and S. Glantz (2009) Civil society and the negotiation of the Framework Convention on Tobacco Control. *Global Public Health* 4(2): 150–68.

Mamudu, H.M., R. Hammond and S. Glantz (2011) International trade versus public health during the FCTC negotiations, 1999-2003. *Tobacco Control*, 20(1): e3.

Mancall, P.C. (2004) Tales tobacco told in sixteenth-century Europe. *Environmental History*, 9(4): 648–78.

Mancuso, S. and A. Viola (2015) *Brilliant Green: The Surprising History and Science of Plant Intelligence*. Washington, DC: Island Press.

Marcus, G.E. (1998) *Ethnography Through Thick and Thin*. Princeton: Princeton University Press.

Marshall, M. (2013) *Drinking Smoke: The Tobacco Syndemic in Oceania*. Honolulu: University of Hawai'i Press.

Marston, J. ([1599] 1991) *Antonio and Mellida*, ed. W. Reavley Gair. Manchester: Manchester University Press.

Martin, E. (2006) The pharmaceutical person. *BioSocieties*, 1(3): 273–87.

Martin, J.J. (2002) The myth of Renaissance individualism. In G. Ruggiero (ed.) *A Companion to the Worlds of the Renaissance*, Oxford: Blackwell, pp. 208–24.

Martin, P. (1973) The discovery of America. *Science*, 179(4077): 969–74.

Marx, K. ([1867] 1977) *Capital: A Critique of Political Economy*, vol. 1, trans. Ben Fowkes. New York: Vintage.

Mathews, D. (2012) Tobacco gift to Durham caused turmoil at the top. *Times Higher Education*, November 8th.

Mathieu, A. (1993) The medicalization of homelessness and the theater of repression. *Medical Anthropology Quarterly*, 7: 170–84.

Matthee, R. (2004) Tobacco in Iran. In S.L. Gilman and Z. Xun (eds) *Smoke: A Global History of Smoking*. London: Reaktion, pp. 58–67.

Matthee, R. (2005) *The Pursuit of Pleasure: Drugs and Stimulants in Iranian History 1500–1900*. Princeton: Princeton University Press.

Matthee, R. (2014) Alcohol in the Islamic Middle East: ambivalence and ambiguity. *Past and Present* 222 (suppl.9): 100–25.

Mabey, R. (2015) *The Cabaret of Plants: Botany and the Imagination*. London: Profile Books.

Meadows, D.H., D.L. Meadows, J. Randers and W.W. Behrens III (1972) *The Limits to Growth: A Report for the Club of Rome*. New York: Universe Books.

Meillassoux, Q. (2006) *After Finitude: An Essay on the Necessity of Contingency*. London: Bloomsbury.

Meltzer, D.J. (2015) Pleistocene overkill and North American mammalian extinctions. *Annual Review of Anthropology*, 44: 33–53.

Merchant, C. ([1980] 1990) *The Death of Nature: Women, Ecology and the Scientific Revolution*. San Francisco: HarperCollins.

Meskell, L. (2010) An anthropology of absence: commentary. In M. Bille, F. Hastrup and T. Flohr Soerensen (eds) *An Anthropology of Absence: Materializations of Transcendence and Loss*. New York: Springer Science and Business Media, pp. 207–13.

Miller, D. (2005) Materiality: an introduction. In D. Miller (ed.) *Materiality*. Durham: Duke University Press.

Miller, D. (2009) *Stuff*. London: Polity Press.

Miller, L. (2000) *Roanoke: Solving the Mystery of the Lost Colony*. New York: Arcade Publishing.

Milne, E. (2005) NHS smoking cessation services and smoking prevalence: observational study. *British Medical Journal*, 330(7494): 760.

Mintz, S. (1985) *Sweetness and Power: The Place of Sugar in Modern History*. New York: Penguin.

Moldenhauer, H. (1970) Webern's death. *The Musical Times*, 111 (1531): 877–81.

Molineux, C. (2007) Pleasures of the smoke: 'Black Virginians' in Georgian London's tobacco shops. *William and Mary Quarterly, Third Series*, 64(2): 327–76.

Monardes, N. (1577) *Joyfull Newes out of the New Found World*, trans. John Frampton. London: Imprinted in Paules Churchyard at the Signe of the Quene's Armes by William Norton.

Morgan, E.S. (1975) *American Slavery, American Freedom*. New York: Norton.

Morgan, P.D. (1998) *Slave Counterpoint: Black Culture in the Eighteenth-Century Chesapeake and Lowcountry*. Chapel Hill: University of North Carolina Press.

Mulligan C.J., A. Kitchen and M.N. Miyamoto (2008) Updated three-stage model for the peopling of the Americas. *PLoS ONE* 3(9): e3199.

Museum of New Zealand, Te Papa Tongarewa (n.d.) Tobacco harvesting, Motueka. F.R. Lamb View-Master reel. https://collections.tepapa.govt.nz/object/1031220 [Accessed 31st August 2018].

Musser, R.O., S.M. Hum-Musser, H. Eichenseer, M. Peiffer, G. Ervin, J.B. Murphy and G.W. Felton (2002) Caterpillar saliva beats plant defences. *Nature*, 416(6881): 599–600.

Nathanson, C. (1999) Social movements as catalysts for policy change: the case of smoking and guns. *Journal of Health Policy, Politics and Law*, 24(3): 421–88.

National Center for Chronic Disease Prevention and Health Promotion (US) Office on Smoking and Health (2014) *The Health Consequences of Smoking – 50 Years of Progress: A Report of the Surgeon General*. Atlanta: Centers for Disease Control and Prevention.

Neuburger, M.C. (2013) *Balkan Smoke: Tobacco and the Making of Modern Bulgaria*. Ithaca: Cornell University Press.

NHS Digital (2017) *Statistics on Smoking, England: 2017*. London: Government Statistical Service.

Nichter, M. (2015) *Lighting Up: The Rise of Smoking on College Campuses*. New York: New York University Press.

Nikogosian H. (2010) WHO Framework Convention on Tobacco Control: a key milestone. *Bulletin of the World Health Organization*, 88(2): 81–160.

Nixon, R. (2011) *Slow Violence and the Environmentalism of the Poor*. Cambridge: Harvard University Press.

Nokes, D. (1995) *John Gay: A Profession of Friendship*. Oxford: Oxford University Press.

Northrop Moore, J. (1984) *Edward Elgar: A Creative Life*. Oxford: Oxford University Press.

Norton, M. (2008) *Sacred Gifts, Profane Pleasures: A History of Tobacco and Chocolate in the Atlantic World*. Ithaca: Cornell University Press.

Novotny T.E. (2006) The 'Ultimate Prize' for Big Tobacco: opening the Chinese cigarette market by cigarette smuggling. *PLoS Med*, 3: e279.

Nowka, S.A. (2006) *Character Matters: Enlightenment Materialism and the Novel*. PhD thesis, University of Iowa.

O'Shea, P.K. (1997) *The Golden Harvest: a History of Tobacco Growing in New Zealand*. Christchurch: Hazard Press.

Opie, J. (1987) Renaissance origins of the environmental crisis. *Environmental Review*, 11(1): 2–17.

Ortiz, F. ([1947] 1995) *Cuban Counterpoint: Tobacco and Sugar*. Durham: Duke University Press.

Otago Daily Times (2011) Hulme to leave 'mcmansion' Okarito. December 22nd. http://www.odt.co.nz/entertainment/books/191953/hulme-leave-mcmansion-okarito, [Accessed 5th January 2014].

Otañez, M., H.M. Mamudu and S.A. Glantz (2009) Tobacco companies' use of developing countries' economic reliance on tobacco to lobby against global tobacco control: the case of Malawi. *American Journal of Public Health*, 99(10): 1759–71.

Outram, D. (1995) *The Enlightenment*. Cambridge: Cambridge University Press.

Owen, W. (1967) *Collected Letters*. Oxford: Oxford University Press.

Oxford English Dictionary (2018) *OED Online*. Oxford: Oxford University Press.

Oyuela-Caycedo, A. and N.C. Kawa (2015) A deep history of tobacco in lowland South America. In A. Russell and E. Rahman (eds) *The Master Plant: Tobacco in Lowland South America*, London: Bloomsbury, pp. 27–44.

Pal, L.A. (1990) Knowledge, power, and policy: reflections on Foucault. In S. Brooks and A.-G. Gagnon (eds) *Social Scientists, Policy and the State*. New York: Praeger, pp. 139–58.

Pampel F.C. (2001) Cigarette diffusion and sex differences in smoking. *Journal of Health and Social Behavior*, 42(4): 388–404.

Panter-Brick, C., S.E. Clarke, H. Lomas, M. Pinder and S.W. Lindsay (2006) Culturally compelling strategies for behaviour change: a social ecology model and case study in malaria prevention. *Social Science and Medicine*, 62(11): 2810–25.

Parsons, R. (1592) An advertisement written to a secretarie of my L. Treasurers of Ingland, by an Inglishe intelligencer as he passed throughe Germanie towardes Italie. [Publisher unknown.]

Pattison, S. and I. Heath (2010) On the irreducible individuality of the person and the fullness of life: Simon Gray's smoking diaries. *Health Care Analysis*, 18(3): 310–21.

Pavord, A. (1999) *The Tulip*. London: Bloomsbury.

Pels, P. (1998) The spirit of matter: on fetish, rarity, fact and fancy. In Spyer, P. (ed.) *Border Fetishisms: Material Objects in Unstable Spaces*. London: Routledge, pp. 91–120.

Pendarvis, J. (2016) *Cigarette Lighter*. New York: Bloomsbury Academic.

Pendergrast, M. (2010) *Uncommon Grounds: The History of Coffee and How it Transformed Our World*. New York: Basic Books.

Penn, W.A. (1902) *The Soverane Herbe: A History of Tobacco*. London: Grant Richards.

Peréz-Mallaína, P.E. (1998) *Spain's Men of the Sea: Daily Life on the Indies Fleets in the Sixteenth Century*, trans. C.R. Phillips. Baltimore: John Hopkins University Press.

Petryna, A. (2003) *Life Exposed: Biological Citizens after Chernobyl*. Princeton: Princeton University Press.

Petticrew, M., K. Lee, H. Ali and R. Nakkash (2015) 'Fighting a Hurricane': tobacco industry efforts to counter the perceived threat of Islam. *American Journal of Public Health*, 105(6): 1086–93.

Peukert, D.J.K. (1987) *Inside Nazi Germany: Conformity, Opposition and Racism in Everyday Life*. London: B.T. Batsford.

Philaretes (1602) *Work for Chimny-Sweepers, or A Warning for Tobacconists*. London: T. Este for Thomas Bushell.

Philip Morris International (Pakistan) Limited (2014) Home page. http://philipmorrispaki stan.com.pk/philip-morris-international [Accessed 11th November 2018].

Philips, J. (1736) *The Rape of the Smock*, 3rd. ed. London: printed for E. Curll, at Pope's Head, in Rose-Street, Covent-Garden.

Pickering, A. (1995) *The Mangle of Practice: Time, Agency and Science*. Chicago: University of Chicago Press.

Pilnick, A. and T. Coleman (2003) 'I'll give up smoking when you get me better': patients' resistance to attempt to problematize smoking in general practice (GP) consultations. *Social Science and Medicine*, 75: 135–45.

Plotnikova, E., S.E. Hill and J. Collin (2014) The 'Diverse, Dynamic New World of Global Tobacco Control'? An analysis of participation in the Conference of the Parties to the WHO Framework Convention on Tobacco Control. *Tobacco Control*, 23: 126–32.

PMI (Philip Morris International) (n.d.) Our manifesto: designing a smoke-free future. https://www.pmi.com/who-we-are/designing-a-smoke-free-future [Accessed 23rd June 2018].

Pollan, M. (2002) *The Botany of Desire: A Plant's Eye View of the World*. London: Bloomsbury.

Pollock, F. (1880) *Spinoza: His Life and Philosophy*. London: Kegan Paul.

Pomeroy, C. (2015) Measles and the Tragic Seduction of Pseudoscience, *Fox News*, February 6th. https://www.foxnews.com/opinion/measles-and-the-tragic-seduction-of-pseu doscience [Accessed 11th November 2018].

Popay, J., M. Whitehead and D.J. Hunter (2010) Injustice is killing people on a large scale: But what is to be done about it? *Journal of Public Health* 32(2): 148–49.

Porter, R. (2000) *Enlightenment: Britain and the Creation of the Modern World*. London: Penguin.

Porter, R. (2003) *Flesh in the Age of Reason: How the Enlightenment Transformed the Way we See our Bodies and Souls*. London: Penguin.

Prettejohn, E. (2012) *The Cambridge Companion to the Pre-Raphaelites*. Cambridge: Cambridge University Press.

Price, J.M. (1964) The economic growth of the Chesapeake and the European market, 1697-1775, *Journal of Economic History* 24(4): 496–511.

Price, J.M. (2007) Tobacco use and tobacco taxation: a battle of interests in early modern Europe. In J. Goodman, P.E. Lovejoy and A. Sherratt (eds) *Consuming Habits: Global and Historical Perspectives on How Cultures Define Drugs* (2nd ed.) London and New York: Routledge, pp. 158–77.

Proctor, R.N. (1996) The anti-tobacco campaign of the Nazis: a little known aspect of public health in Germany, 1933-45. *British Medical Journal*, 313 (7070): 1450–53.

Proctor, R.N. (1997) The Nazi war on tobacco: ideology, evidence, and the possible cancer consequences. *Bulletin of the History of Medicine*, 71(3): 435–88.

Proctor, R.N. (1999) *The Nazi War on Cancer*. Princeton: Princeton University Press.

Proctor, R.N. (2008a) On playing the Nazi card. *Tobacco Control*, 17(5): 289–90.

Proctor, R.N. (2008b) Agnotology: a missing term to describe the cultural production of ignorance (and its study). In R.N. Proctor and L. Schiebinger (2008) (eds) *Agnotology: The Making and Unmaking of Ignorance*. Stanford: Stanford University Press, pp. 1–33.

Proctor, R.N. (2011) *Golden Holocaust: Origins of the Cigarette Catastrophe and the Case for Abolition*. Berkeley: University of California Press.

Proctor, R.N. (2013) Why ban the sale of cigarettes? The case for abolition. *Tobacco Control*, 22(s1): i27–i30.

Proctor, R.N. and L. Schiebinger (2008) (eds) *Agnotology: The Making and Unmaking of Ignorance*. Stanford: Stanford University Press.

Raffles, H., L. Shani, R. Goldstein and K. Wentworth (2015) Writing/power/story: why and how to do ethnography of non-human beings and things. *Cultural Anthropology*, February 12th. http://www.culanth.org/fieldsights/642-writing-power-story-why-and-how-to-do-ethnography-of-non-human-beings-and-things [Accessed 11th November 2018].

Rahman, E. (2015) Tobacco and water: everyday blessings. In A. Russell and E. Rahman (eds) *The Master Plant: Tobacco in Lowland South America*. London: Bloomsbury, pp. 131–52.

Rajan, R. (1999) Bhopal, vulnerability, routinization and the chronic disaster. In A. Oliver-Smith and S. M. Hoffman (eds) *The Angry Earth: Disaster in Anthropological Perspective*. New York: Routledge, pp. 257–77.

Ramos, A.R. (2012) The Politics of Perspectivism. *Annual Review of Anthropology*, 41: 481–94.

Ransome, D.R. (1991) Wives for Virginia, 1621. *William and Mary Quarterly*, 48(1): 3–18.

Read, M.D. (1992) Policy networks and issue networks: the politics of smoking. In D. Marsh and R.A.W. Rhodes (eds) *Policy Networks in British Government*. Oxford: Clarendon Press, pp. 124–48.

Reader, J. (2009) *The Untold History of the Potato*. London: Vintage.

Reed, A. (2007) Smuk is king: the action of cigarettes in a Papua New Guinea prison. In A. Henare, M. Holbraad and S. Wastell (eds) *Thinking Through Things: Theorising Artefacts Ethnographically*. London: Routledge, pp. 47–67.

Reid, L.A. (2014) The spectre of the School of Night: former scholarly fictions and the stuff of academic fiction. *Early Modern Literary Studies*, Special Issue 23. https://extra.shu.ac.uk/emls/journal/index.php/emls/article/view/182/156 [Accessed 11th November 2018].

Reid, R. (2005) *Globalizing Tobacco Control: Anti-Smoking Campaigns in California, France, and Japan*. Bloomington: Indiana University Press.

Reig, A. (2015) Landscapes of desire and tobacco circulation in the Yanomami ethos. In A. Russell and E. Rahman (2015) (eds) *The Master Plant: Tobacco in Lowland South America*, London: Bloomsbury, pp. 167–81.

Reynolds, L.A. and E.M. Tansey (2012) (eds) WHO Framework Convention on Tobacco Control. *Wellcome Witnesses to Twentieth Century Medicine, 43*. London: Queen Mary University of London.

Rhodes, N. (2003) *William Cowper: Selected Poems*. London: Routledge

Rhodes, R. (2002) *Masters of Death: The SS-Einsatzgruppen and the Invention of the Holocaust*. London: Perseus Press.

Rideout, E.H. (n.d.) Unpublished notes for a book on the Liverpool tobacco trade. University of Liverpool Special Collections and Archives.

Riesman, D., N. Glazer and R. Denney (1950) *The Lonely Crowd*, New Haven: Yale University Press.

Rival, L. (2014) Encountering nature through fieldwork: expert knowledge, modes of reasoning, and local creativity. *Journal of the Royal Anthropological Institute*, 20(2): 218–36.

Rivoal, I. and N.B. Salazar (2013) Contemporary ethnographic practice and the value of serendipity. *Social Anthropology/Anthropologie Sociale*, 21(2): 178–85.

Robbins H. and M. Krakow (2000) Evolution of a comprehensive tobacco control programme: building system capacity and strategic partnerships – lessons from Massachusetts. *Tobacco Control*, 9: 423–30.

Robert, J.C. (1949) *The Story of Tobacco in America*. New York: Alfred A. Knopf.

Roberts, A.F. (2004) Smoking in Sub-Saharan Africa. In S.L. Gilman and Z. Xun (eds) *Smoke: A Global History of Smoking*. New York: Reaktion, pp. 46–57.

Roberts, B.W.C. and R.F. Knapp (1992) Paving the way for the Tobacco Trust: from hand rolling to mechanized cigarette production by W. Duke, Sons and Company. *The North Carolina Historical Review*, 69: 257–81.

Robins, N. (2006) *The Corporation that Changed the World: How the East India Company Shaped the Modern Multinational*. London: Pluto Press.

Robinson M. (2014) Alfie Worthington 'Could Have Been Killed' after e-cigarette exploded. *Daily Mail*, October 20th. http://www.dailymail.co.uk/news/article-2799944/toddler-killed-charging-e-cigarette-exploded-like-catherine-wheel-just-inches-played.html [Accessed 21st October 2014].

Roemer, R., A. Taylor and J. Lariviere (2005) Origins of the WHO Framework Convention on Tobacco Control. *American Journal of Public Health*, 95(6): 936–38.

Rogoziński, J. (1990) *Smokeless Tobacco in the Western World, 1550-1950*. New York: Praeger.

Rohatynskyj, M. (2015) Empowering the dividual. *Anthropological Theory*, 15(3): 317–37.

Romaniello, M.P. (2007) Through the filter of tobacco: the limits of global trade in the early modern world. *Comparative Studies in Society and History*, 49(4): 914–37.

Romaniello, M.P. and T. Starks (2009) *Tobacco in Russian History and Culture: From the Seventeenth Century to the Present*. London: Routledge.

Rosenblatt, R. (1994) How do tobacco executives live with themselves? *New York Times Magazine*, March 20th: 22-34.

Rossetti, W.M. (2013) *Some Reminiscences*, Vol. 1. Cambridge: Cambridge University Press.

Roy, A. (2011) Tobacco consumption and the poor: an ethnographic analysis of hand-rolled cigarette (bidi) use in Bangladesh. *Ethnography*, 13(2) 162–88.

Roy, A., D. Efroymson, L. Jones, S. Ahmed, I. Arafat, R. Sarker and S. FitzGerald (2012) Gainfully employed? An inquiry into bidi-dependent livelihoods in Bangladesh. *Tobacco Control*, 21(3): 313–17.

Royal College of Physicians (1962) *Smoking and Health: A Report on Smoking in Relation to Lung Cancer and Other Diseases*. London: Royal College of Physicians.

Royal College of Physicians (2014) *Why Asthma Still Kills – The National Review of Asthma Deaths (NRAD)*. London: Royal College of Physicians.

Rudgley, R. (1993) *Essential Substances: A Cultural History of Intoxicants in Society*. New York: Kodansha International.

Russell A. (2015) Women and smoking in the North East of England. In J. Bissell J. C. Caiado, M. Goldstein and B. Straughan (eds) *Tipping Points: Modelling Social Problems and Health*. Oxford: Wiley-Blackwell, pp. 32–48.

Russell, A. (2017) Smog in a time of tobacco control. *Anthropology Today*, 33(6): 27–9.

Russell, A. (2018) Can the plant speak? Giving tobacco the voice it deserves. *Journal of Material Culture*, 23(4): 472–87.

Russell, A. and E. Rahman (2015) (eds) *The Master Plant: Tobacco in Lowland South America*, London: Bloomsbury.

Russell, A., S. Heckler, S. Sengupta, M. White, D. Chappel, D.J. Hunter, J. Mason, E. Milne and S. Lewis (2009) The evolution of a UK regional tobacco control office in its early years: social contexts and policy dynamics. *Health Promotion International*, 24: 262–68.

Russell, A., M. Wainwright and H. Mamudu (2015) A chilling example? Uruguay, Philip Morris International, and WHO's Framework Convention on Tobacco Control. *Medical Anthropology Quarterly*, 29: 256–77.

Russell, A., M. Wainwright and M. Tilson (2018) Means and ENDS – e-cigarettes, the Framework Convention on Tobacco Control, and global health diplomacy in action. *Global Public Health*, 13(1): 83–98.

Rutter, A. and A. Crossfield (2012) Policy at the front line: the local, sub-national and national divide. In *Fifty years since* Smoking and Health: *Progress, Lessons and Priorities for a Smoke-Free UK*. London: Royal College of Physicians, pp. 47–9.

Ryan, W.F. (1983) Peter the Great's English yacht: Admiral Lord Carmarthen and the Russian tobacco monopoly. *The Marine's Mirror*, 69 (1): 65–87.

Sahlins, M. (1988) Cosmologies of capitalism: the trans-Pacific sector of 'the world system'. *Proceedings of the British Academy*, 74: 1–51.

Sahlins, M. (2008) *The Western Illusion of Human Nature*. Chicago: Prickly Paradigm Press.

Sainsbury, W.N. (1880) (ed.) *Calendar of State Papers, Colonial Series: America and West Indies 1661-1668*. London: Longmans.

Salaman, R.N. (1949) *The History and Social Influence of the Potato*. Cambridge: Cambridge University Press.

Salmond, A. (2017) Uncommon things. *Anthropologica*, 59: 251–66.

Salter, P. (2010) *First, We Take Berlin*. Adam Smith Institute: London.

Samuel, W.W.E. (2002) *The War of Our Childhood: Memories of World War II*. Jackson: University Press of Mississippi.

Sarmiento Barletti, J.-P. (2015) Of tobacco and well-being in indigenous Amazonia. In A. Russell and E. Rahman (eds) *The Master Plant: Tobacco in Lowland South America*. London: Bloomsbury, pp. 183–98.

Sartre, J.-P. ([1943] 1958) *Being and Nothingness: An Essay on Phenomenological Ontology*, trans. H.E. Barnes. London: Methuen.

Sassoon, S. (1930) *Memoirs of an Infantry Officer*. London: Faber & Faber.

Schama, S. (1987) *The Embarrassment of Riches: An Interpretation of Dutch Culture in the Golden Age*. New York: Alfred A. Knopf.

Schatz, E. (2009). Introduction: ethnographic immersion and the study of politics. In E. Schatz (ed.) *Political Ethnography: What Immersion Contributes to the Study of Power*. Chicago: University of Chicago Press, pp. 1–22.

Schivelbusch, W. ([1980] 1992) *Tastes of Paradise: A Social History of Spices, Stimulants, and Intoxicants*. New York: Pantheon Books.

Schneider, N.K. and S.A. Glantz (2008) 'Nicotine Nazis strike again': a brief analysis of the use of Nazi rhetoric in attacking tobacco control advocacy. *Tobacco Control*, 17 (5): 291–96.

Screech, T. (2004) Tobacco in Edo period Japan. In S. Gilman and Z. Xun (eds) *Smoke: A Global History of Smoking*. London: Reaktion, pp. 92–9.

Secretary of State for Health (1992) *The Health of the Nation: A Strategy for Health in England*. London: Her Majesty's Stationery Office.

Sharma, M. (2018) Recasting language of work: Beedi industry in post-colonial Central India. *History and Sociology of South Asia*, 12(1): 32–47.

Shaw, R. (2002) *Memories of the Slave Trade: Ritual and the Historical Imagination in Sierra Leone*. Chicago: Chicago University Press.

Sheffield, H. and A. Jameson (2015) Imperial Tobacco says Isis to blame for falling cigarette sales. *The Independent*, May 6th. http://www.independent.co.uk/news/business/news/imperial-tobacco-says-isis-to-blame-for-falling-cigarette-sales-10228583.html [Accessed 26th June 2016].

Shell, A. (2003) Donne and Sir Edward Hoby: evidence for an unrecorded collaboration. In D. Colclough (ed.) *John Donne's Professional Lives*. Cambridge: D.S. Brewer, pp. 121–32.

Shepard, G.H. (1998) Psychoactive plants and ethnopsychiatric medicines of the Matsigenka. *Journal of Psychoactive Drugs*, 30(4): 321–32.

Shepard, G.H. (2004) A sensory ecology of medicinal plant therapy in two Amazonian societies. *American Anthropologist*, 106(2): 252–66.

Short, T. (1750) *Discourses on Tea, Sugar, Milk, Made-Wines, Spirits, Punch, Tobacco, etc.: With Plain and Useful Rules for Gouty People*. London: Printed for T. Longman, in Paternoster Row, & A. Millar, in the Strand.

Simpson D. (2002) Germany: how did it get like this? *Tobacco Control*, 11: 291–93.

Sims M., R. Maxwell, L. Bauld and A. Gilmore (2010) Short term impact of smoke-free legislation in England: retrospective analysis of hospital admissions for myocardial infarction. *British Medical Journal*, 340: c2161.

Singer, M. and H. Baer (2009) (eds) *Killer Commodities: Public Health and the Corporate Production of Harm*. Lanham: AltaMira Press.

Sloterdijk, P. (2009) *Terror from the Air*. Los Angeles: Semiotext(e).

Sly, D.H., R.S. Hopkins, E. Trapido and S. Ray (2001) Influence of a counteradvertising media campaign on initiation of smoking: the Florida 'Truth' campaign. *American Journal of Public Health*, 91(21): 233–38.

Smart, C. (1752) *Poems on Several Occasions*. London: printed for the author by W. Strahan and sold by J. Newbery.

Smith, C. (2012) History of the Rothman's Factory Recounted. http://www.motuekaonline.org.nz/news/stories12/311012s2.html [Accessed 6th January 2014].

Smith, K. (2013) *Beyond Evidence-Based Policy in Public Health: The Interplay of Ideas*. Basingstoke: Palgrave Macmillan.

Smith, K. E., G. Fooks, J. Collin, H. Weishaar, S. Mandal and A.B. Gilmore (2010) 'Working the System' – British American Tobacco's influence on the European Union treaty and its implications for policy: an analysis of internal tobacco industry documents. *PLoSMedicine* 7(1): e1000202.

Soren, B.J. (2009) Museum experiences that change visitors. *Museum Management and Curatorship*, 24(3): 233–51.

Soto, D.A. (2009) The English tobacco free trade and the Spanish tobacco monopoly during the 18th century: comparison, results and implications. Paper presented at the 8th Conference of the European Historical Economics Society (EHES), Geneva, 3-6 September.

Spivak, G. (1988) Can the subaltern speak? In C. Nelson and L. Grossberg (eds) *Marxism and the Interpretation of Culture*. Urbana: University of Illinois Press, pp. 271–313.

Srinivasulu, K. (1997) Impact of liberalisation on beedi workers. *Economic and Political Weekly*, 32(11): 515–17.

Stanford University (n.d.) Research into the Impact of Tobacco Advertising. http://tobacco.stanford.edu/tobacco_main/index.php [Accessed 22nd October 2018].

Stephens, W.E. (2017) Chemometric and trace element profiling methodologies for authenticating, crossmatching and constraining the provenance of illicit tobacco products. *Tobacco Control*, 26: 502–8.

Stephens, W. E., A. Calder and J. Newton (2005) Source and health implications of high toxic metal concentrations in illicit tobacco products. *Environmental Science and Technology*, 39: 479–88.

Steppuhn, A., K. Gase, B. Krock, R. Halitschke and I.T. Baldwin (2004) Nicotine's defensive function in nature. *PLoS Biology* 2(8): e217.

Sterns, L. (1999) *The Smoking Book*. Chicago: University of Chicago Press.

Steward, J. (1955) *Theory of Culture Change*. Urbana: University of Illinois Press.

Stimson G.V., B. Thom and P. Costall (2014) Disruptive innovations: the rise of the electronic cigarette. *International Journal of Drug Policy*, 25: 653–5.

Stolze Lima, T. (1999) The two and its many: reflections on perspectivism in a Tupi cosmology. *Ethnos*, 64(1): 107–31.

Stone, O.C. (1880) *A Few Months in New Guinea*. London: Sampson Low, Marston, Searle & Rivington.

Stork, W.F.J., A. Weinhold and I.T. Baldwin (2011) Trichomes as dangerous lollipops: do lizards also use caterpillar body and frass odor to optimize their foraging? *Plant Signaling and Behavior*, 6(12): 1893–96.

Strathern, M. (2014) Becoming enlightened about relations. *ASA Firth Lecture 2014*, ASA Conference 'Anthropology and Enlightenment', Edinburgh. https://www.theasa.org/downloads/publications/firth/firth14.pdf [Accessed 11th November 2018].

Stratigakos, D. (2015) *Hitler at Home*. New Haven: Yale University Press.

Stubbs, J. (2012) El Habana: the global luxury smoke. *Commodities of Empire* Working Paper No. 20. Milton Keynes: The Ferguson Centre for African and Asian Studies, Open University.

Studlaw D. (2005) The political dynamics of tobacco control in Australia and New Zealand: explaining policy problems, instruments, and patterns of adoption. *Australian Journal of Political Science*, 40(2): 255–74.

Sugg, R. (2007) *Critical Issues: John Donne*. London: Palgrave Macmillan.

Sullum, J. (1999) *For Your Own Good: The Anti-Smoking Crusade and the Tyranny of Public Health.* Glencoe: Free Press.

Suzuki, B.T. (2004) Tobacco culture in Japan. In S. Gilman and Z. Xun (eds) *Smoke: A Global History of Smoking.* London: Reaktion, pp.76–83.

Svevo, I. (2001) *Zeno's Conscience,* trans. W. Weaver. London: Penguin.

Synge, F.M. (1908) *Albert Maclaren, Pioneer Missionary in New Guinea: A Memoir.* Westminster, Scotland: Society for the Propagation of the Gospel in Foreign Parts.

Tamm E., T. Kivisild, M. Reidla, M. Metspalu, D.G. Smith, C.J. Mulligan et al. (2007) Beringian standstill and spread of native American founders. *PLoS ONE* 2(9): e829.

Tate, C. (1999) *Cigarette Wars: The Triumph of the Little White Slaver.* Oxford: Oxford University Press.

Tatham, W. (1800) *An Historical and Practical Essay on the Culture and Commerce of Tobacco.* London: Vernor and Hood.

Taylor, G., A. McNeill, A. Girling, A. Farley, N. Lindson-Hawley and P. Aveyard (2014) Change in mental health after smoking cessation: systematic review and meta-analysis. *British Medical Journal,* 348: g1151.

Thirlway, F. (2015) *The Persistence of Memory: Mobility, Family, Class and Smoking in a Durham Coalfield Village.* PhD thesis, Durham University.

Thirsk, J. (1974) New crops and their diffusion: tobacco-growing in seventeenth century England. In C.W. Chalklin and M.A. Havinden (eds) *Rural Change and Urban Growth 1500-1800: Essays in English Regional History in Honour of W.G. Hoskins.* London: Longman, pp. 76–103.

Thomé, O.W. (1885) *Flora von Deutschland, Österreich und der Schweiz.* Gera, Germany: Köhler.

Thompson, L., J.R. Barnett, and J.R. Pearce (2009) Scared straight? Fear-appeal anti-smoking campaigns, risk, self-efficacy and addiction. *Health, Risk and Society,* 11(2): 181–96.

Thompson, L., J. Pearce and J.R. Barnett (2007) Moralising geographies: stigma, smoking islands and responsible subjects. *Area,* 39: 508–17.

Thompson, L., J. Pearce, J., and R. Barnett, (2009) Nomadic identities and socio-spatial competence: making sense of post-smoking selves. *Social and Cultural Geography,* 10(5): 565–81.

Thompson, R. (2012) Foreword. *Fifty Years Since 'Smoking and Health': Progress, Lessons and Priorities for a Smoke-Free UK.* London: Royal College of Physicians.

Thompson, R.W. (1900) *My Trip in the "John Williams".* London: London Missionary Society.

Thomson, B.H. (1889) New Guinea: Narrative of an exploring expedition to the Louisiade and D'Entrecasteaux islands. *Proceedings of the Royal Geographical Society* N.S. 11: 525–42.

Thwaites, R.G. (1809-1901) (ed.) *The Jesuit Relations and Allied Documents* (73 volumes). Cleveland: Burrows Brothers.

Timmermann, C. (2014) *A History of Lung Cancer: The Recalcitrant Disease.* London: Palgrave Macmillan.

Tinkler, P. (2006) *Smoke Signals: Women, Smoking and Visual Culture in Britain.* Oxford: Berg.

Tobacco Free Kids (2014) You're the Target: New Global Tobacco Campaign Found to Target Teens. https://www.tobaccofreekids.org/assets/global/pdfs/en/yourethetarget_report.pdf [Accessed 28th June 2018].

Toll B.A. and P.M. Ling (2005) The Virginia Slims identity crisis: an inside look at tobacco industry marketing to women. *Tobacco Control,* 14: 172–80.

Tomkis, T. (1607) *Lingua, or, The Combat of the Tongue and the Five Senses for Superiority: A Pleasant Comoedy.* London: Printed at G. Eld for Simon Waterson.

Travers, J. (2003) *James I: The Masque of Monarchy.* Kew: The National Archives.

Treanor, P. (2005) *Neoliberalism: origins, theory, definition.* http://web.inter.nl.net/users/Paul. Treanor/neoliberalism.html [Accessed 11th November 2018].

Trench, C.C. (1978) *Charley Gordon: An Eminent Victorian Reassessed.* London: Allen Lane.

Trewavas, A. (2012) Plants are intelligent too. *EMBO reports,* 13(9): 772–3.

Trewavas, A. (2014) *Plant Behaviour and Intelligence.* Oxford: Oxford University Press.

Trewavas, A. and F. Baluška (2011) The ubiquity of consciousness. *EMBO Reports,* 12(12): 1221–5.

Trotta Borges, M. and R. Simoes-Barbosa (2008) Cigarette as 'companion'. A critical gender approach to women's smoking. *Cadernos de Saude Publica,* 24 (12) 2834–42.

Tsing, A. (2014) Strathern beyond the human: testimony of a spore. *Theory, Culture and Society,* 31(2/3): 221–41.

Tuinstra, T. (2015) A compelling intersect. *Tobacco Reporter,* November: 14–26.

Tupper, J. (1849) Papers of the M.S. Society No. 4, Smoke. *The Germ,* (4): 183–5.

Turner, T.S. (2009) The crisis of late structuralism. Perspectivism and animism: rethinking culture, nature, spirit, and bodiliness. *Tipití: Journal of the Society for the Anthropology of Lowland South America,* 7(1): 3–42.

Tye, L. ([1998] 2002) *The Father of Spin: Edward L. Bernays and the Birth of Public Relations.* New York: Henry Holt.

UCSF Library (n.d.) Truth Tobacco Industry Documents, https://www.industrydocument slibrary.ucsf.edu/tobacco [Accessed 23rd October 2018].

UCSF Library (1981) Minutes of the 35th meeting of the Public Relations Committee of the T.A.C. https://www.industrydocumentslibrary.ucsf.edu/tobacco/docs/#id=yqkb0131 [Accessed 11th January 2018].

Ugen, S. (2003) Bhutan: the world's most advanced tobacco control nation? *Tobacco Control,* 12: 431–3.

Ulucanlar, S., G. J. Fooks and A.B. Gilmore (2016) The policy dystopia model: an interpretive analysis of tobacco industry political activity. *PLoS Medicine* 13(9): e1002125.

Unruh, P. (1983) *'Fumeur' Poetry and Music of the Chantilly Codex: A study of its meaning and background.* MA thesis, University of British Columbia.

US Department of Health, Education, and Welfare (1964) *Smoking and Health: Report of the Advisory Committee of the Surgeon General.* Washington, DC: US Government Printing Office.

Van De Poel-Knottnerus, F. and J.D. Knottnerus (1994) Social life through literature: a suggested strategy for conducting a literary ethnography. *Sociological Focus,* 27(1): 67–80.

Varma, S., K. Choi, M. Koo and H. Skinner (2005) China: tobacco museum's 'smoky' health information. *Tobacco Control,* 14: 4–5.

Vaughan, W. (1600) *Naturall and Artificiall Directions for Health, Derived from the Best Philosophers, as Well Moderne, as Auncient,* London: Printed by Richard Bradocke.

Vilaça, A. (2005) Chronically unstable bodies: reflections on Amazonian corporalities. *Journal of the Royal Anthropological Institute,* 11: 445–64.

Viveiros de Castro, E. (1998) Cosmological deixis and Amerindian perspectivism. *Journal of the Royal Anthropological Institute,* 4(3): 469–88.

Viveiros de Castro, E. (2012a) *Radical Dualism: A Meta-Fantasy on the Square Root of Dual Organizations or a Savage Homage to Lévi-Strauss* (100 Notes/100 Thoughts Documenta 13). Ostfildern: Hatje Cantz.

Viveiros de Castro, E. (2012b) *Cosmological perspectivism in Amazonia and elsewhere*. Masterclass Series 1. Manchester, HAU Network of Ethnographic Theory.

Von Gernet, A. (2000) North American indigenous *Nicotiana* use and tobacco shamanism: the early documentary record, 1520–660. In J.C. Winter (ed.) *Tobacco Use by Native North Americans*. Norman: University of Oklahoma Press, pp. 59–80.

Wakefield. M., K. Coomber, M. Zacher, S. Durkin, E. Brennan and M. Scollo (2015) Australian adult smokers' responses to plain packaging with larger graphic health warnings 1 year after implementation: results from a national cross-sectional tracking survey. *Tobacco Control*, 24: ii17–ii25.

Walker, R.B. (1980) Medical aspects of tobacco smoking and the anti-tobacco movement in Britain in the nineteenth century. *Medical History*, 24: 391–402.

Walkley, A.B. (1915) Tobacco in peace and war. *The Times Literary Supplement*, December 2nd. 724: 439.

Walsh, L.S. (2001) The Chesapeake slave trade: regional patterns, African origins, and some implications. *William and Mary Quarterly*, 58(1): 139–170.

Walton, J. (ed.) (2000) *The Faber Book of Smoking*. London: Faber.

Wandersee, J.H. and E.E. Schussler (1999) Preventing plant blindness. *The American Biology Teacher*, 61(2): 84–86.

Wang, F., S. Sun, X. Yao and H. Fu (2016) The museum as a platform for tobacco promotion in China. *Tobacco Control*, 25: 118–21.

Ward, E. (1745) *A Compleat and Humorous Account of All the Remarkable Clubs and Societies in the Cities of London and Westminster*. London: Printed for the author and sold by Joseph Collier at Shakespear's Head in Ludgate-Street.

Warman, A. (2003) *Corn and Capitalism: How a Botanical Bastard Grew to Global Dominance*, trans. N.L. Westrate. Chapel Hill: University of North Carolina Press.

Warner, W. (1606) *A Continuance of Albions England*, 1st edition. London: F. Kyngston for G. Potter.

Wasson, R.G. (1968) *SOMA, Divine Mushroom of Immortality*, Ethnomycological studies No. 1. New York: The American Museum of Natural History.

Watry, M. (2002) *Smokescreen: The Victorian Vogue for Tobacco*. Liverpool University Special Collections and Archives. https://libguides.liverpool.ac.uk/library/sca/smokescreenexhib [Accessed 11th November 2018].

WCTOH (World Conference on Tobacco or Health) (2018) 17th World Conference on Tobacco or Health: Registration - Eligibility. https://wctoh.org/register/eligibility [Accessed 28th April 2018].

Weishaar, H., J. Collin, K. Smith, T. Grüning, S. Mandal and A. Gilmore (2012) Global health governance and the commercial sector: a documentary analysis of tobacco company strategies to influence the WHO Framework Convention on Tobacco Control. *PLoS Medicine*, 9: e1001249.

Welshman, J. (1996) Images of youth: the issue of juvenile smoking 1880-1914. *Addiction*, 91(9): 1379–86.

Wertenbacker, T.J. (1922) *The Planters of Colonial Virginia*. Princeton: Princeton University Press.

Whif, W. (1788) *Gentleman's Magazine* (February) 58(2):122.

Whitlock, B.W. (1962) Donne's university years. *English Studies*, 43: 1–20.

WHO (World Health Organization) (1970) WHA23.32 Health Consequences of Smoking. http://www.who.int/tobacco/framework/wha_eb/wha23_32/en [Accessed 11th November 2018].

WHO Committee of Experts (2000) *Tobacco Company Strategies to Undermine Tobacco Control Activities at the World Health Organization.* Report of the Committee of Experts on Tobacco Industry Documents, July. Geneva: WHO.

WHO (2003) *WHO Framework Convention on Tobacco Control.* Geneva: WHO Framework Convention on Tobacco Control.

WHO (2006) *Rules of Procedure of the Conference of the Parties.* Geneva: WHO Framework Convention on Tobacco Control.

WHO (2012) *Confronting the Tobacco Epidemic in a New Era of Trade and Investment Liberalization.* Geneva: World Health Organization.

Wiener, J. (2010) My favorite Doonesbury character: Mr. Butts. *The Nation*, November 10th.

Wiist, W.H. (2010) (ed.) *The Bottom Line or Public Health: Tactics Corporations Use to Influence Health and Health Policy, and What We Can Do to Counter Them.* Oxford: Oxford University Press.

Wikipedia (2014a) 5th Dalai Lama. http://en.wikipedia.org/wiki/5th_Dalai_Lama [Accessed 10th January 2019].

Wikipedia (2014b) Tulku Dragpa Gyaltsen. http://en.wikipedia.org/wiki/Tulku_Dragpa_Gyaltsen [Accessed 10th January 2019].

Wikipedia (2014c) Keri Hulme. http://en.wikipedia.org/wiki/Keri_Hulme [Accessed 10th January 2019].

Wilbert, J. (1972) Tobacco and shamanistic ecstasy among the Warao Indians of Venezuela. In P.T. Furst (ed.) Flesh of the Gods: The Ritual Use of Hallucinogens. London, George Allen and Unwin, pp. 55–83.

Wilbert, J. (1987) *Tobacco and Shamanism in South America.* New Haven: Yale University Press.

Wilbert, J. (2004) The order of dark shamans among the Warao. In N.L. Whitehed and R. Wright (eds) *In Darkness and Secrecy: The Anthropology of Assault Sorcery and Witchcraft in Amazonia.* Durham: Duke University Press, pp. 21–50.

Wilbert, J. and K. Simoneau (1990) (eds) *Folk Literature of the Yanomami Indians.* Los Angeles: UCLA Latin American Studies Center.

Wild, A. (2010) *Black Gold: The Dark History of Coffee.* London: Harper Perennial.

Wilf, P., M.R. Carvalho, M.A. Gandolfo and N. Rubén Cúneo (2017) Eocene lantern fruits from Gondwanan Patagonia and the early origins of Solanaceae. *Science*, 355(6320): 71–75.

Willburn, S.A. (2006) *Possessed Victorians: Extra Spheres in Nineteenth-Century Mystical Writings.* London: Routledge.

Williams, E. (1964) *Capitalism and Slavery.* London: Andre Deutsch.

Williams, L. (2011) 'So shall the Muse from Smoke elicit Fire': The Poetics of Tobacco in England, 1700-1740. *Digital Miscellanies Index.* http://digitalmiscellaniesindex.blogspot.com/2011/07/so-shall-muse-from-smoke-elicit-fire.html [Accessed 11th November 2018].

Willis, S. (2009) The archaeology of smuggling and the Falmouth King's Pipe. *Journal of Marine Archaeology*, 4: 51–65.

Wilson, N., G.W. Thomson, R. Edwards and T. Blakely (2013) Potential advantages and disadvantages of an endgame strategy: a 'sinking lid' on tobacco supply. *Tobacco Control*, 22 (s1): i18–i21.

Wiltshire, S., A. Bancroft, A. Amos and O. Parry (2001) 'They're doing people a service': qualitative study of smoking, smuggling, and social deprivation. *British Medical Journal*, 323 (7306): 203–7.

Winsor, M. (2015) ISIS beheads cigarette smokers: Islamic state deems smoking 'slow suicide' under Sharia law. *International Business Times*, February 12th.

Winter, J.C. (2000) Traditional uses of tobacco by Native Americans. In J.C. Winter (ed.) *Tobacco Use by Native North Americans: Sacred Smoke and Silent Killer.* Norman: University of Oklahoma Press, pp. 9–58.

Wipfli, H. (2015) *The Global War on Tobacco: Mapping the World's First Public Health Treaty.* Baltimore: Johns Hopkins University Press.

Withey, A. (2014) The great Georgian snuff debate. https://dralun.wordpress.com/2014/09/15/the-great-georgian-snuff-debate.

Withington, P. (2010) *Society in Early Modern England: The Vernacular Origins of some Powerful Ideas.* Cambridge: Polity Press.

Withington, P. (2011) Intoxicants and society in early modern England. *The Historical Journal*, 54(3): 631–57.

Wolff, L. (2007) Discovering cultural perspective: the intellectual history of anthropological thought in the age of Enlightenment. In L. Wolff and M. Cipollini (eds) *The Anthropology of the Enlightenment.* Stanford: Stanford University Press, pp. 3–32.

World Bank (1999) *Curbing the Epidemic: Governments and the Economics of Tobacco Control.* Washington, DC: World Bank.

Worth Estes, J. (2000) The reception of American drugs in Europe, 1500-1650. In S. Varey, R. Chabrán and D.B. Weiner (eds) *Searching for the Secrets of Nature: The Life and Works of Dr. Francisco Hernández.* Stanford: Stanford University Press, pp. 111–21.

Wright, R. (2013) *Mysteries of the Jaguar Shamans of the Northwest Amazon.* Lincoln: University of Nebraska Press.

WTO (World Trade Organization) (2011) Members debate cigarette plain-packaging's impact on trademark rights. http://www.wto.org/english/news_e/news11_e/trip_07jun11_e.htm [Accessed 15th July 2013].

Yach, D. (2008) Food companies and nutrition for better health. *Public Health Nutrition*, 11(2): 112–13.

Yach, D. (2017) Foundation for a smoke-free world. *Lancet*, 390: 1807–10.

Yach, D. and D. Bettcher (2000) Globalisation of tobacco industry influence and new global responses. *Tobacco Control*, 9: 206–16.

Yates, J. (2006) What are 'things' saying in Renaissance studies? *Literature Compass* 3(5): 992–1010.

Yuhl, S.E. (2013) Hidden in plain sight: centering the domestic slave trade in American public history. *The Journal of Southern History*, 79(3): 593–624.

Zhou, S.Z., J.D. Liberman and E. Ricafort (2018) The impact of the WHO Framework Convention on Tobacco Control in defending legal challenges to tobacco control measures. *Tobacco Control*, Epub ahead of print: doi: 10.1136/tobaccocontrol-2018-054329.

Zieger, S. (2014) Holmes's pipe, tobacco papers and the nineteenth-century origins of media addiction. *Journal of Victorian Culture*, 19(1): 24–42.

Ziser, M. (2013) *Environmental Practice and Early American Literature.* Cambridge: Cambridge University Press.

Zola, I. (1973) Pathways to the doctor: from person to patient. *Social Science and Medicine*, 7(9): 677–89.

Index

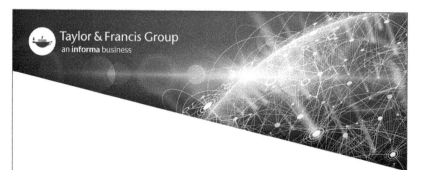